The 21st Century
Health Care Leader

Emory University School of Medicine
Center for Healthcare Leadership

Roderick W. Gilkey, Editor

Introduction by James C. Collins

The 21st Century
Health Care Leader

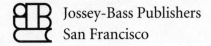 Jossey-Bass Publishers
San Francisco

Jossey-Bass books and products are available through most bookstores.
To contact Jossey-Bass directly, call (888) 378–2537, fax to (800) 605–2665,
or visit our website at www.josseybass.com.

Substantial discounts on bulk quantities of Jossey-Bass books are available to
corporations, professional associations, and other organizations. For details
and discount information, contact the special sales department at Jossey-Bass.

 Manufactured in the United States of America on Lyons Falls Turin Book.
This paper is acid-free and 100 percent totally chlorine-free.

Library of Congress Cataloging-in-Publication Data

The 21st century health care leader / Roderick W. Gilkey, editor.
     p.   cm.
  Includes bibliographical references and index.
  ISBN 0-7879-4157-3 (alk. paper)
  1. Health services administration.   2. Health services
administration—United States.   I. Gilkey, Roderick W.
  [DNLM: 1. Delivery of Health Care—organization & administration.
2. Delivery of Health Care—trends.   3. Health Facility
Administrators.   4. Leadership.   W 84.1Z13 1998]
RA971.A12   1998
362.1—dc21
DNLM/DLC
for Library of Congress   98-39561

FIRST EDITION
HB Printing   10 9 8 7 6 5 4 3

~~~ Contents

Preface   xi
Roderick W. Gilkey

Acknowledgments   xv

The Editor   xvii

Introduction   xix
James C. Collins

Part One: Navigating to a New Century   1

1 The Three C's: Consumerism, Cyberhealth,
and Co-Opetition   3
Russell C. Coile Jr.

2 Forces and Scenarios That Will Shape
Health Services Delivery   22
Joe Flower

3 Policy Challenges   39
Joel Shalowitz

4 Ethical Values for a New Century   51
Lawrence O. Gostin

5 Preparing for the Global Health Transition   74
Kent Glenzer, Maurice I. Middleberg

6 Public and Community Health   85
William H. Foege, Mark Rosenberg

Part Two: The New Health Care Organization   91

7 What Comes After Consolidation?   93
Jeffrey C. Barbakow

 8 Growing Effective Leadership in New Organizations   101
     John D. Henry Sr., Roderick W. Gilkey

 9 Reinventing the Academy   111
     Darrell G. Kirch

10 Leading Academic Health Centers   117
     Michael Johns, Thomas J. Lawley

11 Decisions for Insurers   124
     Patrick G. Hays

12 Seeing Insurance Through the Customer's Eyes   132
     Leonard D. Schaeffer, L. Carl Volpe

13 Leadership Skills and Strategies for the
     Integrated Community Health System   142
     Paul K. Halverson

14 Alliances in a Changing Industry   149
     Arnold D. Kaluzny, Howard S. Zuckerman

Part Three: Serving Special Populations   159

15 Challenges for Women's Health   161
     Gloria Feldt

16 Fulfilling a Women's Health Agenda   171
     Wanda K. Jones

17 Caring for an Aging Population   178
     Martha A. McSteen

18 Geriatric Care   186
     William L. Minnix Jr.

19 New Perspectives for Long-Term Care·   199
     Lorraine Tarnove

20 Rural Health Systems   205
     Jon B. Christianson, Anthony L. Wellever

Part Four: Technology Leaders   217

21 The Evolving Role of Health Information   219
     Charles W. McCall, Ellen S. Dodson

22 Wiring the Health Revolution   231
    Morton H. Meyerson

23 Strategic Health Care Computing   242
    Russell J. Ricci

24 Technology-Induced Ethical Questions   250
    Stephen R. Latham

Part Five: Clinical Leaders   259

25 Challenges to Physician Leaders   261
    Thomas R. Reardon

26 Core Competencies for Physicians   269
    Edward O'Neil

27 The Future of Nursing   278
    Marjorie Beyers

28 Transforming Nursing Leadership   290
    Marilyn P. Chow, Janet M. Coffman, Robin L. Morjikian

Part Six: Gaining New Skills   299

29 Leading Across the Network   301
    Marshall Goldsmith

30 Four Dimensions of Lasting Change   308
    Karen Golden-Biddle, R. Mark Biddle

31 Developing Organizations by Developing Individuals   316
    Elaine Franklin, Robbin M. Moore

32 The Changing Dynamics of Customer Satisfaction
    and Its Measurement   323
    Charles D. Frame

33 Blending Health Care Organizations   331
    Roderick W. Gilkey, Gary R. Lieberman

Part Seven: Managed Care: Answers and Questions   345

34 Regaining the Public's Trust in Managed Care   347
    David M. Lawrence

35 The New Health Economics   355
    Merrill Matthews Jr.

36 Managed Care and the Black Physician   368
    Randall C. Morgan Jr.

37 Leading Behavioral Health Services   376
    Keith Dixon

Name Index   387

Subject Index   393

~~~ Preface

The exploding costs of health care in the industrialized world have created a challenge of unprecedented proportion. Although the economic and political mandates for decreasing costs and increasing quality are apparent, what is not obvious is how current and future health care leaders can respond effectively to these developments. What is clear is that this new environment will significantly alter the requirements for effective organizational leadership in health care. This book explores the profound implications of these changes, as health care leaders are called upon to create new kinds of organizations and systems that can provide higher-quality and lower-cost clinical care to a broader population of Americans with long life expectancies. Although the need to do more with less is a general leadership requirement in an increasingly competitive world, this requirement creates altogether new dilemmas for health care leaders. The skill sets required to address and manage these disparate dilemmas are vastly different from those used by the preceding generation.

James Collins, in the Introduction, tells us that right now is a very exciting time to be taking a leadership role in health care. He reminds us that even though there are many changes to be made in health care today, we have to be selective. We cannot simply change for the sake of change: the reason to change must be to create better systems of delivering health care to people.

AUDIENCE FOR THIS BOOK

This book is written primarily for practitioners in the health care industry, although the quality and rigor of the work reflected in this volume will undoubtedly contribute to the sizable stream of leadership research that is growing year by year. We hope that this book will be of particular value to health care professionals, executives, consultants, academics, and journalists. The authors represent the broadest range of health care–related professions and sectors: HMOs, insurers, providers, special populations, information technology, academic medical centers, and public health and global health organizations.

OVERVIEW OF THE CONTENTS

This book is divided into seven parts. Part One, "Navigating to a New Century," begins as Russell C. Coile Jr., Joe Flower, and Joel Shalowitz, in Chapters One, Two, and Three, respectively, present broad and multifaceted views of the health care opportunities and challenges that lie ahead of us in the next century. In Chapter Four, Lawrence O. Gostin explores the specific ethical dilemmas we face in the changing health care environment. In Chapter Five, Kent Glenzer and Maurice I. Middleberg consider the effects of the changing U.S. health care delivery system on the delivery of global health care. And in Chapter Six, William H. Foege and Mark Rosenberg examine the significance of that changing system on public and community health.

Part Two, "The New Health Care Organization," begins with a look at the pieces of the whole pie of health care delivery systems: Jeffrey C. Barbakow discusses consolidation and the hospital of the future in Chapter Seven, John D. Henry Sr. and I describe a method of developing leaders by empowering employers in Chapter Eight, Darrell G. Kirch considers the need to reinvent academic medical centers in Chapter Nine, and Michael Johns and Thomas J. Lawley analyze the leadership challenges unique to academic medical centers in Chapter Ten. In Chapters Eleven and Twelve, we hear the insurer's point of view about future ways of both controlling costs and improving quality, with observations from Patrick G. Hays and from Leonard D. Schaeffer and L. Carl Volpe. Part Two ends with two discussions that examine the structure of health care organizations and the creation of an effective, integrated delivery system, as Paul K. Halverson, in Chapter Thirteen, describes a community health system and Arnold D. Kaluzny and Howard S. Zuckerman, in Chapter Fourteen, discuss health care alliances.

Part Three, "Serving Special Populations," focuses on how the delivery of health care differs from one population segment to another, depending on each segment's special needs. In Chapters Fifteen and Sixteen, Gloria Feldt and Wanda K. Jones, respectively, describe specific issues leadership must address in women's health care. As our nation's baby boomers age, more attention will be focused on their special health care needs including long-term care, and Martha A. McSteen, William L. Minnix Jr., and Lorraine Tarnove examine these needs in Chapters Seventeen, Eighteen, and Nineteen, respectively. Jon B. Christianson and Anthony L. Wellever present the various roles of insider and outsider leadership in rural health systems in Chapter Twenty.

The role of technology in health care is the focus of Part Four, "Technology Leaders." Is more better? Not necessarily; not when it leads to exponential growth in costs without corresponding benefits and eventual cost reductions. Charles W. McCall and Ellen S. Dodson in Chapter Twenty-One, Morton H. Meyerson, in Chapter Twenty-Two, and Russell J. Ricci, in Chapter Twenty-Three, report on the progress made and the substantial work still to be done by health care organizations in using information technology to improve not only business practices but also patient services and outcomes. In Chapter Twenty-Four, Stephen R. Latham offers thoughts on technology-induced ethical problems.

What new roles will the providers of health care face in the twenty-first century? Part Five, "Clinical Leaders," opens with the different perspectives of Thomas R. Reardon, in Chapter Twenty-Five, and Edward O'Neil, in Chapter Twenty-Six, on the new skills needed by physician leaders in the future. Nurses will face new challenges as well, requiring expanded roles and changes in nursing education, and these ideas are explored in Chapters Twenty-Seven and Twenty-Eight by Marjorie Beyers and by Marilyn P. Chow, Janet M. Coffman, and Robin L. Morjikian, respectively.

What are the new leadership skills that will be required in the twenty-first century? Part Six, "Gaining New Skills," investigates them. Marshall Goldsmith, in Chapter Twenty-Nine, describes skills future leaders will need for leading across health care networks. Karen Golden-Biddle and R. Mark Biddle, in Chapter Thirty, present four dimensions leaders should consider in order to sustain organizational changes. Elaine Franklin and Robbin M. Moore, in Chapter Thirty-One, focus on the importance of developing individuals' competencies to ensure the future of the organization. Charles D. Frame defines some dynamics and measurement issues in customer satisfaction in Chapter Thirty-Two, and Gary R. Lieberman and I close Part Six (in Chapter Thirty-Three) with a discussion of the consequences of mergers and acquisitions in health care.

The central focus in Part Seven, "Managed Care: Answers and Questions," is leadership in the new world of managed care. In Chapter Thirty-Four, David M. Lawrence considers the importance of trust as a component of the managed care leadership needed in the future. Will managed care survive into the twenty-first century? That is the question Merrill Matthews Jr. poses in his discussion of health care economics in Chapter Thirty-Five. Randall C. Morgan Jr., in Chapter Thirty-Six, addresses the needs of minority populations within managed care systems and the need to involve many more black physicians in managed care programs. Finally, in Chapter Thirty-Seven, Keith Dixon delves into the concerns faced by leaders in mental health coverage and services under managed care.

Atlanta, Georgia   RODERICK W. GILKEY
November 1998

~~~ Acknowledgments

A project of this magnitude is the product of the work and dedication of many individuals. The idea and inspiration came from conversations with Marshall Goldsmith. The editor of previous volumes in this leadership series, Marshall saw the need to address the health care leadership challenges of the future and prompted those of us working in the field to create this book. He is an inspired and inspiring teacher, executive educator, colleague, and friend. Thank you, Marshall; I owe you a debt of gratitude for your key role. My consultations with Frances Hesselbein of the Drucker Foundation during the formative phase of this book also proved invaluable.

At Jossey-Bass, Andy Pasternack's belief in the value of this book; his steadfast support of all involved; and his patience, insight, and wise counsel established a high standard of editorial excellence. Adrienne Chieng, editorial assistant for the Jossey-Bass health series during the time this book was developed, demonstrated her commitment and competence daily. My respect for Andy, Adrienne, and all their Jossey-Bass colleagues is abiding and deep.

Within the Center for Healthcare Leadership Sheryl Tomberlin was the driving source and orchestrator of all collective efforts. She performed the monumental tasks of coordinating, integrating, and editing with great skill and commitment and her devotion to this effort was unswerving and inspiring. I offer my thanks and gratitude.

Past and present members of the Emory Healthcare Learning Council provided invaluable inspiration and continued support for this project. I would like to thank Peg Bloomquist and Robbin Moore in particular for their dedicated leadership, as well as Mary Capka, Joan Chioffe, Linda Espinosa, Elaine Franklin, Deborah Mills, and Rick Springfield.

Finally, and most important, I am indebted to the many insightful and generous individuals who contributed to this book. It is a product of both their profound insight and their generosity of spirit. In addition to contributing their valuable time and insights, they have contributed their royalties to fund medical research, making their chapters an expression of their profound commitment to the advancement of health care and of their own leadership. I thank them for their wisdom and generosity; they are living examples of the kind of leadership and commitment required to enhance the quality of our health care systems for future generations.

As this book is being written, my father, Dr. Wallace Gilkey, has been struggling with a series of life-threatening illnesses. He has been in the care of the administration and staff of the Lane wing of the Pardee Memorial Hospital, with Joanne Helppie, M.D., as his primary physician. Together they have provided a level of innovative and effective care that has been in every way exemplary. This is a reminder that the highest expression of leadership in a health care organization is the quality of individual care provided to patients and their families. It is also a reminder that health care leadership can make a difference.

R.W.G.

⚡ The Editor

Roderick W. Gilkey is associate professor in the Practice of Organization and Management Goizueta School of Business, Emory University. He is the recipient of the university's highest teaching honor, the Emory Williams Award. Gilkey's research writing is focused on leadership, change management, and international negotiation. He is coauthor of *Joining Forces: Successfully Managing Mergers and Acquisitions* (with Joseph McCann, 1998) and a contributor to *Organizations on the Couch* (edited by Manfred Kets de Vries, 1991). He holds a Ph.D. degree from the University of Michigan, and has provided consulting and executive education service to a broad array of global and Fortune 500 companies.

THE CENTER FOR HEALTHCARE LEADERSHIP EDITORS

Charles Frame
Elaine Franklin
Gary Lieberman
Sheryl Tomberlin

Introduction

James C. Collins

*James C. Collins is founder and executive director
of the Advanced Management Research Laboratory
in Boulder, Colorado. He has coauthored three books
and published over forty articles. His most recent book,
Built to Last (with Jerry Porras, 1994), has generated
over sixty printings worldwide and been translated into
fourteen languages. He has held faculty positions at
the Stanford University Graduate School of Business,
where he received the Distinguished Teaching Award,
and the University of Virginia. He has taught senior
executives and CEO at over one hundred corporations.
He has also worked for such nonprofit health care
organizations as the Johns Hopkins University School
of Medicine, the Healthcare Forum, and the University
Health Consortium.*

—∾∾∾— Ⅰf you are investing your time in reading this book, you already recognize the fact of change within the health care industry. This volume will help you better grasp the depth, extent, and speed of that change, and it will provide tools and alternatives you can apply within your own span of responsibility. Yet even given the magnitude of the changes facing health care, it would be a mistake to embark upon change just because your environment demands that you do so. You must undertake change within a context, change without abandoning what you stand for, change toward exciting aspirations, not merely change in response to external conditions. In this Introduction, I offer four basic precepts that I hope you will keep in mind as you act on the learning gleaned from reading this volume.

1. CLARIFY WHAT SHOULD NEVER CHANGE

The proper response to a changing world for any great institution is *not* first to ask, What should we change? Rather the proper first question is, What do we stand for and why do we exist? The values this question identifies should never change. And *then* we can feel liberated to change everything else. All great organizations have a set of timeless core values that they cherish and hold sacred. They also have an enduring core purpose—a fundamental reason for being beyond just making money—which they relentlessly pursue for decades or centuries, like a guiding star on the horizon. Taken together, the core values and purpose form the bonding glue and guiding philosophy that preserve the essence and spirit of the organization as it changes in adapting to an ever-changing world. Only by managing this dual dynamic of continuity and change—of preserving the core and stimulating progress—can you hope to create enduring prosperity amid the seismic changes discussed in this volume.

You must distinguish with great clarity your core values and core purpose (which should not change) from your practices, strategies, norms, mechanisms, policies, systems, and structures (all of which should be open to change) (see Figure I.1). For example, "freedom of inquiry" might be a core value that should never change; academic tenure, in contrast, is a practice, a manifestation of the core value, that should be open to change. "Improving the health of our community" might be a core value; tax status (nonprofit or for-profit) is merely a strategy that should be open to change. "The interest of the patient is the only interest to be considered" might be a core value; inpatient and outpatient services are simply practices. A shift from inpatient to outpatient services, if done properly, can be a change consistent with the core value.

As a health care executive, you face decades of accumulated practices, strategies, and norms. The vast majority are not—and should not be considered—sacred. Yet they can *feel* sacred. And the only way to break beyond them and also preserve the integrity of the institution is to pin down the very few core principles that should never change, leaving everything else open for evolution. There are no universally *right* core values nor one single *correct* core purpose for all health care organizations. Even though your institution's core probably resembles the cores of other health care institutions, careful reflection will likely reveal idiosyncrasies. Even similar institutions in the same industry can have different core values and purpose.

The key is not to look outside to identify the right core for today's world but to reflect *inside* to discover your institution's enduring and authentic core (for this process, see Collins and Porras, 1994, 1996).

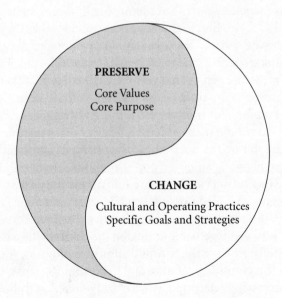

PRESERVE

Core Values
Core Purpose

CHANGE

Cultural and Operating Practices
Specific Goals and Strategies

Figure I.1.   **What to Preserve and What to Change.**

Even at this time of great change—indeed, especially at this time— you must clarify what your institution holds to be core, *independent* of the current environment, competitive pressures, or management fads. You must be relentlessly honest as you push to discover what is truly core to your institution—not what you think *ought* to be core, or what industry experts think your core *should* be, or what a ranting management guru proclaims you *must embrace.* Yes, your institution needs new practices and strategies, but you do *not* need to corrupt or abandon its core values.

How do you distinguish between a core value and a practice? You should be able to answer with a resounding yes the following question about a core value: If circumstances changed and *penalized* us for holding this core value, would we still keep it? Only values that pass this test qualify as core values; those that fail it should be relegated to the category of noncore practices open to change.

It is particularly important to clarify the difference between your institution's core purpose (fundamental reason for being) and its business strategies—a common point of confusion in health care institutions. Academic medical centers, for example, frequently speak of their *three missions*—clinical work, research, and teaching. Yet clinical work and research are not intrinsically core values. They are methods, strategies. Indeed, as former Stanford Medical School dean David Korn (1996) has made clear, many academic medical centers have become so wedded to their clinical and research strategies that they have lost sight of why they exist in the first place. A great organization does not exist to pursue specific strategies; it exists to fulfill a purpose, and its strategies must be open to change within the context of that purpose. Your institution's core purpose, as distinct from its strategies, should remain intact for centuries. Yet even though that core purpose does not change, it should inspire change. The very fact that purpose, like that guiding star on the horizon, can be pursued but never fully realized means that you can never stop stimulating change and progress so that the institution can live more fully to the purpose.

I find many so-called mission statements to be a muddled stew of purpose, values, aspirations, goals, practices, behaviors, tactics, and strategies, jumbled together and lacking the clarity to be a useful tool. To successfully preserve the core and stimulate progress, you have got to unravel this confusing mixture and gain ruthless clarity. Only then can you successfully decouple what is truly sacred and should never change from that which should be open to change.

2. PROMULGATE THE GENIUS OF *AND*

Health care institutions attract people motivated in their work by deeply held values and a noble cause—people like you. Yet this motivation can block productive change and progress if adapting to increasing competitive market pressures produces fear that "we will become just like any other profit-making business" or that "we will run the risk of losing our sense of social mission." I am struck by how many health care professionals fall prey to the tyranny of *or*—the false belief that they face such choices as gaining efficiency *or* gaining quality, fulfilling a higher purpose *or* making money, preserving core values *or* creating success in a changing market place, and so on.

The trick, of course, is to reject the tyranny of *or* and embrace the genius of *and*. An organization can be efficient *and* deliver exceptional quality, pursue a noble purpose *and* make money, preserve core values *and* create success in a rapidly changing world. Health care institutions have the great advantage of being engaged in work that directly affects the well-being of people. It would be tragic to see these institutions capitulate their core values and noble purpose in the false belief that they must choose their economic viability over their principles. It would be equally tragic if they undermined their ability to thrive and function in the false belief that they must choose core principles over economic strength. No, they must do all these things, and as a health care executive, one of your great tasks is to help those around you to live by *and*, not die by *or*.

3. DECIDE NOT ONLY WHAT TO ADD,
BUT ALSO WHAT TO REMOVE

In our hyper-action-oriented Western culture, we respond to challenge and change primarily by adding stuff—new initiatives, new programs, new strategies, new policies, new goals, new imperatives. We add, we clutter, we pile on. And in so doing we neglect the critical question of what to *not* add and what to remove. Let me use a personal example to illustrate. I love to read books and reflect thoughtfully on what I have read. So to stimulate progress in reading and reflection, I set a goal to read and reflect on one hundred books a year. Being a typical American, I launched this effort by adding to an already cluttered life: stacks of new books; long to-read lists; and new reading lamps, desks, chairs, and so on. And yet I continued to fall far short of my reading and reflection goals. Then it dawned on me: the television. Get rid of the television! And so my wife and I unplugged our TV. We no longer have a television set in our home. The silence is blissful, and my reading productivity (not to mention my time to listen to great music) has soared—not quite to one hundred books a year, but about double what it was before.

As a health care executive you probably have a healthy to-do list and a lengthy list of new priorities and initiatives for your organization. But have you paused to ask explicitly, What should we *stop* doing? What should we unplug? Unplugging is one of the most catalytic steps you can take. And it applies across the board, from unplugging business strategies to unplugging policies, procedures, practices, systems, and mechanisms of all types. Health care organizations are in the business of *doing good* for people. Yet this very fact makes it difficult to decide what to not do and what to stop doing. A core value to "be of service" or a purpose "to improve human health in our community" does not mean that an organization should provide *all* services and improve *all* human health. A great organization says no to products and services that simply do not fit, no matter how common at other companies in its industry. In thinking about what strategies to keep, to add, to reject, and remove, you can use a simple three-circle model (Figure I.2), adding or keeping those activities that fit in the intersection of all three circles. Great organizations pay equal attention to their core values and core purpose, linking all three circles together into an integrated whole.

4. REJECT SURVIVAL AS YOUR PRIMARY GOAL

At times of great change, challenge, and struggle, organizations of all types can fall prey to a debilitating survival mentality. Health care institutions today face such substantial external changes that some executives, in their more honest reflections, wonder if their institutions can survive in anything resembling their current incarnations. Yet mere survival seldom inspires as a goal. It conveys no sense of forward movement, no feeling of hope for the future, no sense of shaping one's own destiny. The key is to shift the psychology from a survival mentality to a prevail mentality.

Let me use a favorite historical example. In August 1940, Great Britain stood alone. France had fallen to Hitler and his Nazi war

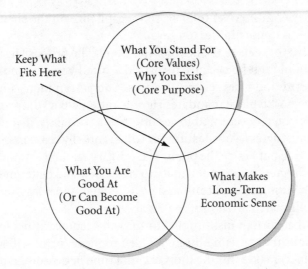

Figure I.2. Three-Circle Model.

machine, as had Belgium, Luxembourg, Holland, Denmark, Norway, and most of Eastern Europe. Hitler had not yet turned against Russia and was concentrating on the planned invasion of the British Isles. The United States stood on the sidelines, and would not enter the war until the attack on Pearl Harbor, sixteen months in the future. As British pilots flew to meet swarms of German bombers and fighters, the world watched and wondered—Can Britain survive? Winston Churchill, who at age sixty-five had shouldered the dual responsibilities of Prime Minister and Minister of Defense, rejected the question. The goal is not to survive, he retorted. The goal is to *prevail.*

Churchill's shifting of people's thoughts from surviving to prevailing played a huge role at a pivotal point of the war, giving the world hope and Hitler pause. It is one of the great lessons of leadership from history. Another part of the lesson is that Churchill adopted and adhered to a straightforward yet inspiring definition of *prevail.* For him it meant, "cleansing Europe from the Nazi pestilence and saving the world from the new Dark Ages." As a health care executive, you have to define what prevail means for your institution. You have to *create* a goal. By setting forth an audacious ten-to thirty-year Big Hairy Audacious Goal (not merely a five-year strategic objective) that is rooted in your institution's core values and purpose, you can do much to shift your organization's focus from How do we react to the changes facing us so we can survive? to How do we capitalize on the changes in front of us as opportunities to prevail?

And indeed that gets to the heart of this book. The primary reason to change should not be because the world around you demands it. Yes, your institution faces seismic changes. And yes, an increasingly competitive marketplace mandates significant efficiency improvements, higher-quality care, and lower prices. And certainly, if you do not stimulate progress, your institution will eventually cease to exist. All of this is true but beside the point. The primary reason to stimulate change and progress is the opportunity to create new and better methods of contributing to the health and well-being of those you serve. And *that* is ultimately what this book is about.

The fact that current institutional forms will become extinct (and the institutions that remain blindly wedded to those forms will also become extinct) makes this the most exciting time in decades to play a leadership role in health care. It gives you the opportunity to apply the consummate human skill—creativity combined with foresight— to *invent* new institutional forms at a pivotal point in history. Those who make the biggest impact on health care in the twenty-first century will be those who apply creative imagination not just to crafting new business strategies but to inventing entirely new organizational forms. So, as you harvest the insights of the impressive array of thinkers and experts assembled expressly for this volume, keep in mind that the ultimate solutions will not come from the pages of a book. They will come from people like you—people ferociously committed to preserving the timeless core values and enduring core purpose of their institutions and equally dedicated to demolishing dysfunctional structures and inventing new institutional forms that can flourish in a new era.

References

Collins, J. C., and Porras, J. I. *Built to Last.* New York: Harper Business, 1994.

Collins, J. C., and Porras, J. I. "Building Your Company's Vision." *Harvard Business Review,* Sept.–Oct. 1996, pp. 65–77.

Korn, D. "Reengineering Academic Medical Centers." *Academic Medicine,* 1996, *71*(10), p. 1033.

PART ONE

Navigating to a New Century

The Three C's: Consumerism, Cyberhealth, and Co-Opetition

Russell C. Coile Jr.

Russell C. Coile Jr. is managing partner of the Strategic Planning Practice of Chi Systems (based in Dallas), a division of Superior Consultant Company, Inc. He is the author of The Five Stages of Managed Care *(1997) and four other books on the future of the health field, and editor of the monthly newsletter* Russ Coile's Health Trends. *In 1996 and 1997, his annual forecast of the top ten trends in health care was 100 percent accurate.*

Think of it . . . massive movements of Americans of every stripe, embracing fitness, sound diets, stress management, positive thinking, personal responsibility and related constructive practices—a revolution in health status leading to substantial increases in optimal functioning and life satisfaction. And all this during the right-here-on-earth lifetime.

> Donald B. Ardell, "Health, Wellness and
> Secular Humanism" (1997, p. 2)

A new era is emerging in U.S. health care. Beyond the current era of managed care, the concerns of consumers, a spate of governmental regulation, and new attitudes about health improvement are combining to fuel a fundamental rearrangement of the financing and delivery of health care in the United States in the twenty-first century. Seven critical components mark this watershed in the evolution of U.S. medicine:

- Third-party payers are relinquishing their efforts to control health costs, focusing narrowly on marketing and customer service to demonstrate their value as more traditional intermediaries.

- Providers are assuming financial, professional, legal and moral risk for patient care in capitated payment arrangements.

- Consumers with access to extensive on-line information and patient support groups take an active role in their own health improvement.

- Information systems are linking highly decentralized provider networks to integrated care systems by providing real-time information on patient health status, clinical care, and financial costs.

- The health system is refocusing on health promotion for the 85 percent of the population who are the *worried well* and the 15 percent who are at risk or are already chronically ill.

- On-line nurses and home health workers are providing day-to-day management for high-risk patients and the chronically ill.

- Public *report cards* are supplying detailed information on clinical outcomes and patient satisfaction for each health plan and provider network.

This chapter outlines major changes occurring in health care, revealing the opportunities and challenges that face health care organizations and practitioners who must learn to practice co-opetition, use technology wisely and effectively, and meet the needs of people as both patients and consumers.

With managed care in the United States now entering a stage in which 25 to 40 percent of residents are enrolled in health maintenance organizations (HMOs), very large provider organizations are going head-to-head with the biggest health plans in the market (Coile, 1997). HMOs are in retreat, suffering declining public relations as well as profitability. Provider sponsored organizations (PSOs) are tightening their grip on market share, building bigger networks that cover entire market regions. Dominant providers are stretching the definition of cooperation. Connecticut's Hartford Health Care Corporation, for example, is a statewide network of community hospitals, physician organizations, and an academic medical center that is based on partnering, not merger (Droste, 1997b).

Health care providers are retaking control of the health system. The assumption of risk for comprehensive care is transforming providers from fee-for-service vendors into cost-accountable care systems. Employer coalitions could play an important role in the transition. Some employers are banding together in powerful coalitions, like the San Francisco–based Pacific Business Group on Health, in order to demand better deals from HMOs. Other employer groups, like Minnesota's Buyers Health Care Action Group (BHCAG), are making an end run around traditional HMO plans and their capitated gatekeeper models. These groups are working directly with providers in new ways to lower costs and improve care, creating an opening for the provider networks efficient and gutsy enough to step in (Meyer, 1996). Now Medicare is offering provider sponsored organizations the opportunity to participate in managed Medicare, with qualified PSOs federally certified to sign up seniors at the local Medicare capitation rate.

Southern California's PacifiCare has offered to provide administrative services for local provider sponsored organizations that assume Medicare risk. Today's competitors are finding new common ground for business collaboration tomorrow, a revolutionary concept labeled *co-opetition* (Brandenburger and Nalebuff, 1996). When competitors reach a standoff in market advantage, they can switch to cooperation to increase their mutual strengths and benefits. In Houston, Terry Ward, of the Ward Group, is working to develop a local cooperative joint venture involving some of the market's biggest competitors. By refocusing these traditional competitors into a shared business alliance, Ward (1997) hopes they will reduce their development and operating costs and share a better level of profitability than any could have achieved independently. Co-opetition is one of the emerging themes for the decade ahead.

REINVENTING HMOS

The HMO industry is entering a "rocky new phase," according to a recent front-page story in the *New York Times* (Kilborn, 1997, p. A1). The HMO industry is under continuous attack from consumer groups, plaintiffs' attorneys, and the media. Stock prices are slumping, with New York's Oxford Health Plans plunging more than 60 percent in one day, after reports of computer problems and underestimated medical expenses. The spate of criticism comes even though HMOs have signed up more than sixty-six million Americans and are holding national health care inflation under the Consumer Price Index.

Rising *medical loss ratios* signal that HMOs are losing their grip on provider utilization and health care expenditures. The plans continue to hold a dominant position because they have millions of enrollees, but employers are openly questioning whether HMOs should be taking 15 to 20 percent off the top of the premium for administration, marketing, and medical management. A growing number of HMOs are abandoning efforts to compete with providers as *integrated delivery networks.*

Evidence from a number of markets around the nation suggests that HMO initiatives in vertical integration are failing (Kilborn, 1997). In the West, California's Kaiser Permanente is contracting out hospital services to community facilities. In Kansas City, in the country's heartland, the local Blue Cross and Blue Shield organization is closing eleven of its twenty-two clinics, and laying off half of its sixty-five primary care practitioners. Crosstown rival Humana is also dismissing physicians and will slash salaries of cardiovascular surgeons by 40 to 50 percent next year.

Employers are rethinking their reliance on HMOs, and adopting more flexible, provider-friendly arrangements. Electronics giant Motorola launched a nongatekeeper preferred provider organization (PPO) last year, with 100,000 participating physicians and 450 hospitals. In the first open enrollment, 59 percent of employees dumped their HMOs and switched to the company-backed PPO, which is managed by a third-party administrator (TPA), Private Health Care Systems (Meyer, 1996).

Employer discontent is not the end of the line for health maintenance organizations. HMOs can stay in the managed care game by
broadening their product lines: for example, by providing TPA services.
In Illinois, United Healthcare set up a self-insured point of service plan
for the Whitman Corporation in Rolling Meadows. The plan offers an
unusually high level of payment (80 percent) for services provided out
of network.

MANAGED MEDICARE

The nation's number one health care consumers—Medicare's thirty-
five million seniors and disabled—are shifting to managed Medicare.
Some 12.6 percent of Medicare beneficiaries have already switched to
managed care, the number doubling in the past five years, according
to St. Paul, Minnesota–based InterStudy, a managed care think tank
and market research organization that tracks the HMO industry
(Hamer, 1997a). Enrollment in Medicare HMOs is climbing rapidly,
up 27.8 percent in 1997, and could reach 11.6 million enrollees, about
one-third of all seniors, by the end of 2001 (see Figure 1.1). Only four
states still have no Medicare HMOs: Alaska, Missouri, Tennessee, and
South Carolina. That should change swiftly now that the 105th Congress has boosted Medicare HMO reimbursement for many areas.

Seniors accustomed to choice of providers and easy access will
demand similar accommodation from Medicare HMOs. Planning
consultant Dan Beckham predicts that "the elderly will receive whatever they want. There is no way this group isn't going to vote for their
interests when it comes to healthcare. . . . Baby Boomers also have the
clout to ensure their parents are treated well by health plans" (Droste,
1997a, p. 2).

HEALTH CARE SPENDING FORECAST: LOW INFLATION

Despite rising HMO premiums the likelihood of double-digit increases
in health spending is low. The core rate of health care inflation will
remain low to moderate, in the range of a 3 to 4 percent annual
increase. The economics of competitive managed care will ensure that
health care expenditures do not rise out of control in the near future.
Health economist Paul Ginsburg (1997) credits employer willingness

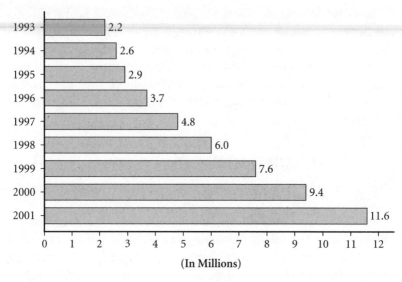

Figure 1.1.   Medicare HMO Enrollment Forecast.
Source: Hamer, 1997a, p. 6.

to switch health plans to get a competitive price as a major factor ensuring low inflation.

Inflation concerns arise from the current status of the HMO industry. Slumping profits in publicly traded HMOs are worrying Wall Street and HMO executives. The pall on managed care plans is affecting even successful HMOs like California's Wellpoint, despite its recently reported 24 percent net income growth (Freudenheim, 1997). Wellpoint's good news came a day after the Oxford Health Plans share price fell 60 percent. HMOs will attempt to boost prices 4.6 percent, according to the Sherlock Company's annual HMO pricing survey (McGuire, 1997), but they will run into price resistance from major employers, predict industry observers, with actual increases more likely to fall in the range of 2 to 3 percent.

HMOs are caught in the six-year insurance pricing cycle, in which, on average, three years of premium competition and lower prices are followed by three years of rising premiums to improve profits. The current pricing pattern appears to be part of a rising premium cycle. The 651 HMOs in the United States are being squeezed between slowly rising medical expenses and employer resistance to price hikes. According to InterStudy the medical loss ratio for HMOs is now averaging 86 percent, up almost 3 percent in three years (Hamer, 1997a).

HMO profits are slumping. The top 25 percent of HMOs, generally larger, more efficient plans, are still making money, in the range of 1 to 2 percent, but smaller, newer HMOs are experiencing losses ranging from 5 to 9 percent. The arrival of 53 new HMOs, many established by providers, ensures continuing price competition.

MANAGED CARE REFORM

A *patient bill of rights* drafted by a presidential commission on consumer protection and quality is likely to become federal law (Rodrigue, 1997). The proposal guarantees that health plans must pay for prudent emergency care, supply an adequate number of primary care and subspecialty physicians, and eliminate *gag rules* that prevent doctors from discussing treatment options with patients. Managed care industry opposition to this new "ClintonCare" proposal is already forming, and the Health Insurance Association of America has fired back with a threat to "trash" the proposal. Republican lawmakers like Richard Armey (R-TX) have predicted that employers could drop their health coverage rather than comply and have criticized the commission for potentially driving up the costs of health insurance and increasing the number of medically uninsured.

The threat of congressional action comes at the time when HMOs have already signed up sixty-six million Americans, predicted to grow to more than one hundred million enrollees by January 2001, according to InterStudy (Hamer, 1997a) (see Figure 1.2). HMOs have become the health plan choice of the middle class and of growing numbers of Medicare and Medicaid beneficiaries. The public may fear governmental regulation even more than tight-walleted HMOs and insurers. Although people overwhelmingly favor placing more controls on health plans—84 percent to 16 percent—they are divided on who should exercise these controls. A recent survey by the Henry J. Kaiser Family Foundation found that only one in five Americans favors federal regulation. Twenty percent want states to take a role, and another 33 percent want an independent oversight commission (Rodrigue, 1997). Support for regulation dropped to 52 percent when survey interviews told consumers that regulation could raise health care prices.

Patient concerns about privacy and security are likely to regulate the use of electronic medical records by managed care organizations. The American Psychiatric Association is concerned that "electronic

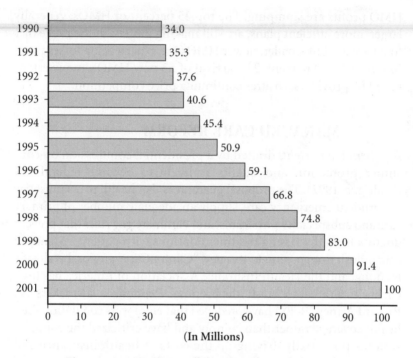

Figure 1.2.   HMO Enrollment Forecast, 1997 to 2001.

Source: Hamer, 1997a, p. 2.

peeping Toms" in managed care organizations and government will have access to patients' confidential records (Wechsler, 1997, p. 16). The Clinton administration has a medical records privacy proposal, and twelve health information security measures were introduced in Congress in 1997. Some federal legislation is likely in 1999, possibly teamed with antidiscrimination protections. A number of the proposals would require managed care organizations to record information disclosures and make that record available to patients, a costly process for the plans to administer. The debate is complicated by the fact that federal action would be an effort to preempt existing state laws, and argument over it could tie up medical confidentiality issues in the courts for years to come.

To help reduce the threat of regulation, the managed care industry is responding actively to consumer concerns. After years of frustration, health care patients are getting what they want in the managed care era: access to specialists, fewer gatekeeper requirements and HMO hassles, and new benefits like alternative medicine and podiatry. Stingy

HMO attitudes and limited provider panels are being replaced by consumer-friendly service and open-access products.

DIRECT CONTRACTING

Provider sponsored organizations have a window of opportunity for direct contracting in Medicare, Medicaid, and self-insured ERISA (Employee Retirement Income Security Act) health plans. Congressional action on PSOs has opened the door for providers to participate directly in managed Medicare, signing up seniors and assuming risk at the local Medicare capitation rate. Midsized and small markets may be the best targets for PSOs. Big HMOs already dominate large markets, increasing their market from 23.2 to 31.2 percent in just the last three years (Hamer, 1997c). HMOs have much lower penetration (20.8 percent) in midsized markets of about 500,000 people. In local markets, PSOs have the advantages of high visibility and market recognition, potentially reducing their selling costs to recruit seniors.

Employer health care coalitions could become "wholesale" customers for direct contracting. Business coalitions unhappy with HMO price increases in 1998 could turn to provider sponsored organizations, just as BHCAG in Minneapolis-St. Paul did in 1997. Stanford economics professor Alain Enthoven (1997), who serves on an advisory board to the California Public Employee Retirement System (CalPERS), the largest managed care buyer in California, has championed a market-based solution he calls *managed competition*. In California, market forces have produced six employer sponsored purchasing groups, including three for small, one for midsized, and two (one public, one private) for large employers.

The trend to direct contracting is still more potential than actual, but signs of employer discontent are widespread. Employer groups in Wisconsin, Iowa, Illinois, and Texas, for example, are rethinking their reliance on HMOs. Corporate health benefits managers are unhappy with HMO premium increases, which are averaging 5 percent in 1998 for large employers and 6 to 12 percent for smaller firms (Kilborn, 1997). In Houston the Health Care Purchasing Organization represents 40 large companies and 2,500 smaller ones and contracts directly with a network of providers. Organization president Ralph Smith argues that "the HMO middleman sets a fixed premium for employers, pushes the risk onto the providers, and then any gain goes to the

HMO while providers and employers take all of the downside risk"
(Meyer, 1996, p. 36).

MARKET CONSOLIDATION

The market consolidation of health plans and providers is leading to
a new phase of market competition, sometimes called sumo wrestling,
in which very large plans bargain hard with provider networks of
dozens of hospitals and thousands of doctors. For plans and providers,
consolidation seeks economies of scale; it can slash overhead and
operating costs and gain market leverage for contracting. Hospitals
and physicians are consolidating at an ever-increasing pace. Regional
markets are shaking down to two to three competing provider sponsored networks, each controlling a share of the market ranging from
25 to 35 (or more) percent. They are facing three to four dominant
health plans that collectively control 70 to 80 percent of HMO local
market share (Hamer, 1997b).

Economics is driving the increased concentration of power in the
hands of a few provider sponsored organizations. In a national survey by TriBrook/AM&G, the top five reasons for consolidation were
reducing operating expenses, attracting more managed care contracts,
improving community health, reducing capital expenditures, and
responding to employer and business coalition pressures (Japsen,
1997). Industry consolidation is rolling up U.S. hospitals, physicians
and health plans into large, regionally integrated systems and networks. Hospital mergers, for example, went up by 44 percent from
1994 to 1995 (Monroe, 1996). In trend-setting Southern California, a
record twenty-nine hospitals completed mergers, acquisitions, or formal affiliations in 1996, a pace twice that of consolidations in 1995. A
survey indicated that another twenty-eight hospitals planned to affiliate or merge in 1997 (Wall, 1997). In more than half of these transactions, for-profit hospitals became part of larger chains. Five hospitals
converted from nonprofits to for-profits, and two from for-profits to
nonprofits.

Vertical integration is still a prominent strategy driving health organization merger mania. A recent industry survey showed that hospitals, physicians, and managed care organizations are planning to
acquire each other in record numbers (see Table 1.1). Nearly one-third
of the surveyed hospitals had been part of a consolidation in the past

five years, and one-third of the health plans had acquired another HMO in the same period (Greene, 1997). Half of the surveyed medical groups had been involved in a transaction with a for-profit physician company or nonprofit hospital or health system. Hospitals were still interested in buying medical group practices, despite reports that 80 percent of hospitals were losing money on the physician deals.

MEDICAL MEGA-GROUPS

A new generation of very large physician organizations is rising to take charge of some markets. Compared to their predecessors, these *medical mega-groups* are not only larger but better capitalized and managed and more broadly distributed to provide regional coverage. Many more physician organizations are now taking capitation. A growing number of them are owned or managed by Wall Street–financed physician practice management companies, which provide capital, systems, and management expertise.

Large, market-savvy medical groups have many capabilities that managed care organizations are seeking (Holm and Zuza, 1997):

• A geographical distribution that puts physicians within ten to fifteen minutes of all enrollees

• The ability to manage risk for professional services and, in some plans, global risk for inpatient and outpatient services

• Effective governance and management systems

	Organizations		
Strategy	Hospitals	Managed Care Organizations	Medical Groups
Buy a hospital	47 percent	32 percent	27 percent
Buy a group practice	23	23	63
Ally with a managed care organization	33	42	23

Table 1.1.   Who Plans to Do What with Whom?
Future Partnership Strategies.

Source: Data from Jay Greene, "1997 Leadership Survey," cited in Greene, 1997, p. 8.

- The financial strength to accept capitation and various payment options
- A primary care orientation
- The ability to document quality indicators, including patient satisfaction and clinical outcomes

Physician groups are merging to create market-dominating organizations that swing real clout. In the past three years linkages between physician groups have risen 58 percent (Monroe, 1996). Bigger medical groups have more leverage in managed care contracting, but there are additional reasons for physician consolidation. Sharing the cost of upgrading information systems is a major factor, cited by 61 percent of the groups. Only 4 percent of physicians were submitting claims electronically in 1996, mostly larger groups (Slepin, 1996). Another benefit is the ability to compare practice patterns, lowering costs and improving productivity.

A second generation of independent practice associations (IPAs), medical mega-groups of another kind, is demonstrating that the network model of organization can successfully assume and manage capitation for large enrolled populations (Lowes, 1997). In San Francisco an IPA originally started by the California Pacific Medical Center and later restructured as a physician-owned entity, the Brown & Toland Medical Group, now has 1,250 physicians and 172,000 covered lives under capitation. Brown & Toland recently became the first IPA in California to obtain a state license (known in California as a limited Knox-Keene license) to accept global capitation for both inpatient and outpatient services.

And it's not happening just in California. In Milwaukee the Wisconsin Independent Physicians Group has organized 1,050 physicians to service forty-five thousand Medicaid patients under a global risk contract. The IPA is capitated, but physicians are paid on a fee-for-service basis. The group is using a population health approach to reduce risks and utilization. To control costs, the doctors own a free-standing imaging center and channel all testing through a commercial lab. The IPA describes its physician fee schedule as "generous" and relies on education rather than discipline to manage costs. It also uses peer pressure as another method of controlling utilization. Physician performance data systems regularly profile every doctor's costs, and physicians' names appear on reports so that colleagues can compare performance.

FOR-PROFIT BACKLASH

Wall Street may no longer be welcome on Main Street, at least not in the operation of hospitals and health plans. A growing backlash composed of media criticism, public concern, and state regulation is slowing the growth of for-profit health care companies. Public confidence in for-profit HMOs and health care companies is dropping. A random poll of one thousand Americans by the Henry J. Kaiser Family Foundation showed that the percentage who thought for-profit organizations provided better care fell from 55 percent to 42 percent in 1997 (Walker, 1997).

Columbia/HCA's troubles with the FBI and the Justice Department have been widely chronicled in the *Wall Street Journal* and *New York Times*. Under the twin clouds of massive Medicare fraud investigation and falling profits, the dismemberment of Columbia and the sale of all but its core hospitals is now underway, with two or more new companies likely to result (Sharpe, 1997). Columbia has now announced plans to spin off some 108 hospitals that do not fit Columbia's long-term strategy (Woodyard and Findlay, 1997). Columbia facilities outside the markets in which Columbia now has a critical mass could also be sold. Columbia/HCA suffered another blow when several states joined a shareholders' lawsuit against it. California, New York, Louisiana, and several municipalities have entered the fray, charging that Columbia management had allowed Medicare fraud to "flourish" (White and Lagnado, 1997, p. B5). California's Public Employee Retirement System suffered a $50 million loss when Columbia's shares sank in the wake of the fraud investigations.

Troubles for the for-profit health care industry are far from over. There are echoes of the *Wal-Mart wars* in the rising public antipathy toward for-profit health care companies. Even well-managed companies like Tenet, HealthSouth, and PhyCor may find growing opposition to acquisitions and new development. State attorney generals have discovered the publicity value of opposing for-profit takeovers of nonprofit providers. Several states, including California, Rhode Island, and Nebraska, have recently passed legislation making for-profit conversions subject to state review.

Despite the negative publicity and regulatory hurdles for-profits face, CEOs of nonprofit hospitals expect that for-profit hospital chains will expand their market share to 20 percent by the year 2000, rising to 29 percent within ten years, according to a national survey (Greene, 1997).

CYBERHEALTH

Information technology is the fastest-growing U.S. industry. According to *Cybernation*, a national study by the American Electronics Association and the NASDAQ stock exchange, computing and telecommunications have grown 57 percent since 1990 (Lohr, 1997). The high-tech sector generates 6.4 percent of the U.S. gross domestic product (GDP) and employs 4.2 million workers. *Cyberhealth* information systems today include electronic medical records, enterprisewide information linkages, Internet and intranet connections, data warehouses, distributed PC networks, remote-site telecommunications, and even in-home patient monitoring systems.

Health care information systems are essential to managing costs through disease management programs. In Falls Church, Virginia, the Innova Health System is creating a data repository to track more than 500,000 inpatient and outpatient visits per year (Hornung, 1997). The primary end products will be clinical analysis, quality assurance, and outcome assessment. Financial connectivity is another important goal of automation. Providers are learning to make effective use of their information system investments in such areas as claims processing and electronic data interchange (EDI). Submitting claims electronically can save $2.00 to $4.00 per claim, with some integrated systems experiencing savings of 75 to 90 percent in business office claims costs, which average $7.50 per bill (Slepin, 1996).

Information systems are expensive, and many buyers are still skeptical of the return on investment. The payoff comes from doing things differently, not just faster. Computerized analysis of cost variation can help repay information system investments. In South Bend, Indiana, the Holy Cross Health System saved $4.5 million by reducing variations in the pattern of care for thirty-six case groups (Appleby, 1997). Holy Cross information specialists also predicted the impact of managed care on the system's eleven facilities, finding that the system had to cut $80 million out of operating expenses or suffer major losses. The wake-up call was painful but timely.

Although most health care providers still only dream of a paperless information system, electronic medical records are making headway. A national survey of nearly five hundred physician group practices found that 22 percent of the groups had some or all of their records computerized (Montague and Pitman, 1996). Managed care transactions such as claims processing, eligibility verification, access to health plan enrollment lists, and submission of monthly encounter lists are fast-growing targets for automation. For capitated physicians, automating to reduce the cost of these backroom functions means more net income for themselves.

The application of cybernetics to patient care and also patient satisfaction is widening rapidly. In the area of physician-patient communication, for example, computers can insert instructions in electronic medical records to remind physicians to respond to patient concerns. Doctors at the William N. Wishard Memorial Hospital in Indianapolis respond to cues embedded in the hospital's intranet-enabled clinical information network. The messages are based on patient satisfaction surveys that identified disease-specific communication concerns. For example, doctors treating colonoscopy patients are reminded, "Before you order this colonoscopy, consider that patients often report they were not warned a test might cause pain or discomfort" ("Hospital to Test Use of Computer-Based Reminders," 1997, p. 5).

CONSUMERISM

Consumers have more choices in health care today, and retail marketing strategies are targeting them like Patriot missiles. Media campaigns by hospitals and health plans are reviving market warfare in their appeals to consumers' preferences. In New York, Aetna US Healthcare (1997) purchased a full-page advertisement in the *New York Times*. Showing a photo of a large apple dominating a table of oranges, Aetna boasted that it was the first HMO in New York City to win both full accreditation from the National Committee for Quality Assurance and the Sachs "seal of excellence" awarded for consumer satisfaction.

Retail marketing gives providers opportunities to *grow* their businesses with creative approaches to revenue growth and customer trends. Marketing consultant Ellen Goldman, of GrowthPartners in Reston, Virginia, and Karen Corrigan, of Sentara Health System in Norfolk, recommend three retail marketing strategies (Goldman and Corrigan, 1997):

- *Enhance the customer's experience.* Focus on the "atmospherics" of the point of service, creating an environment in which people want to purchase services. Attend to decor, displays, signage, selling techniques, and customer service. For example, offer waiting rooms that look like hotel lobbies, not airport holding areas. Winners of Modern Healthcare's 1997 design awards for health facilities were praised for their "patient-driven architecture," which featured residential characteristics and a family orientation (Pinto, 1997, p. 47).

- *Meet the customer's related needs.* Take opportunities to present and sell related products or services. Stimulating additional spending responds to customers' needs for convenience. For example, situating a home health agency outlet adjacent to heavy hospital patient and visitor traffic may stimulate additional business.

- *Segment products and markets.* Identify the unmet needs of people by age, sex, ethnicity, income, or other demographically defined subgroup. Marketers look for product or service variations that are tailored to a specific set of customers, for example, small businesses. Market gaps are unrecognized segments or products. In health care services, for example, adolescent medicine is aimed at youths aged fourteen to nineteen who may be too old to be pediatric patients but who do not want to share their parents' practitioners.

COMPLEMENTARY MEDICINE

Alternative medicine has almost reached mainstream acceptance. Its latest name is *complementary medicine,* a new label for treatments once called *unconventional.* Acupuncture, biofeedback, chiropractic, herbal remedies and homeopathy, nutrition, osteopathy, and yoga have arrived to join mainstream medical care. A marketing blitz by health plans and hospitals intends to capture consumers who have been spending $10 billion a year of out-of-pocket cash for health promotion and wellness.

Complementary medicine is popular with managed care enrollees, and a half-dozen national HMOs have begun to offer some complementary medicine benefits. National health plans, for example, have begun running multipage advertisements in newspapers such as the *New York Times* to announce this different philosophy and new attitude toward the delivery of health care services. HMOs are trumpeting newly credentialed networks of alternative medical providers.

In Dallas the "new medicine" was the subject of a widely attended medical conference sponsored by the University of Texas's Southwest Medical School and drawing 1,200 participants (Peterson, 1997).

The payoff in offering complementary medicine may be more than a marketing advantage. HMOs experimenting with alternative therapies are finding real cost benefit. According to Herbert Benson, M.D., head of Boston's Mind/Body Medical Institute, HMOs can experience a 50 percent reduction in stress-related injuries and 30 percent fewer visits for chronic back pain by training patients in self-relaxation and stress management (Montague, 1996).

Finally, the public's current high interest in health and wellness may have profit potential. For example, former Columbia/HCA executive Richard Scott is reentering the health industry from an unexpected direction—consumer health information. Scott and former second-in-command David Vandewater have purchased a majority stake in America's Health Network, a Florida-based cable channel that was the target of a Columbia acquisition offer until Richard Scott's departure as head of Columbia. The network features such programs as "Ask the Doctor" and currently reaches about 6.5 million households (Lagnado, 1997).

References

Aetna US Healthcare. "The More You Compare Health Care Companies, the More You Realize There Is No Comparison." Advertisement. *New York Times,* Nov. 12, 1997, p. A15.

Appleby, C. "Payoff @ InfoTech.Now." *Hospitals & Health Networks,* 1997, *71*(19), 59–60.

Ardell, D. B. *Health, Wellness and Secular Humanism.* Amherst, N.Y.: Council for Secular Humanism, 1997.

Brandenburger, A. M., and Nalebuff, B. J. *Co-Opetition.* New York: Doubleday, 1996.

Coile, R. C., Jr. *The Five Stages of Managed Care.* Chicago: Health Administration Press, 1997.

Droste, T. M. "Health System Marketers Must Learn from Past Mistakes So History Won't Repeat Itself." *Medical Network Strategy Report,* Sept. 1997a, pp. 1–4.

Droste, T. M. "One System Relies on Partnering as a Strategy to Build a State-wide Network." *Medical Network Strategy Report,* 1997b, *6*(10), 1–3.

Enthoven, A. "There's Gold in Them Thar' Coalitions." *Managed Health-care,* 1997, *10*(7), 21–24.

Freudenheim, M. "Wellpoint Shares Sink Despite Profit Gain." *New York Times,* Oct. 31, 1997, p. C2.

Ginsburg, P. B., and Pickreign, J. D. "Tracking Health Care Costs: An Update." Cited in *Medical Benefits,* 1997, *14*(17), 7.

Goldman, E. F., and Corrigan, K. V. "'Thinking Retail' in Healthcare: New Approaches for Business Growth." *Healthcare Strategist,* 1997, *1*(1), 1–9.

Greene, J. "1997 Leadership Survey." Cited in *Medical Benefits,* 1997, *14*(17), 8.

Hamer, R. L. "HMO Facts and Trends." Presentation materials. St. Paul, Minn.: InterStudy, 1997a.

Hamer, R. L. "HMO Regional Market Analysis." *InterStudy Competitive Edge,* 1997b, *7*(2), 1–138.

Hamer, R. L. "Small Markets Present Opportunities for Provider-Sponsored Networks." Cited in *Healthcare Leadership Review,* 1997c, *16*(9), 9.

Holm, C. E., and Zuza, D. J. "Positioning Primary Care Networks: Understand What Managed Care Organizations Really Want." *Health Care Services Strategic Management,* 1997, *15*(8), 1, 22–23.

Hornung, K. "Tap into Patient Data to Bolster Your Disease Management Program." *Healthcare Demand & Disease Management,* 1997, *3*(7), 97–101.

"Hospital to Test Use of Computer-Based Reminders." *Health Data Network News,* 1997, *6*(10), 5, 7.

Japsen, B. "Survey: Money, Not Mission, Driving Mergers." *Modern Healthcare,* 1997, *27*(41), 14.

Kilborn, P. T. "Health Care Plans Are Seen Entering Rocky New Phase." *New York Times,* Nov. 22, 1997, pp. A1, A11.

Lagnado, L. "Ousted CEO of Columbia Leads Cable Buy." *Wall Street Journal,* Nov. 12, 1997, p. B10.

Lohr, S. "Information Technology Field Is Rated Largest U.S. Industry." *New York Times,* Nov. 18, 1997, p. C12.

Lowes, R. L. "The Second-Generation IPA: Will It Save Independent Practice?" *Medical Economics,* 1997, *74*(16), 182–191.

McGuire, J. "HMOs Expect Significant Premium Hikes for 1998." *Managed Care Outlook,* 1997, *10*(20), 7.

Meyer, H. "Beyond HMOs: The Tide of the Times." *Hospitals & Health Networks,* 1996, *70*(8), 34–40.

Monroe, S. "Health Care Merger and Acquisition Report." New Canaan, Conn.: Irving Lewis Associates. Cited in "Mergers: The Center of the Storm." *Hospitals & Health Networks,* 1996, *70*(8), 10.

Montague, J. "Mind over Maladies." *Hospitals & Health Networks,* 1996, *70*(8), 26–27.

Montague, J., and Pitman, H. "Currents: Information Systems." *Hospitals & Health Networks,* 1996, *70*(8), 10–11.

Peterson, S. "Can the New Medicine Heal You?" *D,* Nov. 1997, pp. 80–91.

Pinto, C. "1997 Design Awards." *Modern Healthcare,* 1997, *27*(41), 47–62.

Rodrigue, G. "Panel Calls for HMO Changes." *Dallas Morning News,* Nov. 20, 1997, pp. A1, A12.

Sharpe, A. "Columbia/HCA Weighs Plan to Spin Off One-Third of Company's 340 Hospitals." *Wall Street Journal,* Nov. 11, 1997, p. B13.

Slepin, R. E. "EDI Translates into Big Savings." *California HFMA Journal,* 1996, *9*(4), 48–49.

Walker, T. "Kaiser Poll Pans For-Profit Plans." *Managed Care,* 1997, *10*(7), 8.

Wall, P. "Consolidations Accelerate, Nearly Double in 1996." *California HFMA Journal,* 1997, *10*(1), 34–36.

Ward, T. *Co-Opetition: An Innovative Strategy Which Combines Cooperation and Competition.* Houston, Tex.: Ward Group, Oct. 1997.

Wechsler, J. "Proposal Struggles with Privacy and Practicality." *Managed Healthcare,* 1997, *7*(10), 15–16.

White, J. B., and Lagnado, L. "Columbia/HCA Dealt Sharp Blow by CalPERS Move." *Wall Street Journal,* Oct. 21, 1997, p. B5.

Woodyard, C., and Findlay, S. "Columbia to Dump a Third of Hospitals." *USA Today,* Nov. 18, 1997, p. B1.

CHAPTER TWO

Forces and Scenarios That Will Shape Health Services Delivery

Joe Flower

Joe Flower is principal of the Change Project in Larkspur, California. He writes, speaks, and consults about health care, high technology, and the management of change in chaotic environments. Author of several books and several hundred articles, a contributing editor for Wired, Health-care Forum, *and* Physician Executive, *and a founding member of the International Health Futures Network, he has been writing about the management of health care for over fifteen years.*

Health care leaders of the future must be prepared to respond to the wide array of forces already changing the shape of health care. These forces include stunning medical and technological achievements that are completely reshaping how we deliver health care, national and global social trends that heighten the burden on health care, and shifts within the health care industry itself in response to such achievements and trends. In addition, leaders will have to contend with social forces—not the least of which is the aging of the baby boom generation.

MANY MEDICAL ADVANCES— AND ONE RETREAT

Every area of medicine is moving forward with incredible speed, from our capabilities in diagnostics and imaging to the ways in which we organize the day-to-day practice of medicine. In fact I have room here to mention only a few of the most interesting advances.

Diagnostics

Technologies such as polymerase chain reactors (PCRs) allow rapid, certain, inexpensive identification of particular bits of DNA and thus of the pathogens that carry the DNA, putting great diagnostic power in the hands of machines and the technicians that operate them and reducing reliance on the highly trained (and expensive) judgment of physicians (*Genome Research,* 1995–1998). Biosensor chips—computer chips that can positively identify the presence or absence of particular proteins or chemicals in any sample dropped on them—promise similar certainty, speed, and low cost, replacing much of today's lab work with small handheld or minimally invasive devices based on nanoscale ion switches (Olson and others, 1997). The University of Pennsylvania Medical Center has developed a sensor that can actually smell a number of different infections ("Brave New Medicine," 1997). Expert systems using *fuzzy logic* can also assist clinicians in the complex and crucial business of diagnostics. Some (such as the emergency room computer program APACHE) have already demonstrated remarkable abilities useful in both diagnostics and triage.

Genetic identification of diseases will lead to a whole new taxonomy based not on similarity of symptoms but on genetic subtypes of pathogens (Olson and others, 1997). The increasing identification of human genetic markers, often as early as in utero, that can tell clinicians that this person is predisposed to, say, breast cancer or diabetes or that person is predisposed to a heart condition will guide lifelong preventive care programs, tailor-made for each individual.

Imaging

New types of imaging are greatly expanding the clinician's ability to see inside and analyze the body. A number of new methods have emerged for using magnetic resonance imaging (MRI) and for extracting more data from it, such as magnetic resonance angiography (MRA) and magnetic resonance spectroscopy (MRS). A number of techniques (such as MRI/EEG, SPECT/MR, PET/MR, T2-weighted MRI, and HMPAO-MR) enhance magnetic resonance images by combining them with other sources of imagery. Other techniques, such as MRI with echo-planar imaging (EPI), boast remarkable speed. New types of sonography use the entire sonogram signal in ways that give a moving, real-time sonogram the precision of a good x-ray image.

Surgery

In the past few years *minimally invasive* techniques have revolutionized medical interventions from knee surgery and gall bladder removals to cardiac artery bypass grafts and pacemaker insertions. As these techniques continue to be adapted to more areas, a number of laboratories, private companies, universities, and groups like SRI International and also the U.S. Defense Department are moving to the next stage: handlike servo probes, capable of many degrees of freedom, slaved to the hand movements of a surgeon sitting at a console watching a three-dimensional video display. The surgeon will not have to enter the sterile field, and the instruments will be vastly easier to manipulate than today's "two-foot chopsticks" (SRI, 1998).

The next step is robotic assistance. A robotic industrial machine tool adapted to medical use and dubbed Robodoc, already on the market, drills the sockets for hip replacements faster, more precisely, and with less incidence of fracture than any human surgeon can. Another robot surgeon's assistant on the market, Aesop, responds to the surgeon's voice commands for precise placement of instruments, lighting, or video lenses in laparoscopic surgery (Computer Motion, 1998). Minerva, a French robotic neurosurgeon, operates inside a CT scanner, computer driven by the scanner's output. NASA's Jet Propulsion Laboratory (1998) in Pasadena, California, has been refining a robotic neurosurgeon that can tell the difference between soft and firm tofu, which mimics the difference in density between healthy brain tissue and tumors.

Current experiments in miniaturization will likely result in tiny, tractorlike micro-robots capable of being inserted into the body through small incisions or of simply driving in through an available orifice. Such micro-robots will perform a variety of tasks such as angioplasty, gall bladder removal, and biopsy retrieval.

The final stage in surgical miniaturization will be nanotechnology, the invention of machines so tiny they likely will not be visible to the naked eye, injected into the body by the hundreds of thousands, built and programmed to perform specific tasks such as destroying tumor cells or rebuilding bone tissue.

In fact, advanced pharmaceuticals and nanotechnology may render much surgery unnecessary. Advanced radiology may come to perform much of what we consider surgery without any incision at all. The time may come in which today's surgical interventions seem barbaric, in which we need never cut through healthy tissue to get to damaged tissue, in which the only people who go under the surgeon's knife are those whose tissue has already been ruptured by trauma.

Pharmaceuticals

Pharmaceuticals are advancing even more quickly than surgery. Genetically engineered vaccines are beginning to appear. According to the Institute for Alternative Futures (IAF), "DNA vaccines will begin to be available over the next five to ten years, and are likely to be universally adopted before 2020. They will be far superior to traditional vaccines, safer, and more effective at conferring both humoral and cellular immunity" (Olson and others, 1997, p. 1–8).

The new range of pharmaceuticals also includes such genetically engineered cytokines as EPO and granulocyte colony-stimulating factor (G-CSF) (Zeng and others, 1997) and new, more precisely targeted immunosuppressants such as rapamycin (Senft, 1996). Anti-sense RNA compounds, exact complements of the RNA sequences produced by viral (or cancer) genes within a cell, lock onto "bad" RNA and prevent it from directing undesired protein production within the cell. Anti-sense RNA compounds are so individual to each cell type that (in concept) they will stop the disease process cold without destroying cells' natural chemical process (Normanno and others, 1995). Anti-angiogenesis drugs such as TNP-470, which selectively inhibit the growth of blood vessels that feed tumor cells, show promise of actually turning into the long-elusive cure for cancer (Folkman, 1997).

Whole new strategies are arising, such as gene transfer therapy. HV-tk gene therapy, for instance, plants the markers of the herpes virus on tumor cells, then uses herpes drugs to kill the tumor cells (Davidson, 1995). The IAF expects the field of gene therapy over the next twenty years to be "comparable in its impact to past changes such as the introduction of microscopy, anesthesia, vaccination, and antibiotics" (Olson and others, 1997, p. 1–8).

Even the methods by which we find and manufacture drugs are radically changing. Pharmaceutical chemists have traditionally simply tested thousands of naturally occurring chemicals and compounds to see how different kinds of cells and pathogens react to them. With the advent of inexpensive, powerful computers and imaging techniques capable of actually seeing molecules, we have entered the age of rational drug design. Experimenters can, for instance, discover the exact shape of a pathogen's docking mechanism, or the site at which it attaches to the cell, and then design a molecule that will exactly fit that shape (like a jack in a plug) to block the interaction. Experimenters can test these designs in virtual reality, "pushing" giant molecules into place, and "feeling" whether they snap in or are rejected by molecular forces.

Another strategy, directed molecular evolution, uses the techniques of bioengineering (in its rough outlines not unlike beer making or other large-scale bioindustrial processes) to push a selected type of bacteria or other organism down an accelerated evolutionary path toward a particular end (Joyce, 1992).

These new strategies and breakthroughs put an increasingly wide array of tools in the hands of clinicians. Some of these tools are expensive, but most pharmaceuticals cost far less than the surgical alternative—an important factor in an increasingly cost-conscious age.

Results-Driven Medicine and Practice Guidelines

Under a number of different names, including *evidence-based medicine* and *outcomes management*, everyday medical practice is coming under the kind of statistical scrutiny that can finally tell us what works and what doesn't. The great majority of medical practices have never been submitted to double-blind scientific study. Because of the wide variations between and complications in individual cases and because of ethical concerns, it is not possible to put most medical practice under a rigorous scientific microscope. But with the appearance of inexpensive, powerful computing and the rapid increase in electronic patient records, it has become possible to aggregate data retrospectively from hundreds or even thousands of very similar cases—say, women between forty-five and fifty with nonmetastatic breast cancer—and then query these data with highly specific questions: Does drug X or drug Y work better? In what dosages? Which sequence? For how long? Whether the data have been gathered within an institution, within a local population, or across large numbers of affected people across the continent, the goal will be the same: to design practice guidelines that embody the best of current knowledge about each particular condition.

These are deeply important clinical studies, but they are also driven by today's overarching concern for cost. The golden path to low cost in medicine is high quality: do it right the first time. As such studies spread and are iterated, their findings will force enormous changes in the day-to-day practice of medicine.

Antibiotics

The one great medical retreat is the rapid decline in the effectiveness of antibiotics as multi-drug-resistant pathogens appear. Most people now alive have grown up during the brief period in human history when bacteria could be readily defeated by antibiotics. That era appears to be ending. The huge need for research into substitutes, vaccines, and other public health measures that this fact implies arises at the precise moment when funding can be expected to become scarcer and resources more stretched.

TECHNOLOGY

Technology is changing the shape of health care in areas beyond the practice of medicine. Communications and computing technologies, especially, are at the core of coming major shifts. And at the root of these technologies we find four machine abilities: *sensing, computing, remembering,* and *connecting.* Each of these abilities has grown enormously in power and dropped precipitously in price over the last three decades. These trends show every sign of continuing until all four abilities become both cheap and ubiquitous—they will cost almost nothing and be almost everywhere.

The possible results range from surgery at a distance to bed sheets that can notify the laundry by radio that they need changing, from interactive, customized personal health training on a Web TV to real-time mentoring of emergency medical technicians and battlefield medics by physicians ensconced miles away. One way to look over the future is to look at every part of your environment, from your shoes and pocket pen to the patient's medical chart to the surgical suite, and ask yourself: What if this object had intelligence? What if it could remember? What if it could sense something about its environment and respond to that information? What if it could communicate with us or with other objects in the environment?

Communications and computing technology are affecting health care in four major areas: administrative, professional, clinical, and public.

Administrative

Cheap computing and communications, especially in the form of the Internet (and its subsets, intranets and extranets), make it possible to decentralize health care organizations and to make them larger in any shape desired, stringing together concatenations of home health services, hospitals, pharmacies, multispecialty practices, insurance firms, laboratories, bookstores, surgicenters, and doc-in-the-box clinics. What makes these strange, hurly-burly systems work is the massive amount of information—clinical, administrative, and billing—that travels back and forth among the different elements in perfect security and at high speed; these systems are not possible without high-speed computers and telecommunications.

Professional

The Internet and other communications networks make it possible for health care professionals to link together much more readily than ever before. A family physician confronted with a rare condition can easily and quickly query the world's medical libraries, locate and contact colleagues who are leading the research effort and trying new techniques anywhere in the world, and join in ongoing discussions with physicians, other professionals, and informed laypeople—all through e-mail, mail lists, and the World Wide Web.

Physicians can increasingly use the judgment and creative thought of far-flung experts by simply e-mailing them the relevant images,

EKGs, and other information or by engaging in real-time video-conferencing over the Internet.

Clinical

New technologies make it possible for health care administrators, insurance companies, medical committees, and others to endlessly massage the available data to improve care and lower costs, driving the construction and use of institutionwide and industrywide clinical protocols.

They make it easier to concatenate and distribute information about the quality of each institution and physician in order to weed out those who are not up to standards and to allow the rest to compete not just on price but on quality.

They make it possible to target particular subpopulations with preventive messages and care, so that the next century's public health care can be custom-made private health care.

They change the relationship between the physician and the patient. Those patients who choose to immerse themselves in the rapidly growing electronic infosphere, through home computers, Web TV, or connections at work, school, or their local library, can discover enormous amounts about their particular conditions—in some cases more than their doctor may know—and can take a much more active part in managing their own therapy. Physicians' roles with patients will tend to become much more flexible.

Public

New technologies, from the Internet and computers to telephone messaging systems, fax-back systems, CDs and CD-ROMs, make it far easier and cheaper to involve people in lifelong, wide-ranging, interactive discussions about their personal health, their habits, their lifestyles and diets. Web TVs, CD-ROMs, interactive television, and other technologies can bring people easy-to-use health risk assessments, along with personal contact with nurses, nutritionists, and other health advisers. People who otherwise might be institutionalized simply to be monitored can stay home, take their own vital signs, and stay in touch with the monitoring organization through personal computers, alphanumeric pagers, or Touch-Tone telephones.

INDUSTRY FORCES

Several forces within the health care industry are of particular importance for the future. In addition to continuing issues of cost and access, health care leaders must consider the changes driven by increasing clinical knowledge and use of alternative therapies and also the effect of turbulent change on the health care organizations and professionals.

Continuing Concern over Cost and Access

Historically high levels of health care costs combined with growing class gaps, the aging of the population, changes in job structure, and other social changes mean that the concern that health care costs too much and is not readily available to many people is going to be a long-term part of the U.S. political landscape. The demand for services will likely increase heavily in the coming decades, but the willingness to fund those services, whether through federal or state government, through business, or out of people's pockets, will not increase. It is likely that the percentage of the economy dedicated to health care will be forced down, whether by a rational plan or chaotically. Any scheme or business initiative that promises to do this as it maintains quality and broadens access will likely find public or private funding.

Proliferation of Clinically Useful Knowledge

Clinically useful knowledge—information that improves the prognosis for real cases—is estimated to have doubled twice since 1986. This rate of growth is far faster than any clinician can keep up with using traditional methods such as reading journals and going to conferences. Doctors and other medical professionals increasingly depend on medical review writers and other experts, who themselves are often several years behind in recommending changes in practice. In the face of this we are seeing an explosion of *expert systems,* systems for gathering information off the Internet and other silicon *doc extenders.* We are likely to see the rapid development of other similar tools and their integration into standard clinical practice.

Mainstreaming of Alternative Therapies

In a pivotal 1993 article in the *New England Journal of Medicine,* David Eisenberg, M.D., established the enormous size of the market for alternative therapies in the United States. According to his research, in 1990, Americans made more visits to unconventional therapists (425 million) than to primary care doctors (388 million) and spent an out-of-pocket amount ($10.3 billion) on such therapists and therapies comparable to their out-of-pocket expenses on hospitalizations. Twenty-five percent of Americans who visit an M.D. for a serious health problem are also using an unconventional therapy for the same problem, and 70 percent of them do not tell the doctor about that therapy (Eisenberg and others, 1993).

These figures would not be a force in the future of health care except for three important facts:

• Alternative therapies such as chiropractic, acupuncture, naturopathy, and meditation are often effective (especially as part of a comprehensive, integrated therapeutic protocol) and typically have less potential for harm than medical techniques.

• Alternative therapies are often much less expensive than the medical therapies (such as surgery and pharmaceuticals) that they replace or supplement.

• Cost is a major driver of change in health care.

Taken together these facts suggest that the clinical and funding mechanisms of health care will increasingly shift to incorporate a number of alternative therapies in a new, *integrated* regime.

Industry Turbulence and Physicians' Dissatisfaction

The 1990s have seen patient bed days per thousand members of the population (a key figure for the hospital industry) drop from a nationwide peak of 1,130 in the early 1980s to less than 200 in some jurisdictions now, and the number is expected to bottom out at that level nationwide. The number of hospital beds in actual use continues a rapid decline as the amount of inpatient acute care falls.

Many doctors, especially in ophthalmology, urology, and certain other specialties, have seen serious declines in their incomes, in their control over their professional lives, and sometimes even in their social status. One 1996 American Medical Association survey showed that 63 percent of M.D.'s would not recommend clinical medicine to their children as a career, as many as 40 percent are thinking of leaving the field, and 92 percent of those under forty years of age would not choose it again for themselves.

Hospitals have responded to these changes throughout the 1990s, but increasingly since 1993, by consolidating and integrating both vertically and horizontally, in the widely shared but untested belief that the stand-alone acute care hospital is a doomed institution. Increasing amounts of care have been shifted from the relatively high-cost (and usually not-for-profit) hospital environment into lower-cost (and usually for-profit) ambulatory facilities, clinics, and physicians' offices. Although the number of hospitals has dropped only slightly over the past two decades (from 6,707 in 1975 to 6,376 in 1996), the number of inpatient hospital beds per thousand people has tumbled by 45 percent (51.5 beds per thousand in 1975; 28.4 beds per thousand in 1996) (Health Care Financing Administration, 1998). Throughout the 1990s, cash flows increasingly shifted from the cash-strapped not-for-profit sector, represented largely by public, private, and community hospitals, to the flush for-profit sector, represented by a small percentage of hospitals and almost all other organizations and professionals in the industry.

The 1990s also showed a steady movement of power from doctors and providers to insurance entities, a movement only accelerated by the failure of the Clinton administration's proposed health care reforms in 1993. This power shift was accompanied by the rapid spread of capitated models—and their most prominent avatar, the health maintenance organization—along with other forms of managed care. For the most part these organizations were interested in controlling the behavior of doctors in their role as the chief drivers of costs.

There were only two problems with this trend. One, and perhaps the less severe one, was that it set the industry on the opposite side from the public and business (the two ultimate payers) on every basic choice about the shape of health care. The members of the public and most business leaders wanted their choice of doctors, stability in their relationship with their doctors, a voice in their therapy, full information, and access to complementary therapies—in general, that is, some sense of control and access in return for a decent and predictable price. What the industry offered was restricted access, restricted information, restricted physician panels, and denial of claims for seemingly arbitrary reasons, all in return for prices that still climbed or fell only incrementally.

The second and more severe problem with the trend was that it did not work. It usually did not expand access or lower prices by very much—and when it did, it accomplished this feat by turning into a Soviet-style health care system whose chief marks seemed to be interminable lines, vast forms to fill out, and arbitrary bureaucratic control over intimate, life-and-death matters.

Increasingly in 1997, major industry figures paid attention to data showing that the only way to control costs through physicians was not to control physicians from afar but to make the physician practice the risk-bearing entity. The most vigorous HMOs had been able to push patient bed days per thousand people per year in the Medicare population from the 2,400 range down only to the 1,600 range. Risk-bearing physician organizations were routinely able to drive that number down to the range of 700, through medically sound early interventions, prevention, education, and a wide range of techniques that lowered costs not by weakening the patient's bond with the physician and denying care but by strengthening that bond and increasing the quality and timeliness of care.

SOCIAL FORCES

These technological, medical, and industry forces meet and fuse in the cauldron of far larger, sometimes global, social forces.

World Population

The population of the world continues to grow and continues to get younger. According to the consensus of the most recent estimates, world population is expected to nearly double once more within the next generation before leveling off near eleven billion (Lutz, 1996). This growth and juvenilization has predictable results:

• Greater instability in less developed nations (leading to more revolutions, and more wars with neighbors)

• Increased famine

• Increased cases of communicable diseases (as people experience weakened immune systems, heightened contact, increased stress, and exposure to increasingly polluted water supplies)

• Increased death and injury tolls from natural disasters
(as greater numbers of people are forced to live in more
marginal places)

In the more developed, population-stable countries such as the
United States, world population growth is leading to greater immigration pressures and an increased level of fear (as opposed to optimism), which has been repeatedly shown to be a vector for weakened
immune systems.

Globalization

The continuing and rapid increase in international travel and trade,
mega-urbanization, small-scale warfare, and displaced populations
leads to a variety of health effects, especially environmental devastation across borders and regions and the rapid spread of such "new"
infectious diseases as AIDS, Argentine hemorrhagic fever, the Hanta
virus, and new types of influenzas.

The Aging U.S. Population

In the United States, Canada, and Australia, the leading edge of the
postwar baby boom generation turns fifty-four years old in the year
2000, and those at peak of that wave will be about forty-eight. In these
societies, which have a powerful effect on other cultures around the
globe, for the past half century whatever was important to this generation, from the family-centered stability of the 1950s to the questioning of the Vietnam War in the 1960s to the career focus and money
making of the 1980s and 1990s, has become a major part of the
agenda of the times. Now this massive generation is rapidly progressing into middle age and toward retirement. At the same time, their
parents are becoming the frail elderly, moving toward end-stage illness and death. This tells us that in the coming decade or so, we will
be faced with

• A rapidly growing burden on health care

• An increased focus on home health care, skilled nursing
facilities, and all the other ways we give long-term care

• A relatively smaller working population to support increased
health care needs

A Change in Social Structure

Over the past few decades, we have witnessed a long-term, relatively permanent change in family and social structure in the United States and many other countries, one that shows up in population statistics as shorter marriages, more divorces, more (and smaller) households, later dates of first marriages, increased numbers (and decreased ages) of single mothers, increased mobility (with more changes of domicile in each lifetime), and increased numbers and percentages of women and children in poverty. At the same time, the mass media have become more immediate and personal (as we read fewer newspapers and watch more cable and satellite television), and personal contacts have tended to shift from the face-to-face, routinized, and daily to the electronically mediated (telephone, pager, e-mail), random, and sporadic. The resulting social fragmentation leads to greater stress, fewer and more frail support networks, less contact with mainstream health structures (like personal physicians), and increased difficulty in paying for health care. At the same time, we see a greatly increased number of socially induced health problems, including trauma from street and domestic violence and problems with substance abuse (accompanied by developmental problems in the children of substance abusers).

Demographic Fragmentation

In less media aware times, people tended to think of themselves as part of a single large (and fairly homogenous) population, focusing less on whatever differences they personally carried. New media realism and the social history of the last few decades increasingly encourage people to emphasize differences, dividing populations by ethnic group, age, class, language, and culture. This is contributing to an increase in fear and a drop in optimism, the rise of radical social movements of fragmentation and blame on both the right and the left, and a decrease in wide civic awareness and sense of responsibility, and all these results increase the burden on health care by feeding the behaviors that are vectors for ill health.

Rise of the McJob

Under cover of its long-term strength, the U.S. economy (followed by a number of other national economies) has changed the shape of the average job. Lifetime employment by large, stable corporations has increasingly given way to serial employment in *McJobs*—lower paying, less secure, often less than full-time, and often without health benefits (which are job based in the United States). For many people this instability undercuts the stability of their relationships with their doctor and other health care providers. Steadily increasing numbers of working people are cut off from health care entirely.

Health Awareness

In the last few decades, in the one major social development with positive effects on health, public awareness about the true vectors of health and disease has clearly shifted. People are far more aware of the roots of health in behavior, diet, habits, and family than they were a generation ago—and far more likely to take action based on that awareness.

The Disappearance of the Deficit

By late 1997, it began to appear that because of the continued steady growth of the U.S. economy, the federal deficit might disappear of its own accord before too long, that in fact a surplus might appear in the budget. In reality, if Social Security funds, in surplus for years in an attempt to build against the baby boomers' retirement, were subtracted from the equation, tax receipts would still fall far short of funding the operations and borrowing of the federal government. But the perception of a looming surplus is as important as its reality.

Political forces are balanced over how to spend this perceived surplus. Most conservatives, in their quest to shrink the government, favor cutting taxes. Some economists favor paying off the debt. Many liberals hope for at least modest increases in spending for health care, education, and other soft public investments. Public polls seem largely to side with the liberals: shrinking the federal government is not a consensus goal. Taxes are bearable in a booming economy, the federal debt seems rather abstract, but the problems in health care and education seem immediate and real to the average American. Weighing against this perception is the still-smarting memory of the political cost of the failed Clinton reforms and the widespread perception that health care has a lot of fat still to lose.

With all these factors pushing and pulling on the future of health care, we could make a wide range of credible scenarios for that future, asking ourselves which forces or developments seem most crucial, most likely to make a large difference. For instance, physicians' ability to consult with other physicians over the Internet, shipping images back and forth with ease, seems bound to make a big difference in clinical practice. But this innovation is so certain (in fact, it is already operating to some degree in most environments) and so useful that it is difficult to imagine a scenario that would *not* use it. However, researchers' ability to find replacements for today's antibiotics and the world economy's general ability to support continued growth and avoid a spiral into depression are not certainties but large questions whose answers we cannot now know, even though those answers will profoundly effect the future of health care.

Scenarios that posit answers to such questions are guaranteed not to be exact descriptions of the future. But the process of asking the questions and searching for the answers will leave us more informed about the possible shapes that our future could take and about the hinge points where forces moving one way or another make a real difference.

References

"Brave New Medicine," *U.S. News & World Report,* Dec. 1, 1997, p. 82.

"Computer Motion." [www.computermotion.com]. Jan. 1998.

Davidson, S. "Technological Cancer: Its Causes and Treatment." *Healthcare Forum,* Mar.–Apr. 1995.

Eisenberg, D. M., and others. "Unconventional Medicine in the United States: Prevalence, Costs, and Patterns of Use." *New England Journal of Medicine,* 1993, *328,* 246–252.

Folkman, J. "New Directions in Angiogenesis Research." Paper presented at the National Institutes of Health (NIH) Director's Lecture, Bethesda, Md., Nov. 19, 1997.

Genome Research. Cold Spring Harbor, N.Y.: Cold Spring Harbor Laboratory Press, 1995–1998.

"Health Care Financing Administration, Bureau of Data Management and Strategy." [www.hcfa.gov/stats/stats.htm]. 1998.

"Jet Propulsion Laboratory." [http://robotics.jpl.nasa.gov/tasks/rams/
    homepage.html]. Jan. 1998.

Joyce, G. "Directed Molecular Evolution." *Scientific American,* Dec. 1992.

Lutz, W. "International Institute for Applied Systems." Paper presented at
    the annual meeting of the American Association for the Advance-
    ment of Science, Baltimore, Md., Feb. 10, 1996.

Normanno, N., and others. "Amphiregulin Anti-Sense Oligodeoxynu-
    cleotides Inhibit Growth and Transformation of a Human Colon
    Carcinoma Cell Line." *International Journal of Cancer,* 1995, *62*(6),
    762–766.

Olson, R., and others. *MHSS 2020: Focused Study on Biotechnology and
    Nanotechnology.* Arlington, Va.: Institute for Alternative Futures,
    for SRA International, for U.S. Department of Defense, Office of
    Health Affairs, 1997.

Senft, J. "Study Confirms New Drug Reduces Organ Rejection in
    Transplants." University of Texas, Houston Online.
    [oac.hsc.uth.tmc.edu/uth_orgs/pub_affairs/news/releases/kahan.
    html]. June 11, 1996.

"SRI International Telepresence Surgery." [http://os.sri.com/medical/
    telepres.html]. 1998.

Zeng, D., and others. "Granulocyte Colony-Stimulating Factor Reduces the
    Capacity of Blood Mononuclear Cells to Induce Graft-Versus-Host
    Disease: Impact on Blood Progenitor Cell Transplantation." *Blood,*
    1997, *90,* 453–463.

CHAPTER THREE

Policy Challenges

Joel Shalowitz

*Joel Shalowitz is professor and director of the health services
management program at the J. L. Kellogg Graduate School
of Management, Northwestern University, and professor
of medicine at Northwestern's medical school. He is the
managing partner for a primary care group with more
than twenty practitioners, and he practices internal
medicine with the group. A Fellow of the American College
of Physicians, he also serves as a board member for the
Academy for Healthcare Organizations, Network for
Healthcare Management and Research, and Alexian
Brothers Medical Center.*

As our society modifies traditional notions of health
care cost, quality, access, and insurance yet retains an ideal of patient
freedom of choice, conflicts are arising that require us to make critical decisions not only about how many resources we can consume but

what trade-offs we can afford. These modifications are examined here, along with the challenges they present and the trade-offs and conflicts that arise from the U.S. public's wanting it all.

INSURANCE BENEFITS

The original purpose of insurance was to indemnify the policyholder against catastrophic risk. Such risk came from acute illnesses or injuries. In keeping with this notion, commercial insurance evolved from covering only hospital care (the most expensive item, as early as the 1930s) to covering physician services and then to paying for medical devices and approved pharmaceuticals. More recently a number of special interest groups have successfully lobbied state legislatures to mandate benefits that do not meet the definition of catastrophic illness. These benefits range from wigs for chemotherapy patients to infertility services. Further, they increase the cost of care for all. The health insurance question of most concern has therefore changed from *what* should be covered (apparently everything politically expedient) to *how much* insurance companies and individuals will pay.

In order to avoid the constraints of such mandatory benefits, many companies have taken advantage of their option under the Employee Retirement Income Security Act (ERISA) to design their own benefit packages for the workers they cover. Realistic policymakers understand that on the one hand, if we are to implement substantial health reform in this country, ERISA exemptions must be challenged; on the other hand, if these exemptions are modified or eliminated, many fear some businesses will eliminate health care coverage entirely.

Challenge.   Reformulate health policy so that basic health insurance can include only those services and products necessary for prevention, treatment, and palliation of illness.

DEMOGRAPHICS

The fastest percentage growth in any age group is in people over eighty-five years old. Further, the first members of the baby boom generation became fifty in 1996. In considering these statistics, we often focus on the health needs of the increasing number of elderly. Equally important, however, is that there are proportionately fewer younger persons to pay for care for the elderly (particularly through the Medicare system) and to provide nonreimbursable caretaking services.

Challenge. Through more efficient use of current resources and targeted research, identify strategies that will prolong the functional life of the elderly. (Cost challenges are discussed later.)

VALUE

The nexus of cost and quality considerations is value. *Value* can be defined as the best quality one can obtain for a given price or as payment of the lowest price for a desired level of quality. In order to gauge whether we are getting value from our health care systems, we need to decide what it is we want to maximize. Our traditional focus has been on acute illness and disease care rather than health care. Early in this century we appropriately devoted resources to public health measures like infection control. When infectious diseases were no longer the chief cause of mortality in this country, resources were directed at and technology was developed to treat the ailments that succeeded infectious diseases as the leading causes of death—heart disease and cancers. Although no one would argue the wisdom of saving the life of a child with leukemia, the public has mixed feelings about bypass surgery routinely performed on octogenarians. The reason for this disparity of feelings is that when we assess value in these cases, we implicitly apply a metric other than mortality reduction—namely, years of life saved. If we carry this argument further and consider such components of value as the costs of prevention or treatment and the number and ages of persons affected and receiving services, we would probably direct more resources to such measures as prenatal care, provision of car seats for infants, and immunizations. In evaluating value we should also take into account such factors as individual patient preferences and quality of life (as measured by quality of life years saved, for example).

Challenge. Define what it is we want to optimize when we design systems to deliver and pay for health care.

In addition to our lack of focus on what we want to optimize, some of us still believe that there must be a *trade-off* between cost and quality. Although quality is not completely free, after a point there is either no correlation between cost and quality or a negative association. For example, if one looks at the published reports of the Pennsylvania Health Care Cost Containment Council and considers the cost and risk-adjusted outcomes data for cardiac bypass surgery for hospitals, one finds in many cases that the higher the cost, the worse the outcome. Poor quality in health care is certainly more expensive than good quality. One of the problems of traditional reimbursement systems is that they reward both efficient, high-quality performance and costly, low-quality performance. Although the more efficient providers may make more money than the inefficient, this may not force the latter to make necessary changes.

Challenge.   Reward high-quality providers and help lower-quality ones to improve. We must realize that as we accomplish this goal, further institutional consolidations may occur and low-volume institutions may close.

COST

The current impetus to examine health care systems in this country comes from the desires of public and private payers to rein in their portion of expenses. These expenses are a function of three elements: price per service, number of services, and intensity of care. Most public and private cost containment strategies have focused primarily on lowering prices. There are several reasons for this approach. First, price regulation is easy. It is accomplished by governmental fiat or by large insurers' market power. Second, basing payments on volume of services smacks of rationing. This technique, though widely practiced in many foreign countries, is anathema to the public in this nation. Finally, regulating costs due to intensity of service is difficult.

Intensity itself has several components. The first is level of service provided. We may ask, for example, whether the patient needs an operation when medication or watchful waiting may provide similar results. Controversies over the most appropriate treatments for angina pectoris and prostate cancer fall into this category. A second component is the coding of the patient's problem. Even though many insurers track frequency distributions of CPT-4 codes by provider, looking particularly for *upcoding*, few follow up on this analysis with actual chart audits to determine codes' accuracy. A third aspect to intensity is the appropriateness of the site of care. For example, we might ask whether an inpatient ought to be in the intensive care unit or on a general floor. Finally, intensity can be viewed as a proxy for the application of technology, defined by the Office of Technology Assessment as drugs, devices, and procedures and the support systems in which they are delivered. Regulating the application of technology is difficult for several reasons. The foremost reason is the absence of a single body with the authority to issue opinions about the cost benefit or cost effectiveness of technology. For example, the federal government has done its best to remove itself from the role of impartial arbiter of technology implementation and evaluation. This abrogation of responsibility was evident when the Reagan administration partially dismantled the aforementioned Office of Technology Assessment and the Clinton administration watched as a Republican Congress cut financial support for the Agency for Health Care Policy and Research after nearly shutting it down. In the absence of a single authoritative body, the legal system has favored plaintiffs in liability suits even when the science supports defendants. Examples range from suits involving silicone breast implants and autoimmune disorders to those involving Bendectin and birth defects. Fear of liability is a potent factor in technology regulation. Finally, withholding technology is akin to rationing, which, as mentioned, is abhorrent to the public.

An example of apparently successful technological control is managed care plans' use of pharmaceutical formularies. The nominal costs of the drugs determine their formulary status, yet little is known about the effects of switching from a nonformulary drug to one on the approved list. Further, the *total* costs of drugs with cheaper purchase prices are not clear; for example, it is not known whether they cause more side effects or require more laboratory test monitoring.

One often cited example of successful rationing is the Oregon Medicaid waiver program. After various constituencies (including those in the medical, political, and religious communities) gave their opinions about which treatments would be efficacious and cost effective for a number of conditions, those treatments were ranked. The state then imposed cutoffs: treatments below certain rankings are not covered. By prioritizing provisions for technology, however, the state covers more beneficiaries than it did before the waiver program began, and the program's total cost has *increased*.

Challenge. Form a consortium of public and private partners with the ability and authority to coordinate technology assessment; the consortium will standardize benefits, and its findings can serve as legal protection to those offering the benefits.

In the public realm, Medicare Part A expenses have rapidly escalated since that program began in 1966. The federal government responded to threats of Medicare Hospital Trust Fund bankruptcy by changing hospital payments from a cost-plus basis to a cost basis to a system linked to patient diagnosis (diagnosis related groups, or DRGs).

As these various measures were failing, more money was put into the fund by eliminating the ceiling on eligible payroll taxes, the fund's principal funding source. When this too failed, the Balanced Budget Act of 1997 moved home health care from the Hospital Trust Fund to Medicare Part B. This shell game merely shifted the financial responsibility for home health services to general revenues, the source of about three-fourths of Part B funds. As more baby boomers become eligible for Medicare and the ratio of working to retired persons continues to shrink, few politically palatable options are left for saving Part A. The proposal that would have the longest and most significant impact on fund solvency is to delay Medicare eligibility. However, this suggestion has been dismissed by a number of legislators as political suicide.

Although Medicare Part B has also experienced financial pressures, its crisis has not been as severe or obvious because payments come largely from general tax revenues. Few beneficiaries realize that in current dollars their out-of-pocket expenses have never been greater. Nevertheless, political pressure to control expenses derives from fears that premiums will need to be increased. Cost-control responses in the past have evolved from using a *customary, prevailing,* or *reasonable* fee schedule to using a resource-based relative value schedule (RBRVS). Although volume-based updates in the RBRVS fees were initially entertained, political pressure by such groups as the American Medical Association eliminated this consideration. The government then stabilized fee costs by redistribution of payments among specialists. However, now that home health care, one of the most rapidly growing components of Medicare Part A, has been shifted to Part B, it is inevitable that costs for Part B will rise considerably.

Challenges.   Ensure long-term viability of the Medicare Hospital Trust Fund and stabilize inevitable escalations in Part B expenses. Such changes may require raising FICA, delaying the age of Medicare eligibility, or making each generation responsible for its own expenses, with a safety net for those who cannot afford care.

The other major public health care program, Medicaid, has become a financial burden for both the federal government and individual states. In order to alleviate this problem the federal government began to allow states to obtain waivers to the traditional program. Problems with enrollment, eligibility, patient education, development of provider networks, and payment procedures are some of the shortcomings of many state waiver programs. The Balanced Budget Act of

1997 allows states to establish alternative Medicaid plans without such waivers, yet states will still face these administrative problems. An additional problem is the repeal of the 1981 Boren Amendment, which required states to provide "reasonable and adequate" payments to Medicaid providers. Lacking this federal protection, these providers now face an uncertain process for payment determination. A further important dilemma facing Medicaid is the demographic disparity between eligible recipients in general and those who receive the most program benefits. Although most eligibles qualify for Medicaid because they meet the criteria for Aid to Families with Dependent Children (AFDC), most of the Medicaid money is spent on nursing home care for the elderly. (AFDC was replaced by the Temporary Assistance for Needy Families program in 1996. Those eligible under AFDC prior to July 16, 1996, can retain Medicaid coverage, however.)

Challenges. States need to develop an organizational infrastructure that allows efficient and effective Medicaid management. Rather than use a traditional public health model, they need to borrow the best features of successful managed care plans, including information systems and customer relations programs. They need to provide adequate funding (and timely payment) to ensure participation by a wide network of qualified providers. And they need to establish fairer systems for allocating resources between AFDC recipients and the elderly.

In the private sector during the 1980s and early 1990s, employers faced double-digit increases in their health insurance premiums. Frequently their health care costs approached net profits. In response to these financial pressures, large employer groups engaged in at least three strategies. First, they took advantage of the flexibility in health plan design and coverage afforded by ERISA. Second, they either bought coverage or contracted for administrative services from managed care plans, particularly health maintenance organizations (HMOs). Finally, they shifted more financial responsibility to workers, in the form of higher cost sharing for premiums or of increased coinsurance and deductibles. As part of this shift, coverage for dependents has diminished, perhaps contributing to the size of the uninsured population, particularly children.

Challenge. Make health insurance more affordable to employers and individuals through benefit redesign, appropriate employee cost sharing, and realistic expectations about the trade-offs involved between cost and quality on the one hand and freedom of choice of providers on the other (as discussed later).

QUALITY

The public and private focus on cost-cutting measures is leading people to direct increased attention toward ensuring that quality is not diminished. Briefly, the public is concerned with at least two dimensions of quality: technical and service (that is, amenities of care). Only the former is discussed here. Scrutiny of the technical dimension impels these questions: Are things done for the right reasons? And are they done correctly? Questions policymakers may ask of the public are whether people know how to evaluate the technical aspect of quality, and if so, will their care-seeking behavior change once they know some answers? The response to both those questions appears to be no, at least for now. For example, published risk-adjusted mortality rates for New York State cardiovascular surgeons had little impact on patients' choices. Likewise, the Pennsylvania cardiovascular data mentioned earlier have not been shown to alter patient decisions. One bright spot in this effort is the work of the Foundation for Accountability (FACCT) that seeks to make valid quality measurements understandable to the average health care consumer. This initiative, however, is aimed at allowing comparison between health plans rather than at evaluating individual providers.

A further problem with evaluating technical quality is that services are frequently required emergently. Even if the quality data could be perfectly understood, time is often not available to gather them. And even if a patient knows the best provider, an emergency situation may allow access only to the closest provider.

Challenge.   Provide more quality information, make it more understandable and accessible to the public, and improve efforts to make *all* providers better, rather than punishing the bad and improving only the best.

ACCESS

Access to health care has a number of dimensions. The first is being able to afford such care. For many services, being able to afford the care translates into being able to purchase a health insurance policy. Currently about forty-one million people are uninsured in this country. The reasons range from inability to purchase a policy because of a preexisting condition to inability to afford a policy to the gamble that coverage will not be needed.

Having insurance coverage is certainly important, but it is not the whole story behind access. For example, in a November 26, 1997, press release, the Agency for Health Care Policy and Research stated that of the 12.8 million families who faced barriers to health care, just 3.3 million were completely uninsured. Perhaps a more telling statistic from the same study was that more than forty-six million persons lacked a regular source of health care. Similarly, as shown by a Rand Corporation health insurance experiment (Keeler, 1992), out-of-pocket expenses, although reducing utilization, did not have a substantial impact on health outcomes.

Certainly several factors in addition to cost and the ability to obtain insurance influence the accessibility of health care. First is the availability of health care providers. Despite the oversupply of physicians in some metropolitan areas, many inner cities and rural areas lack adequate numbers of practitioners. Several reasons for this disparity exist, including practice conditions and differing rates of compensation. Second, transportation is not always easy for those who need care, even when practitioners are available. This holds particularly true for the poor and elderly. Third, scheduling and coordinating multiple diagnostic and therapeutic procedures can be complex and confusing, even for those familiar with the health care field. Facing these challenges, some may wish to forego even needed services as simple and infrequent as screening mammographies. Finally, understanding insurance benefits and proper filing procedures can be daunting, perhaps causing some to avoid needed services.

Some organized delivery systems have addressed these access issues. They have coordinated services among otherwise fragmented system components, recognized the difference between health care and disease care by offering more preventive services, and moved from an acute care model to a continuum of care model.

Challenge. Enhance coordinated systems' efforts by offering incentives for eliminating waste and improving communitywide health outcomes. Such systems do not have to be under a single owner but can comprise a number of community-based organizations, often those competing with one another.

PARADOXES

The one constant and growing desire among members of the public is to choose their own providers. The public and the press trace the blame for many of the "horror" stories about managed care to closed systems. The common refrain is, "If only this person had been allowed to choose his or her own providers, this wouldn't have happened." Those making such statements believe it is possible to have freedom of choice of providers, high-quality medical care, the best access to such care, and low costs. Unfortunately, all these features cannot be optimized simultaneously. The challenge we face is determining how much of each we want and what trade-offs we are willing to accept in order to obtain the desirable mix.

Freedom of Choice and Access

The best feature managed care has to offer, compared to the traditional fee-for-service sector, is enhanced coordination of services. It is difficult for individuals to coordinate their own care across a continuum of needs. Further, if providers' financial incentives are not aligned, there is little reason for those providers to coordinate care. Witness the traditional Medicare system where one practitioner often hands off a case to another; one person's responsibility ends and another person's begins. In typical managed care systems, however, the primary care physician is responsible for coordinating care regardless of the varied needs the patient has. This process is the essence of case management. Conversely, complete freedom of choice implies that the patient is substantially responsible for coordinating his or her own services. Although managed care plans require primary care providers and medical groups (via contracts and financial incentives) to provide timely care, initial appointment delays often exist. Once their problem has been identified, however, many patients find the referral process better coordinated under managed care than in the fragmented fee-for-service environment.

Freedom of Choice and Quality

As pointed out earlier, in the public backlash against the real and anecdotal abuses by managed care plans, the primary solution one hears is to give beneficiaries freedom of choice of their providers. Some states have gone as far as passing laws making freedom of choice a patient right. For example, Illinois allows a woman to see any contracted obstetrician-gynecologist in the plan, and Florida requires plans to provide freedom of choice of dermatologists. Further, some states have passed what is called *any willing provider* legislation. These laws require health plans to accept any provider willing to sign a standard health plan contract. At the same time these measures are being passed, health plans are designing new *open access* products (discussed further later). These give members the opportunity to see a wider network of providers than they can under a more restrictive HMO product. And all these changes are occurring at the same time health plans and their contracted providers are facing increased external scrutiny and accountability for the quality of care they provide, for example, in the form of National Committee for Quality Assurance (NCQA) certification, Health Plan Employer Data and Information Set (HEDIS) reports, and FACCT criteria. The trade-off with respect to freedom of choice and quality is that we cannot expect accountability in a system where plans and providers lose control of their referral choices and hence of the ability to coordinate care. For example, in Illinois it is not uncommon for OB-GYNs to hospitalize a patient at a facility where her primary care physician and other consultants are not on staff. In these cases freedom to choose an OB-GYN has taken precedence over continuity of care.

Freedom of Choice and Cost

As with costs of other insurance products, health care coverage costs depend on the choice the insured makes to pay either low premiums and higher out-of-pocket expenses (like coinsurance and deductibles) or higher premiums and lower out-of-pocket expenses. With the introduction of managed care plans a third dimension was introduced—freedom of choice of providers. In the prototypical HMO, if the insured receives nonemergency services from noncontracted providers, the plan will not pay for that care. Compared to indemnity insurance, however, the HMO premiums are lower, as are out-of-pocket expenses. For example, traditional HMOs may have copayments, but they do not have coinsurance or deductibles. With the evolution of managed care plans to include preferred provider organizations (PPOs), beneficiaries can have some portion of nonemergency services covered when they receive those services from providers who do not contract with their health plan; however, the insured's financial liability is greater. Also, premiums may be higher for these plans than for HMOs. The insured person has therefore traded more freedom of choice for higher costs. Responding to recent public demand for more provider choice, health plans have created hybrids between HMOs and PPOs called Point of Service (POS) plans. Also, the products called open access plans have emerged. In these pseudo-HMOs, beneficiaries can refer themselves to any plan provider without a referral from their primary care physician.

In this evolution of products the trade-off between premiums, out-of-pocket expenses, and freedom of choice has in many cases been lost. The public has demanded open access products at HMO prices. In order to meet this demand and sustain profits, health plans have shifted the cost of these ill-designed products to providers in the form of lower payments. In the past year many major health plans have experienced unexpected losses. Although a number of reasons exist for this phenomenon, like poor information systems, I believe one of the fundamental causes is the failure to realize that low premiums, low out-of-pocket expenses, and freedom of choice of providers cannot coexist to the extent that health plan marketing has promised. A possible first step to solving the freedom of choice dilemma would be to require all employers who provide health insurance for their employees in the form of an HMO to also furnish a freedom of choice product. The companies would not be required to pay extra for this benefit; the difference in premium would be borne by the employee.

—∿∿—

The public wants access to health care coverage; it does not want to be told where it can receive health care. It wants the best quality care and demands that care be affordable. It is impossible to fulfill all these demands simultaneously. The real challenge for the political process is to determine how we can achieve an optimal mix of those features, satisfy the most, disenfranchise the fewest, and return health insurance to its original purpose—indemnification against catastrophic loss.

References

Agency for Health Care Policy and Research. Press release. Agency for Health Care Policy and Research, Nov. 26, 1997.

Keeler, Emmett B. "Effects of Cost Sharing on Use of Medical Service and Health," *Journal of Medical Practice Management,* 1992, *8,* 11–15.

CHAPTER FOUR

Ethical Values for a New Century

Lawrence O. Gostin

Lawrence O. Gostin is professor of law at Georgetown University Law Center, professor of law and public health at the Johns Hopkins University School of Hygiene and Public Health, and codirector of the Johns Hopkins–Georgetown University program on law and public health. He is a Fellow of the Kennedy Institute of Ethics of Georgetown University and a member of the steering and executive committees of the Georgetown University Institute for Health Care Research and Policy. Editor of the Health Law and Ethics section of the Journal of the American Medical Association, *Gostin also serves on the editorial boards of such scholarly journals as the* Yale Journal on Regulation, International Journal of Bioethics, *and* International Journal of Health and Human Rights.

This chapter is based on two earlier articles by the author: "Foreword: Health Care Reform in the United States—The Presidential Task Force," *American Journal of Law & Medicine*, 1993, *19*, 1–20, and "Securing Health or Just Health Care? The Effect of the Health Care System on the Health of America," *St. Louis University Law Journal*, 1994, *39*, 7–43. The author would like to thank Lance Gable and Imron T. Aly for their invaluable help with chapter preparation and research.

T here are troubling paradoxes in the U.S. health care system. According to the U.S. Department of Health and Human Services, this country spends approximately 13.6 percent of its gross domestic product on health care (Pear, 1998). Yet more than forty million Americans, including some ten million children, have no health insurance. "In comparison with other major industrialized countries, health care in the United States costs more per person and per unit of service, is less accessible to a large portion of its citizens, is provided at a more intensive level, and offers comparatively poor gross outcomes" (Schieber and others, 1991). U.S. spending on health care per capita is over double the average in twenty-four developed countries (Schieber and others, 1991). Yet despite such spending there remain troubling concerns about the fairness and quality of the U.S. health care system and its ability to serve the entire population.

What is absent is a social ethic of what the nation wants to achieve in health care and a method of achieving better health in the population as a whole (Reinhardt, 1997). In this chapter I offer six ethical values for the U.S. health care system: *access, equity, justice, choice, quality,* and *cost.* All these values are important, although not all of equal importance. At the same time, it will be obvious to any thoughtful observer of the health care system that promotion of one or more of these values results in diminution of other values. How is it possible, for example, to expand access without incurring additional cost? Can society ensure a more equal distribution of services for all without diminishing choice or quality for some? Can society, moreover, provide an entitlement to services for all, regulate quality, or guarantee justice without interfering with a free market or redistributing economic resources? There are no easy answers, and I do not intend to offer a systematic theory of health system reform. Rather, I will examine these six ethical values in light of the fact that it will be necessary to measure future reform efforts against a reasonable set of ethical standards.

ACCESS

Although methods of measurement vary, data suggest, as I have mentioned, that over forty million people in the United States lack health insurance coverage at any given time (Thorpe, 1997; Levit and others, 1992). This represents approximately 15 percent of the population. Different methodologies yield significantly higher estimates. According to some researchers, for example, nearly sixty million Americans have no health insurance for at least one month in any given year (Lewin/VHI for Families USA Foundation, 1993; Donelan and others, 1996). The number of uninsured and underinsured, moreover, is likely to grow (Schroeder, 1996) as employers drop health care benefits (Employee Benefit Research Institute, 1996) and as cutbacks in Medicaid and welfare reduce coverage for low-income Americans (Davis, 1997).

When researchers refer to the point-in-time estimate of more than forty million uninsured, they are counting people who are chronically uninsured (about 60 percent of the total uninsured) plus those who are uninsured only for certain periods during the year. The finding that a proportion of uninsured spells end within six months reinforces the perception that the harm of uninsurance is exaggerated. Yet even short exposures to risk can lead to large numbers of people who experience serious health consequences during a period in which they are not covered by insurance (Swartz, 1994). Moreover, the basic characteristics of persons without insurance remain constant: the uninsured are more likely to be young, poor or near poor, nonwhite, unmarried, poorly educated, unemployed, or employed in low-wage jobs.

The uninsured are not the only persons who have difficulty obtaining access to health care. Nearly thirty million more people are considered underinsured (Short and Banthin, 1995). Underinsurance is a concept hard to define or to quantify (Bipartisan Commission on Comprehensive Health Care, 1990). Persons may be underinsured due to insufficient overall insurance coverage (for example, they may have capitations on coverage that limit their costs or service usage), due to exemptions for certain conditions (for example, preexisting conditions or mental health or childbirth services), or due to low reimbursement rates that result in denials of service.

Individuals' lack of health insurance, of course, does not mean that they are entirely without health care. Persons who become acutely ill can seek, and usually receive, treatment on a voluntary basis at hospital emergency departments, clinics, and physician offices. This is a form of catastrophic health insurance paid for by shifting the cost of such charity care to those who pay for health services (privately or publicly insured patients) or to taxpayers through public funding of municipal trauma centers and public health clinics.

The irony of current cost containment methods is that health care providers are becoming less able to transfer the economic burden of charity care to paying patients. As managed care constricts payments to hospitals and health care professionals, it will become increasingly more difficult for these providers to cost shift. This will either threaten the economic viability of many public and nonprofit institutions or significantly curtail their ability to serve persons without insurance, or both (U.S. General Accounting Office, 1989).

Does health insurance make a difference? Data suggest that persons without insurance, despite the existence of charitable care, receive considerably fewer health services than those with insurance (Long and Marquis, 1994). Indeed, socioeconomic factors being equal, persons without insurance experience triple the mortality rate for similarly situated insured persons, dying at an earlier age (Hadley, Steinberg, and Feder, 1991; Franks, Clancy, and Gold, 1993).

Lack of insurance, of course, is not the only barrier to health care. In addition to this financial barrier, there are also structural, personal, and cultural barriers. Structural barriers are impediments to health care arising from the number, type, concentration, location, or organization of health care providers. Personal and cultural barriers may inhibit people who need medical care from seeking it or, once they obtain care, from heeding recommended clinical advice and following up (Institute of Medicine, 1993).

Primacy of Universal Access as a Value

Universal access to health care is often regarded as the preeminent ethical standard for evaluating the health care system. The very purpose of government is to attain through collective action human goods that individuals acting alone could not realistically achieve (compare Walzer, 1984). Chief among those human goods is the assurance of conditions under which people can be healthy (Institute of Medicine, 1988). Although the government cannot ensure health, it can, within the reasonable limits of its resources, organize its activities in ways that best prevent illness and disability and that promote health among the population.

Health is basic to all human endeavor, and that fact may be regarded as a foundational justification for governmental action (Brock and Daniels, 1994; President's Commission . . ., 1983;

Dougherty, 1992; Daniels, 1985). First, health is necessary for the pursuit of livelihood. Without a certain level of health a person cannot train, develop skills, or employ existing qualifications and skills in income-producing activities. Lack of good health not only impedes individuals in obtaining the basic necessities of life such as food, shelter and clothing but reduces their capacity to contribute to the production of goods and services in society generally. Second, a certain level of health is a necessary condition for the exercise of fundamental rights and privileges. Persons with severe physical or mental disabilities or with acute or chronic diseases may not be able to exercise their rights to liberty (for example, travel), autonomy (for example, decision making in personal and financial affairs), or the franchise. Third, health is of overriding importance in the achievement of personal satisfaction, happiness, and personal relationships. Human fulfillment is much more difficult to achieve when human beings experience unremitting pain and suffering, when they cannot meet their basic self-care needs, and when they lose mental and physical functioning. A person's self-dignity, self-identification, and status in society are often connected with that person's vitality and ability to function (Priester, 1992). When illness or disease is preventable or when pain and disability can be alleviated, the government's failure to act is conspicuous. Persons whose morbidity and suffering could have been prevented or lessened through reasonable governmental assistance may understandably claim that they count less, that their dignity is undermined by governmental inaction.

Equitable Access

Access to health care is measured by the use of health services, the quality of those services, and health outcomes (Institute of Medicine, 1993). The test of equity asks whether there are systematic differences in access and whether these differences result from financial or other barriers to health care. Using these objective measures of equitable access to health care, researchers have been able to demonstrate persistent and sometimes remarkable differences among groups in the United States.

There is a powerful and growing literature on inequitable access to health care (see Feinstein, 1993). On each of the three dimensions just discussed—use (Wenneker and others, 1990), quality (for example,

Burstin and others, 1992), and health outcomes (for example, Wise, 1985)—considerable data demonstrate significant differences among groups, related to their personal, social, and economic status (Ayanian and Epstein, 1991; Merton, 1993). The disparities in access to care are particularly sharp and enduring (Rosenberg, 1974; Eyler, 1989) for persons of low socioeconomic status (the poor or near poor) (Adler and others, 1993; Wise, 1985), the uninsured (Brown, 1990; Hadley, Steinberg, and Feder, 1991; Burstin and others, 1992; U.S. General Accounting Office, 1989), those in public programs such as Medicaid (Wenneker and others, 1990; Medicaid Access Study Group, 1994), and persons in minority racial and ethnic groups (for example, Council on Ethical and Judicial Affairs, 1990; LaVeist, 1993).

Health disparities between poor people and those with higher incomes are almost universal across all dimensions of health (see U.S. Department of Health and Human Services, 1991). For virtually all the chronic diseases that are leading causes of mortality, low income is a special risk factor (Amler and Dull, 1987). Thus the incidence of heart disease and most forms of cancer (lung, esophageal, oral, stomach, cervical, prostate) is significantly higher among persons in poverty than among the rest of the population (U.S. Department of Health and Human Services, 1991; National Heart, Lung, and Blood Institute, 1990). The poor also suffer disproportionately from infectious diseases such as HIV and respiratory diseases such as tuberculosis (Bor and Epstein, 1991). Similar vulnerability to traumatic injuries and death is found among the poor (U.S. Department of Health and Human Services, 1991). Finally, a higher rate of developmental and other disabilities, especially among children, is associated with poverty (National Center for Children in Poverty, 1990; National Center for Health Statistics, 1990).

The association between economic disadvantage and ill health is manifested most strongly in strikingly poor pregnancy outcomes (for example, prematurity, low birthweight, birth defects) and higher infant mortality (Institute of Medicine, 1985); in limitations in life activities due to ill health (National Institute on Disability and Rehabilitation Research, 1989; U.S. Department of Health and Human Services, 1991); and elevated mortality rates. Low-income people have death rates by age twice the rates for people with incomes above the poverty level (Amler and Dull, 1987).

Compared to other groups in society, African Americans and other racial and ethnic minorities are three times more likely to live in poverty (U.S. Department of Health and Human Services, 1991) and to lack health insurance (Cornelius, 1991; Institute of Medicine, 1993; Butts, 1992). They also are subject to discrimination in health care (Randall, 1993; Watson, 1994). The effects of these burdens are borne out in poorer utilization of services, outcomes, and health status "virtually across the board" (Institute of Medicine, 1993). A major study on health and medical care for African Americans concluded that "of all the inequalities in the distribution of health, one of the most pronounced is the distribution by race. . . . African-Americans are not as healthy as white Americans, and they do not live as long" (Reed, 1993, p. xvii). Recent studies have further demonstrated this disparity, indicating that the health care gap between African Americans and white Americans exists not only in higher incidence of disease but also in shorter life expectancy after diagnosis of serious medical conditions (Kilborn, 1998).

Virtually all health status indicators for African Americans and other ethnic minorities are dire when compared with those for white Americans. African Americans have considerably elevated rates of childhood diseases such as measles and chickenpox (Bueler and others, 1989); chronic diseases such as diabetes, heart disease, and cancer (Kilborn, 1998; U.S. Dept. of Health and Human Services, 1986; Institute of Medicine, 1993; Reed, 1993); and communicable diseases such as HIV and tuberculosis (Gostin, 1991, 1995; Reed, 1993). Similarly, the rates of infant and maternal mortality are significantly higher for African Americans in comparison to white Americans (Kilborn, 1998).

Plainly the reasons for the pronounced differences in health status and mortality rates between poor people, particularly racial minorities, and the rest of the population are attributable to many factors unrelated to health care, such as environment, housing, behavior, and nutrition. Yet most thoughtful observers conclude that barriers to access to health services, measured by utilization of services and health outcomes for equivalent conditions, remain significant contributing factors explaining the increased morbidity and mortality among the poor and minorities (Institute of Medicine, 1993; U.S. Department of Health and Human Services, 1991; Amler and Dull, 1987). For example, the Institute of Medicine (1993) estimates that one-third to one-half of the gaps in mortality rates are attributable to difficulties in obtaining access to health care.

EQUITY

What ethical values support the claim that equity should be observed in the distribution of health services, and what exactly is the equity claim being made? To many, it is not intuitively obvious that equity is a principle that deserves general recognition in society. Americans are prepared to tolerate significant and pervasive inequalities in wealth and in the distribution of most social goods (Bayer, 1983). A theory of equity in health care must provide an account of why health care deserves special treatment, unless the advocate is prepared to defend a considerably broader view of distributive justice for all goods and services (Gutmann, 1981).

One theory of the need for equity in health care, examined previously, relies on the special importance of health care in providing a necessary condition for the fulfillment of human opportunity. Daniels (1981, 1983, 1985) observes that pain and disability, limitation of function, and premature loss of life all restrict human opportunities. If it is accepted that a certain level of health services is a precondition to affording human beings reasonable life opportunities, then some equitable access to those services is warranted.

Government is prepared to provide a public education to all children of school age. Access to education is presumably justified by the importance of education in furnishing fair opportunities for all children, irrespective of their social or economic class. Like education, a certain level of health care is essential to a person's ability to pursue life's opportunities on some roughly equitable basis (Rawls, 1971; Brock and Daniels, 1994). Whereas education provides opportunities by facilitating basic knowledge and skill, health care provides opportunities by enabling a person to function mentally and physically in the application of that knowledge and skill (Rawls, 1971).

A healthy population, like an educated population, is much more likely to be socially and economically productive and less dependent. A multitiered system of health care, in which those in the lower tiers receive clearly inferior and lower-quality services, perpetuates inequalities among individuals and groups. These inequalities affect not only attaining health but, indirectly, attaining status, acceptance, and livelihood in society. As various inequalities among individuals and groups expand, society must deal with the consequences of social unrest, alienation, and dissatisfaction. Strikingly disparate standards of health care for different social, economic, and racial groups, then, are unjust to individuals and to society.

JUSTICE

A just health care system incorporates both substantive and procedural justice. Thus, distributive justice requires a fair sharing of benefits and burdens, but a just distribution of benefits and burdens does not require an equal sharing; when individuals with different needs receive the same services or when individuals with different means pay the same, the system is distinctly unjust.

How would an ethically ideal system determine the distribution of health benefits? Benefits of health care should be distributed on the basis of need; those with greater needs should receive greater services. A needs-based system ensures that those who are ill receive all reasonable services necessary to alleviate their ill health. If the foundational value of health care is to restore functioning and relieve pain and suffering so that individuals can achieve a sense of well-being and contribute to their families and society, then distribution of services according to need is ethically warranted. Distribution of services based, for example, on the ability to pay, places health care in the same position as virtually all other goods and services in society. Distribution by the ability to pay means that more services are provided to those who may need them less. The same services provided to those with more acute needs would achieve greater overall health benefits for the population.

How would an ethically ideal system determine the distribution of payment for health services? Ideally a progressive system of financing is preferred. Persons who can most afford to pay for health services should pay a greater share. This method assigns the greatest burdens of paying the costs of care to those who will experience the cost as less sacrifice in their lives because it is a smaller proportion of their overall incomes. Most countries use progressive systems of general taxation to finance the health care system. The United States finances its health benefits programs, such as Medicaid and Medicare, much in the same way. Even in the realm of private insurance, financing is, in theory, supposed to be fair. Community rating is a method of spreading the risk across a broad population. Thus each person, irrespective of her risks for ill health, pays the same. Even though person X (who is ill) is likely to utilize a far higher proportion of services than person Y (who is healthy), both pay the same premium.

Assume, as Rawls (1971) does, that none of us knows whether she will be rich or poor, sick or healthy. Given this state of ignorance, most would want a health care system that provided benefits for all those in need, and payment by all those who could best afford the economic burden. In this way benefits and burdens are distributed according to principles of justice. Each person pays according to her ability to afford the payment, and each person receives services according to her needs.

Principles of justice entail procedural as well as substantive standards. Consequently, a just health care system must be open and accountable and provide due process for individuals or groups who are denied benefits. An open and accountable health care plan must structure its services in ways that are easily understood by consumers and that ensure needed services are in fact delivered. Therefore consumers have a legitimate claim to full disclosure of information concerning their benefits and treatments (Kinney, 1996): credentials of physicians in the network, including their qualifications, experience, and disciplinary records; capitation agreements and physician incentives that may affect referrals to specialists; rules for access to hospital emergency care; and plan performance indicators, including consumer satisfaction.

Fair procedures suggest that if a person claims an entitlement to a health benefit and it is rejected, fair methods should exist for adjudication. Most health insurance plans provide services for "medically necessary and appropriate" treatments. They can, and do, use this contractual provision to deny services. Managed care organizations also typically devise a variety of methods to restrict services (see Kinney, 1996). Various methods of structuring capitations and incentives may lead primary care physicians to refuse to make a requested referral. Utilization reviewers may also deny care because it is cost ineffective. Fair health care plans would review contested decisions with procedures that are impartial and rigorous. For example, the patient should receive timely notice that an appealable claim exists and the procedures of the appeal process should be easily understandable to the patient (Kinney, 1996). Contested decisions could be reviewable by an independent body, comprising experts in the field, that gives the consumer a full and fair opportunity to present his case.

Determining whether a particular dispute should come under the grievance procedures within the health care plan or should be adjudicated through more formal procedures presents another difficult problem. The process used, whether prescribed by health care plan procedures or by other administrative or judicial procedures, will be adequate provided that the aforementioned procedural safeguards are in place (Kinney, 1996). Additionally, contractual limitations on patients' ability to challenge health care plan policies and care decisions in court should be clear to the patient upon enrollment. Conflict between health care plans and the courts can also arise when courts impose judicial orders for treatments or procedures for which the health plan will not pay (Petrila, 1998).

The idea of open, accountable, and procedurally fair decision making is, however, far from simple. Managed care organizations were formed, in substantial part, to facilitate cost-conscious decisions to allocate health care dollars where they will do most good. At the same time, managed care plans are usually for-profit entities that prosper economically by limiting service. It is possible to envisage a poor, inarticulate consumer being denied such basic services as standard prevention and curative services. In such cases the merits of fairer review criteria and procedures are unmistakable. It is also possible to envisage a well-off consumer being denied a very expensive procedure that offers little evidence of efficacy but is the person's last hope. A person with terminal AIDS or cancer seeking a bone marrow transplant with little evidence of efficacy may have a very different view of the desired treatment than the health care plan. In these circumstances an independent review may be costly to the plan, and outside reviewers may be more inclined to empathize with the terminally ill patient. Courts, for example, have awarded inordinate damages in cases of treatment refusal even when the chance of success was negligible. Thus procedural fairness may result in greater costs, but this may be a trade-off that most consumers would be willing to make.

CHOICE

Patient choice of health care plan and physician, often thought of as an unadulterated good, is in fact a complex value and requires significant trade-offs with other ethical values. Although an ethically sound health care system must have regard for patient choice of health care plans, physicians, and treatments, it also must balance enhanced choice with the values of access, cost, and quality. The importance of protecting, respecting, and making effective individual choices has strong ethical roots in the literature of health care and ethics. No study has definitively linked choice to quality of care, insofar as quality is taken to mean better outcomes for the physical and mental health of patients (Brook, 1997). Yet enhanced choice does appear to have an association with consumer satisfaction in health care, which itself has intrinsic value (Schmittdiel, Selby, Grumbach, and Quesenberry, 1997; Weyrauch, 1996).

Choice can refer to access to health care generally, to health care plans, to physicians and other clinicians, or to treatments. In each case, the concept of choice is fraught with complexity and trade-offs.

Choice, in its most fundamental sense, refers to a person's ability to gain access to the health care system. Choice of whether or not to obtain health care services is, however, restricted by a person's ability to pay and by nonfinancial barriers. The choice of health care plans, providers, or treatments can arise only after a person gains access to the health care system. If guaranteeing such choice to all patients who already have health care means limiting access to others, would this provide a net increase or diminution of choice? Managed care, for example, often diminishes a person's choice of physicians and treatments (Emanuel and Dubler, 1995), but it may cost less than fee-for-service plans. Arguably, if managed care could reduce costs, it would increase affordability and access to health care. Seen in this way, cost-conscious health care plans may reduce choice for some but increase it for others.

Choice can also be measured by the number of health plans available and the number of opportunities to choose among competing health plans. Many Americans do not have a robust choice among health care plans; employers may restrict employee choices to one or more options, the market for health care in some geographical areas may not support more than one plan, and the cost of some health plans may be unaffordable for poorer consumers. In these situations employer cost consciousness, marketplace forces, or financial constraints may deny patients a realistic choice among health care plans.

If choice is to be effective, the consumer must have some reasonable basis upon which to select a health care plan. Consequently, as suggested earlier, full and fair information must be provided by health care plans that permit prospective purchasers to accurately evaluate critical factors such as quality, cost, and patient satisfaction (Longo and others, 1997).

Most people define choice as the right to select a primary care physician or a specialist when they need medical attention. Managed care systems, depending on how they are structured, may substantially decrease choice of providers. This may affect continuity of care if the patient changes health care plans or the physician leaves the network. Even when a health care plan has many physicians in the network, patients may be unfamiliar with those physicians or the HMO may assign patients to available physicians. Limitation on access to specialists is frequently a design feature of managed care plans. This access may be controlled by primary care physicians and utilization reviewers, and compensation arrangements may provide disincentives for referrals to specialists. From the perspective of managed care organizations, these reductions in choice may be necessary to provide cost-effective care. The struggle over patient choice of physician is often represented by *any willing provider* laws that require managed care organizations to include any qualified provider who seeks entry into the network (Marsteller, Bovbjerg, Nichols, and Verrilli, 1997; McCarthy, 1997; Einhorn, 1996).

There are a number of reasons for believing that choice of physicians is an ethical value of some importance, although perhaps not of transcending importance. Patients personal preferences for a clinician deserve respect. A variety of factors such as sex (Elstad, 1994), ethnicity, and socioeconomic status (Temkin-Greener and Winchell, 1991) affect patients' physician preferences. Patient satisfaction with visits in a managed care setting is often less than that in fee-for-service settings (Rubin and others, 1993), and satisfaction with physician performance in HMOs increases when patients are given access to the physician they wish to see (Weyrauch, 1996). Patients who chose their personal physician appear to be substantially more satisfied with their health care than those who do not (Schmittdiel, Selby, Grumbach, and Quesenberry, 1997). Patient satisfaction with their physicians is also likely to increase trust, which is an essential part of the physician-patient relationship (Mechanic and Schlesinger, 1996).

At first glance, giving patients a choice among treatments may appear relatively uncontroversial. The doctrine of informed consent appears to guarantee patients full information about treatment alternatives and the right to determine their preferred course of treatment. Although it may be true that competent patients have the right to decline any treatment, it does not follow that informed consent affords a right to any treatment that the patient chooses. In fact a patient's treatment choice is constrained by many factors: the Food and Drug Administration must approve pharmaceuticals, the physician must believe the treatment is beneficial, and insurers must agree to pay for the treatment (for example, companies may refuse to reimburse for *experimental* treatments).

Conflicts over patients' treatment choices occur in a variety of settings. Some have involved persons with AIDS or other incurable conditions who were seeking access to therapies that offered only a slim hope of recovery (for example, *Weaver* v. *Reagan*, 886 F.2d 194 [8th Cir. 1989]). Affording patients or family members the choice of any possible treatment, irrespective of the expense or the likelihood of success, requires a trade-off with cost, resulting in greater overall cost for the health care system. A health care plan designed to save money by limiting the use of less effective and more costly treatments (for example, limiting treatment to that which is medically necessary or appropriate, implements practice guidelines, and is established by utilization reviews), restricts choice to some extent. However, the resources that are saved may afford greater choice in other areas and improve overall quality.

QUALITY

The value of health care is based on the assumption that medical treatment is effective in preventing, ameliorating, and curing illness. There is an inherent value, therefore, not just in access but in quality. But before discussing definitions and measures of quality, it is important to understand that there are deficiencies in science and in practice.

There is a dearth of evidence for the efficacy of most clinical treatments. The bulk of clinical practice is not built on a strong scientific foundation. Clinical trials supporting the efficacy of treatment are available for a relatively small proportion of medical procedures (Office of Technology Assessment, 1994). And even when research data demonstrate treatments that work, clinicians do not invariably follow these findings (Laffel and Berwick, 1992).

Definitions of quality necessarily reflect the views and values of those who define the term. A physician may evaluate quality of care by the degree to which that care provides a medical cure for a specific ailment. A patient, meanwhile, may evaluate quality of care by the level of attention and concern she receives from her provider during her illness. A third-party payer may define quality of care by the degree of economic efficiency, that is, by the cost-effective allocation of services (Donabedian, 1988). The Institute of Medicine (1990) offers a more scientific definition of quality as the degree to which, given the state of medical knowledge, health interventions increase the probability of desired patient outcomes and reduce the probability of undesired outcomes.

Several areas of research have generated concern about quality. First, iatrogenic injury (for example, illness or disease resulting from, or occurring during the course of, professional medical activities) is a significant problem in hospital care (Bedell and others, 1991). Second, in 10 to 30 percent of cases, providers perform unnecessary or inappropriate diagnostic tests, procedures, and hospitalizations (Institute of Medicine, 1992). Finally, extensive variations exist in practice patterns (for transfusions, caesarean sections, breast cancer and heart disease treatments, for example) and in health services utilization (hospitalizations, for example) (Cleary and others, 1991).

Investigations with findings like these have challenged health care providers and regulators to develop reliable and inexpensive methods to understand, detect, and prevent medical error. The scope of activities implemented in the name of quality management is too extensive to examine comprehensively here, but briefly, they include (Jost, 1988) providing consumer information that promotes informed choice based on quality and cost (Longo and others, 1997); using computerized information systems for health services research, diagnostic assistance, and systematic examination of practice patterns (Schriger, Baraff, Rogers, and Cretin, 1997); licensing physicians and other health care professionals; practicing risk management and reforming the medical malpractice system (Sage, Hastings, and Berenson, 1994); and conducting outcomes research (Mariner, 1994; Ellwood, 1988) and developing clinical practice guidelines (Institute of Medicine, 1992).

Given the ethical importance of quality and the extant problems in health care delivery, quality assessment and systems to encourage more effective treatment have substantial and enduring importance in health care.

COST

The United States spends a larger share of its GDP on health care than any other industrialized nation does (Council of Economic Advisers,

1994). This level of spending has ethical implications because cost has a relationship to health care access and quality, just as it does to many other social goods. Health care is financed in at least three principal ways, and in each one there is a relationship between cost and access: businesses pay for health care by self-insuring or purchasing group health plans; individuals and households pay for health care by contributing to employer-sponsored coverage and purchasing individual (nongroup) plans; and government pays for health care through public health insurance programs (for example, Medicaid and Medicare), direct provision of care (for example, by the Veterans Administration and the Indian Health Service), and indirect subsidies (through the tax system). In each case, greater expenditure results in some diminution of a social function. For example, increases in employer health care costs may result in lower nonbenefit compensation or loss of jobs; increases in household health care costs may result in less income for such other necessities of life as housing, clothing, and food; and increases in governmental health care allocations may result in fewer resources for such other collective goods as environmental protection, transportation, and education. Health care costs, wherever they are incurred, may result in decreased access to health care. As costs and premiums rise, health insurance becomes less affordable and available.

The relationship between cost and quality is more complex. Cost constraints, particularly under managed care, are sometimes assumed to affect quality to some degree (McGraw, 1995). But the question must be asked whether a direct relationship in fact exists between the quantity and cost of health care and its quality. "If we assume that quality and costs are positively related, then it follows that efforts to contain costs threaten quality. If we assume a less linear or even negative relationship, then cost containment and quality improvement may even be complementary" (Wagner, 1994, p. 1951). Economic investments in health care often tend to improve quality. At some point, however, the law of diminishing returns takes hold, and the quality improvements become too small to justify the additional costs.

There is no ideal level of health care spending from an ethical perspective. Yet, within the levels necessary for reasonable quality, health care expenditures should be kept low enough to increase access and to maintain equitable levels of resource allocation.

The U.S. public appears to be caught in a paradox. We value the choice and quality in the current health care system, but we recognize the harm to the economy caused by escalating costs and the harm to the social fabric cultivated through inadequate access and inequitable distribution of services. It appears that each effort to improve one key variable produces a trade-off with another.

Beyond this paradox is the numbing complexity of a pluralistic system that engulfs one-seventh of the nation's economy. The many aspects of the health care system engage our political, social, and economic lives: for example, health care involves benefits, services, governmental regulations, private sector competition, professional standard setting, the tort system, doctor-patient relationships, and public health. All these remain sources of formidable challenges, worthy of rigorous exploration at a theoretical, empirical, and practical level. Above all, as we contemplate private and public sector reforms of the health care system, we must measure these reforms by the core ethical values of access, equity, justice, choice, quality, and cost.

References

Adler, N. E., and others. "Socioeconomic Inequalities in Health: No Easy Solution." *JAMA*, 1993, *269*, 3142.

Amler, R. W., and Dull, H. B. *Closing the Gap: The Burden of Unnecessary Illness.* New York: Oxford University Press, 1987.

Ayanian, J. Z., and Epstein, A. M. "Differences in the Use of Procedures Between Women and Men Hospitalized for Coronary Heart Disease." *New England Journal of Medicine*, 1991, *325*, 221.

Bayer, R. "Introduction." In R. Bayer, A. L. Caplan, and N. Daniels (eds.), *In Search of Equity: Health Needs and the Health Care System.* New York: Plenum, 1983.

Bedell, S. E., and others. "Incidence and Characteristics of Preventable Iatrogenic Cardiac Arrests." *JAMA*, 1991, *265*, 2815.

Bipartisan Commission on Comprehensive Health Care. *A Call for Action: Final Report of the Pepper Commission.* Washington D.C.: U.S. Government Printing Office, 1990.

Bor, D. H., and Epstein, P. R. "Pathogenesis of Respiratory Infection in the Disadvantaged." *Seminars in Respiratory Infections*, 1991, *6*, 194.

Brock, D. W., and Daniels, N. "Ethical Foundations of the Clinton Admin-
    istration's Proposed Health Care System." *JAMA*, 1994, *271*,
    1189–1192.

Brook, R. H. "Managed Care Is Not the Problem, Quality Is." *JAMA*, 1997,
    278, 1612–1614.

Brown, L. D. "The Medically Uninsured: Problems, Policies and Politics."
    Journal of Health Politics, Policy & Law, 1990, *15*, 315.

Bueler, J., and others. "The Reporting of Race and Ethnicity in the National
    Notifiable Diseases Surveillance System." *Public Health Reports*,
    1989, *104*, 457.

Burstin, H. R., and others. "Socioeconomic Status and Risk for Substan-
    dard Medical Care." *JAMA*, 1992, *268*, 2383.

Butts, C. Q. "The Color of Money: Barriers to Access to Private Health Care
    Facilities for African-Americans." *Clearinghouse Review*, May–June
    1992, p. 159.

Cleary, P., and others. "Variations in Length of Stay and Outcomes for Six
    Medical and Surgical Conditions in Massachusetts and California."
    JAMA, 1991, *266*, 73.

Cornelius, L. J. "Access to Medical Care for Black Americans with an
    Episode of Illness." *Journal of the National Medical Association*, 1991,
    83, 617.

Council of Economic Advisers. *Economic Report of the President Transmit-
    ted to the Congress*. Washington D.C.: U.S. Government Printing
    Office, 1994.

Council on Ethical and Judicial Affairs. "Black-White Disparities in Health
    Care." *JAMA*, 1990, *263*, 2344.

Daniels, N. "Health-Care Needs and Distributive Justice." *Philosophy &
    Public Affairs*, 1981, *10*, 146.

Daniels, N. "Health Care Needs and Distributive Justice." In R. Bayer,
    A. L. Caplan, and N. Daniels (eds.), *In Search of Equity: Health
    Needs and the Health Care System*. New York: Plenum, 1983.

Daniels, N. *Just Health Care*. New York: Cambridge University Press, 1985.

Davis, K. "Uninsured in an Era of Managed Care." *Health Services Research*,
    1997, *31*, 641–646.

Donabedian, A. "The Quality of Care: How Can It Be Assessed?" *JAMA*,
    1988, *260*, 1743–1750.

Donelan, K., and others. "Whatever Happened to the Health Insurance
    Crisis in the United States? Voices from a National Survey." *JAMA*,
    1996, *276*, 1346–1350.

Dougherty, C. J. "Ethical Values at Stake in Health Care Reform." *JAMA,* 1992, *268,* 2409–2413.

Einhorn, T. "Reigning in ERISA Preemption? Any Willing Provider Statutes After New York Blue Cross Plans v. Travellers Ins. Co." *Journal of Contemporary Health Law & Policy,* Fall 1996, *13,* 265.

Ellwood, P. M. "Outcomes Management: A Technology of Patient Experience." *New England Journal of Medicine,* 1988, *318*(23), 1549–1553.

Elstad, J. "Women's Priorities Regarding Physician Behavior and Their Preference for a Female Physician." *Women's Health,* 1994, *21,* 1–19.

Emanuel, E. J., and Dubler, N. N. "Preserving the Physician-Patient Relationship in the Era of Managed Care." *JAMA,* 1995, *273,* 323–329.

Employee Benefit Research Institute. *Sources of Health Insurance and Characteristics of the Uninsured: Analysis of the March 1995 Current Population Survey.* Issue brief. Washington, D.C.: Employee Benefit Research Institute, Feb. 1996.

Eyler, J. M. "Poverty, Disease, Responsibility: Arthur Newsholme and the Public Health Dilemmas of British Liberalism." *Milbank Quarterly,* 1989, *67* (Suppl. 1), 109.

Feinstein, J. S. "The Relationship Between Socioeconomic Status and Health: A Review of the Literature." *Milbank Quarterly,* 1993, *71,* 279.

Franks, P., Clancy, C. M., and Gold, M. R. "Health Insurance and Mortality: Evidence from a National Cohort." *JAMA,* 1993, *270,* 737–741.

Gostin, L. O. "The Inter-Connected Epidemics of Drug Dependency and AIDS." *Harvard CL-CR Law Review,* 1991, *26,* 113.

Gostin, L. O. "The Resurgent Tuberculosis Epidemic in the Era of AIDS: Reflections on Public Health, Law, and Society." *University of Maryland Law Review,* 1995, *1,* 54.

Gutmann, A. "For and Against Equal Access to Health Care." *Milbank Quarterly,* 1981, *59,* 546.

Hadley, J., Steinberg, E. P., and Feder, J. "Comparison of Uninsured and Privately Insured Hospital Patients." *JAMA,* 1991, *265,* 374–379.

Hafner-Eaton, C. "Physician Utilization Disparities Between the Uninsured and Insured: Comparisons of the Chronically Ill, Acutely Ill, and Well Nonelderly Populations." *JAMA,* 1993, *269,* 787–791.

Institute of Medicine. *Preventing Low Birthweight.* Washington D.C.: National Academy Press, 1985.

Institute of Medicine. "Public Health Is What We, as a Society, Do Collectively to Assure the Conditions in Which People Can Be Healthy." *The Future of Public Health,* 1988, *19,* 36–38.

Institute of Medicine. *Medicare: A Strategy for Quality Assurance.* Washington D.C.: National Academy Press, 1990.

Institute of Medicine. *Guidelines for Clinical Practice: From Development to Use.* Washington D.C.: National Academy Press, 1992.

Institute of Medicine. *Access to Health Care in America.* Washington D.C.: National Academy Press, 1993.

Jost, T. S. "The Necessary and Proper Role of Regulation to Assure the Quality of Health Care." *Houston Law Review,* 1988, *25* (May), 525–598.

Kilborn, P. T. "Health Gap Grows, with Black Americans Trailing Whites, Studies Say." *New York Times,* Jan. 26, 1998, p. A16.

Kinney, E. D. "Resolving Consumer Grievances in a Managed Care Environment." *Health Matrix: Journal of Law-Medicine,* 1996, *6,* 147.

Laffel, G., and Berwick, D. M. "Quality in Health Care." *JAMA,* 1992, *268,* 407–411.

LaVeist, T. A. "Segregation, Poverty, and Empowerment: Health Consequences for African Americans." *Milbank Quarterly,* 1993, *71,* 41.

Levit, K. R., and others. "Americans' Health Insurance Coverage, 1980–91." *Health Care Financing Review,* 1992, *14,* 31–39.

Lewin/VHI for Families USA Foundation. *Half of U.S. Families Priced Out of Health Protection.* Washington D.C.: Lewin, 1993.

Long, S. H., and Marquis, M. S. *Universal Health Insurance and Uninsured People: Effects on Use and Costs: Report to Congress.* Washington D.C.: Office of Technology Assessment and Congressional Research Service, Aug. 5, 1994.

Longo, D. R., and others. "Consumer Reports in Health Care: Do They Make a Difference in Patient Care?" *JAMA,* 1997, *278,* 1579–1584.

Mariner, W. K. "Outcomes Assessment in Health Care Reform: Promise and Limitations." *American Journal of Law & Medicine,* 1994, *20,* 37.

Marsteller, J. A., Bovbjerg, R. R., Nichols, L. M., and Verrilli, D. K. "The Resurgence of Selective Contracting Restrictions." *Journal of Health Politics, Policy & Law,* 1997, *22,* 1133.

McCarthy, D. "Narrowing Provider Choice: Any Willing Provider Laws After New York Blue Cross v. Travelers." *American Journal of Law & Medicine,* 1997, *23,* 97.

McGraw, D. C. "Financial Incentives to Limit Services: Should Physicians Be Required to Disclose These to Patients?" *Georgetown Law Journal,* 1995, *83,* 1821.

Mechanic, D., and Schlesinger, M. "The Impact of Managed Care on Patients' Trust in Medical Care and Their Physicians." *JAMA,* 1996, *275,* 1693–1697.

Medicaid Access Study Group. "Access of Medicaid Recipients to Outpatient Care." *New England Journal of Medicine,* 1994, *330,* 1426.

Merton, V. "The Exclusion of Pregnant, Pregnable, and Once-Pregnable People (a.k.a. Women) from Biomedical Research." *American Journal of Law & Medicine,* 1993, *19,* 369.

National Center for Children in Poverty. "A Statistical Profile of Our Poorest Young Citizens." National Center for Children in Poverty, 1990.

National Center for Health Statistics. "National Health and Nutrition Examination Survey." NHANES II. Hyattsville, Md.: U.S. Department of Health and Human Services, National Center for Health Statistics, 1990.

National Heart, Lung, and Blood Institute. "National Cholesterol Education Program, Report of the Expert Panel on Population Strategies for Blood Cholesterol Reduction." Bethesda, Md.: National Institutes of Health, National Heart, Lung, and Blood Institute, 1990.

National Institute on Disability and Rehabilitation Research. *Chartbook on Disability in the United States.* Washington, D.C.: National Institute on Disability and Rehabilitation Research, 1989.

Office of Technology Assessment. *Does Health Insurance Make a Difference?* Background paper. Washington, D.C.: Office of Technology Assessment, 1992.

Office of Technology Assessment. *Identifying Health Technologies That Work: Searching for Evidence.* Washington D.C.: Office of Technology Assessment, 1994.

Pear, R. "Health Spending Grew Slowly in '96 but Still Hit $1 Trillion." *New York Times,* Jan. 13, 1998, p. A15.

Petrila, J. "Courts as Gatekeepers in Managed Care Settings." *Health Affairs,* 1998, *17.*

President's Commission for the Study of Ethical Problems in Medicine and Biomedical and Behavioral Research. *Securing Access to Health Care.* Washington D.C.: U.S. Government Printing Office, 1983.

Priester, R. "A Values Framework for Health System Reform." *Health Affairs,* 1992, *11,* 84–90.

Randall, V. R. "Racist Health Care: Reforming an Unjust Health Care System to Meet the Needs of African-Americans." *Health Matrix: Journal of Law-Medicine,* 1993, *3*(127), 144–160.

Rawls, J. *A Theory of Justice.* Cambridge, Mass.: Harvard University Press, 1971.

Reed, W. L. *Health and Medical Care of African-Americans.* Westport, Conn.: Auburn House, 1993.

Reinhardt, W. E. "Wanted: A Clearly Articulated Social Ethic for American Health Care." *JAMA,* 1997, *278,* 1446–1447.

Rosenberg, C. E. "Social Class and Medical Care in 19th-Century America: The Rise and Fall of the Dispensary." *Journal of the History of Medicine,* 1974, *29,* 32.

Rubin, H. R., and others. "Patients' Ratings of Outpatient Visits in Different Practice Settings: Results from the Medical Outcomes Study." *JAMA,* 1993, *270,* 835–840.

Sage, W. M., Hastings, K. E., and Berenson, R. A. "Enterprise Liability for Medical Malpractice and Health Care Quality Improvement." *American Journal of Law & Medicine,* 1994, *20*(1–2), 1–28.

Schieber, G. J., and others. "Health Care Systems in Twenty-four Countries." *Health Affairs,* 1991, *10,* 22–37.

Schmittdiel, J., Selby, J. V., Grumbach, K., and Quesenberry, C. P. "Choice of a Personal Physician and Patient Satisfaction in a Health Maintenance Organization." *JAMA,* 1997, *278,* 1596–1599.

Schriger, D. L., Baraff, L. J., Rogers, W. H., and Cretin, S. "Implementation of Clinical Guidelines Using a Computer Charting System: Effect on the Initial Care of Health Care Workers Exposed to Body Fluids." *JAMA,* 1997, *278,* 1585–1590.

Schroeder, S. A. "The Medically Uninsured: Will They Always Be with Us?" *New England Journal of Medicine,* 1996, *334,* 1130–1133.

Short, P. F., and Banthin, J. S. "New Estimates of the Underinsured Younger Than 65 Years." *JAMA,* 1995, *274,* 1302–1306.

Stoddard, J. J., and others. "Health Insurance Status and Ambulatory Care for Children." *New England Journal of Medicine,* 1994, *330,* 1421–1425.

Swartz, K. "Dynamics of People Without Health Insurance: Don't Let the Numbers Fool You." *JAMA,* 1994, *271,* 64–66.

Temkin-Greener, H., and Winchell, M. "Medicaid Beneficiaries Under Managed Care: Provider Choice and Satisfaction." *Health Services Research,* 1991, *26,* 509–529.

Thorpe, K. E. *The Rising Number of Uninsured Workers: An Approaching Crisis in Health Care Financing.* Washington D.C.: National Coalition on Health Care, Oct. 1997.

U.S. Department of Health and Human Services. Task Force on Black and Minority Health. *Report of the Secretary's Task Force on Black and*

Minority Health. Vol. 7: *Chemical Dependency and Diabetes.* Washington D.C.: U.S. Department of Health and Human Services, 1986.

U.S. Department of Health and Human Services. *Healthy People 2000: National Health Promotion and Disease Prevention Objectives.* Washington D.C.: U.S. Department of Health and Human Services, Public Health Service, 1991.

U.S. General Accounting Office. *Health Insurance: An Overview of the Working Uninsured.* Washington D.C.: U.S. General Accounting Office, 1989.

Wagner, E. H. "The Cost-Quality Relationship: Do We Always Get What We Pay For?" *JAMA,* 1994, *272,* 1951.

Walzer, M. *Spheres of Justice: A Defense of Pluralism and Equality.* New York: Basic Books, 1984.

Watson, S. D. "Minority Access and Health Reform: A Civil Right to Health Care." *Journal of Law, Medicine & Ethics,* 1994, *22,* 127.

Wenneker, M. B., and others. "The Association of Payer with Utilization of Cardiac Procedure in Massachusetts." *JAMA,* 1990, *264,* 1255.

Weyrauch, K. "Does Continuity of Care Increase HMO Patients' Satisfaction with Physician Performance?" *Journal of the American Board of Family Practice,* 1996, *9,* 31–36.

Wise, P. H. "Racial and Socioeconomic Disparities in Childhood Mortality in Boston." *New England Journal of Medicine,* 1985, *313,* 360.

CHAPTER FIVE

Preparing for the Global Health Transition

Kent Glenzer
Maurice I. Middleberg

Kent Glenzer currently is director of the Management Technology Unit of CARE, assisting overseas country offices in strategic and operational planning, leadership development, and organizational change processes. Over the past fifteen years, he has worked in seventeen African countries, assisting nonprofit and public sector organizations in strategic planning and strategy implementation, organizational and management development, training, and organizational restructuring.

As director of the Health and Population Unit of CARE, Maurice I. Middleberg has overall responsibility for CARE's family planning and reproductive health program and for integrating family planning and reproductive health into CARE's health, development, and relief programs. He is also an adjunct faculty member at the Rollins School of Public Health at Emory University, where he teaches the Reproductive Health Program Management course.

T his is a challenging and exciting time for public health professionals working in the developing world. A demographic and epidemiological transformation is underway, creating a more diversified set of health needs in populations traditionally served by international health care nongovernmental organizations (IHNGOs). This shift will redefine the international public health agenda over the next twenty-five years and require health care leaders to, first, adopt fundamentally new approaches in grassroots health programs and, second, make courageous decisions about organizational mission, strategy, structure, skills, and performance measurement.

THE HEALTH TRANSITION

In the 1960s, mortality in the developing nations was highly concentrated, with more than 35 percent of annual deaths occurring in children under five. These deaths were largely attributable to a relatively constrained set of factors: vaccine preventable diseases, diarrheal disease, respiratory infections, short birth intervals, and malnutrition. By 1996, child mortality was down to 22 percent of total deaths (World Health Organization, 1997), and fertility rates, a proxy for obstetric risk, were down in every region except sub-Saharan Africa.

Enter a very different picture of health problems. *The Global Burden of Disease* (GBD; Murray and Lopez, 1996), a study on which the Harvard University School of Public Health and World Health Organization (WHO) collaborated, reveals that developing world health problems are becoming highly differentiated. Here are the trends that will be important over the next twenty years:

- High levels of fertility, child mortality, and maternal mortality are concentrating in sub-Saharan Africa and South Asia; infectious and parasitic diseases remain the most important cause of death in the developing world.
- Mortality percentages are increasing for older age groups.
- Chronic diseases—including cardiovascular diseases, cancers, and respiratory diseases—have become responsible for almost 40 percent of all deaths in developing nations (World Health Organization, 1997).

- Emerging, reemerging, and drug-resistant infectious diseases—of which the most prevalent are HIV/AIDS, tuberculosis, and malaria—are increasing.

- Mortality data are obscuring the larger and more complex issue of the *burden of disease,* a measure that reflects the impact of diseases that seriously hamper economic productivity and quality of life. Table 5.1 shows the long-term trends in the burden of disease. They indicate that no one package of services will uniformly bring down mortality and morbidity. Instead, the developing world faces a *double burden of disease;* as substantial pockets continue to confront the old enemies of childhood disease, unwanted high fertility, and high maternal mortality, many countries and subpopulations will have to grapple with a very different and new disease burden.

A NEW APPROACH TO PROGRAMMING

Increasingly complex health care needs require new operational realities based on new approaches. The *health security framework* (HSF) is a model we have developed to promote the kind of leadership that can respond to the heterogeneous and evolving health care challenges identified by the GBD Study. Health security is achieved when households identify, prevent, and manage significant risks to the health of

1990	2020
1. Lower respiratory infection	1. Unipolar major depression
2. Diarrheal disease	2. Road traffic accidents
3. Conditions arising during the perinatal period	3. Ischemic heart disease
4. Unipolar major depression	4. Chronic obstructive pulmonary disease
5. Tuberculosis	5. Cerebrovascular disease
6. Malaria	6. Tuberculosis
7. Measles	7. Lower respiratory infections
8. Ischemic heart disease	8. War
9. Congenital anomalies	9. Diarrheal disease
10. Cerebrovascular disease	10. HIV

Table 5.1.   Ten Leading Causes of Disease Burden in the Developing World.

household members. Households accomplish this through healthy behaviors, empowered communities, capable institutions, optimal health technologies, and appropriate public policies. The HSF has seven major components, or elements:

• *Household focus.* The framework explicitly ties health status to the overall livelihood security of a household. Poor families face excruciating choices in allocating scarce resources among health care, food, and other basic needs. It follows that health programming should take place within the context of an overall development strategy that brings multiple, mutually reinforcing interventions to bear on the participating households.

• *Risk analysis as basis for programming.* Risk assessment, which includes indicators of disease burden (years of life lost, years lost to disability, quality-adjusted life years, disability-adjusted life years), is the foundation for programs that can be adjusted in response to shifting epidemiology. Levels, causes, and effects of mortality and morbidity must be disaggregated within and among households as well as between genders and among social groups. It is important to combine the tools of epidemiology with the perceptions of the involved households, given the well-known discord between quantitative and subjective risk assessment. Finally, risk assessment is not the sole province of health experts; it must involve the range of legitimate stakeholders and recognize the legitimate diversity of decision-making criteria.

• *Optimal health interventions.* Associated with major causes of mortality and morbidity are what experience and research tell us are optimal health interventions. As principal health risks change over the coming decades, however, optimal health technologies will also change. It is an open question whether the new problems described in the GBD will be amenable to the same technologies used in the past. IHNGOs can play a useful role in testing alternative technical packages.

• *Healthy behaviors within the household.* Many of the current risks experienced by poor households in the developing world can be mitigated at low cost through changes in behavior at the household level. As the nature of health risks changes, however, the costs, benefits, and effectiveness of behavioral change strategies will change. In addition, a household focus reminds us that healthy behaviors, and the opportunity costs they often represent, must be directed at the concerns of the various household members.

- *Community empowerment.* Community norms, social structures, and leadership influence household health behaviors, both positively and negatively. Creating effective, sustainable community-based
organizations (CBOs) that can stimulate institutional and policy
change is key to managing the health transition. Building the skills of
women's groups to mobilize for health care is particularly important,
given the shifting burden of disease.

- *Institutional capacity.* Health security and the management of
health risks also require that health institutions have the requisite
capacity. We use the term *health institutions* broadly. It includes public, private, traditional, nonprofit, and for-profit providers of health
services. Capacity building is an effort to match the skills and systems
of health institutions to the most important health problems. It has
three dimensions. First, capacity building should facilitate *access* to the
services and commodities needed to address current and emerging
health risks. Access encompasses physical proximity to needed services
and the economic means and sociopolitical liberty to seek those services. Second, capacity building should ensure the quality of services,
including the technical competence of providers, adequacy of client
counseling, respect for the dignity and confidentiality of the client,
existence of client follow-up, and appropriate physical setting for care.
Lastly, capacity building must strengthen management systems,
including community health assessment, planning, human resource
management, monitoring and evaluation, drug and commodity supply, equipment and facilities management, and financial management.[1]

- *Appropriate public health policies.* Public policy influences both
the application of appropriate health technologies and the promotion
of appropriate health behaviors relative to the greatest risks to health.
With disease burden changing, IHNGOs must advocate for a review
of public and tacit policies governing health care, to ensure they are
consistent with reducing the shifting risks to health.

The HSF is helping CARE field programs that respond to the reality of heterogeneous and constantly evolving health risks. Concomi-
tant with changes in grassroots programming is the need to develop
an adaptive organizational strategy that responds to epidemiological
transition. This is the first and most fundamental task of the IHNGO
leader who wishes to position the organization for the twenty-first
century.

THE IHNGO LEADER'S WORK: ORGANIZATIONAL STRATEGY, STRUCTURE, SYSTEMS, AND COMPETENCY

The coming health transition requires IHNGOs to reexamine their organizational mission and role. Such hard thinking must then be translated into explicit strategy. New strategy will require new organizational structures, systems, and competencies.

Strategic Options

The shift in the global burden of disease presents a classic example of market redefinition. The IHNGO that wishes to adapt to the health transition has four generic strategy options, as shown in the simple matrix in Figure 5.1.

STICK TO THE KNITTING.   Two factors might lead an IHNGO leader to adopt the strategy of sticking to the knitting. From a resource perspective, few IHNGOs have the capital to invest in experiments. Given that donor and host government priorities lag behind paradigmatic shifts, the cautious IHNGO leader might consciously choose to remain

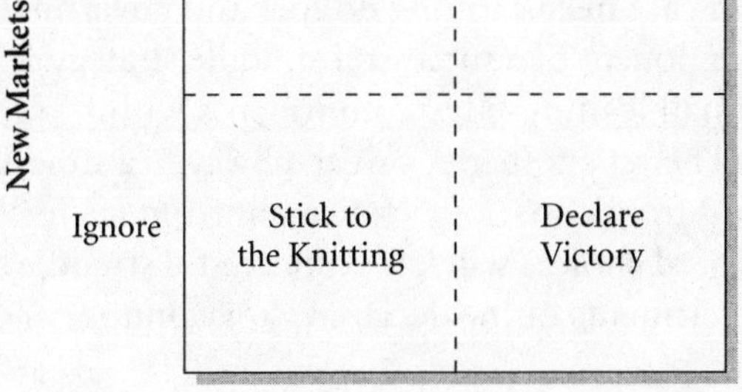

Figure 5.1.   Four Strategy Options for IHNGOs.

in current niches. Second, the emerging disease burden will most negatively affect the relatively wealthy while the old enemies will persist among hundreds of millions of the very poor. Remaining in current niches may very well be more congruent with an IHNGO's existing mission and its culture. This strategy is not without risk, however. Organizations that remain in traditional niches may not have markets for their services ten years from now. Within the foreseeable future, traditional IHNGO health care programs will no longer attract significant donor funding: indigenous NGOs, private providers, and host governments will have the capacity to meet health care needs in a more cost-effective manner. An IHNGO leader who selects this strategy will face obsolescence within two decades.

DECLARE VICTORY—AND GO HOME.   *Declare victory—and go home* is a sound strategic option. For decades we in this field have said that our goal is to work ourselves out of our jobs; this strategy will hold us to this underlying philosophy. To be an effective strategy, however, it requires the IHNGO leader to implement a rigorous, long-term process of phasing the IHNGO out. The IHNGO will need a small number of key, macro indicators of health status; as these country-specific indicators are met or surpassed, the IHNGO can cease the respective programming and focus resources on an ever-diminishing number of country programs.

STRADDLE.   Under the straddle strategy, IHNGOs will adopt a dual track program, continuing to address the enduring problems of child mortality and poor reproductive health and simultaneously developing a more diverse health portfolio. Small and well-monitored pilots will be an important element of such a strategy. Raising awareness of new health care needs among donors and governments will be another key component of a successful straddle strategy. The careful insertion of small leading-edge components within traditional health projects will be yet another. A caveat, however: a straddle strategy that results not from conscious choice but from leaders' simple inability to make hard choices will fail. A successful straddle strategy will also combine elements of the declare victory option, in order to avoid portfolio creep.

REINVENT.   IHNGO leaders have a window of opportunity in the next decade to transform their health portfolios. If done well, such a strategy will position the organization for many more decades of valuable work and will result in extraordinary differences in mission and vision. Yet an IHNGO leader who opts to reinvent faces tremendous obstacles.

The investment needed to build competence is high. The reinvent strategy also brings with it a risk of portfolio proliferation, of trying to do everything and doing nothing well. The successful implementation of a reinvent strategy will demand strong leadership, a firm long-term vision of where the organization's health portfolio should be a decade or more from now, and tangible investment in current staff.

Given that the reinvent strategy will likely be attractive to many IHNGO leaders, the remainder of this chapter turns to the challenges to successful strategy implementation.

Structural, Systems, and Competency Changes Required by Reinvention

IHNGOs will need to be structurally integrated into global surveillance and information systems. Health risk management in a rapidly evolving context requires continuous access to epidemiological information. IHNGOs will require a stronger focus on both accessing information from and providing information to the global network. Such structural integration will demand a great deal of time and effort from IHNGO leaders. A second necessary structural change will be radical decentralization: the GBD study reveals the disintegration of monolithic, globally applicable health approaches and the growth of fragmented, localized *micro-markets*. Such decentralization requires decision-making authority close to the customer. IHNGO leaders face a particularly difficult challenge given that their current financial, decision-making, and administrative systems are defensive, more rooted in ensuring compliance than in promoting decentralized initiative. This challenge pales, however, in comparison to the need for sober, clear-headed performance indicators for decentralized operations, an area in which IHNGOs have a genuinely appalling record. Fortunately, there is nothing mysterious or difficult about such indicators; our real challenge is having the courage to hold ourselves accountable for changes in health status and centering reward systems around the measures of change.

Finally, IHNGO leaders face a tremendous competency gap. IHNGO staff have backgrounds in child survival, reproductive health, water and sanitation, and related primary care fields. These were appropriate competencies under the old paradigm of developing world health concerns. It is less clear that they are important for the future.

PRACTICAL IMPLICATIONS FOR IHNGO LEADERS

IHNGO leaders wishing to reinvent their organizations can take six practical steps.

1. *Raise awareness within and outside the organization.* IHNGO leaders will need to devote time and resources to building a critical mass of consensus about the coming health transition and about organizational mission. They should not underestimate the potential resistance to altered mission and must use every available opportunity over the next few years to organize public conversations. Awareness must be extended beyond the organization to donors, local government officials, the poor and vulnerable with whom they work, and local nongovernmental organizations.

2. *Adapt and apply tools for risk analysis.* IHNGO leaders need to encourage the development, adaptation, and implementation of practical tools for assessing and weighting risks. Here we see a marriage among the tools of epidemiology, community participation, and management decision making. Epidemiological data are only inputs into a participatory process that involves all relevant stakeholders. In setting the health agenda all elements of the HSF—behavior, community empowerment, institutional capacity, policies, and so on—should be considered.

3. *Build new skills and reward their use.* Key components in such a strategy are

- Knowledge of emerging health problems
- Skills in participatory approaches to risk analysis, program development, and project monitoring and evaluation
- Knowledge of health security at the household level and skills in applying it
- Capacities to lead institution building and organizational development at the grassroots level

- Concrete and visible promotion of innovators (a basic responsibility of organizational leadership), providing them with money, encouragement, and political protection

4.   *Select partners for strategic alliances and build long-term relationships.* Given the coming heterogeneity of health problems, it is unlikely that any organization will be able to advance health security without drawing on the skills and resources of other organizations. Strategic alliances will help IHNGOs acquire short-term competence and augment their capital and are attractive to donors and host governments. Strategic alliances are excruciatingly difficult to develop, however; relationships must be nurtured slowly and empathetically, and partners need to decelerate the implementation process if they are to build trust and understanding.

5.   *Strengthen linkages with global surveillance systems.* Because of their deep roots in local communities, IHNGOs can play a vital role in building local capacity to carry out surveillance, detect anomalies and trends in a pattern of disease, and feed this information into global systems. This will be a vital function of the twenty-first century IHNGO. IHNGO leaders must also invest in information technology so staff can make more effective use of the global surveillance data.

6.   *Design performance indicators, reward systems, and management information systems to meet the health transition.* IHNGO leaders must establish concrete, tangible measures of program performance, overhaul internal reward and recognition systems accordingly, and construct global management information systems that adequately track both organizational and individual performance. At the individual and project level, novel measures are particularly needed for community ability to manage health risks and mobilize around health problems, health institutions' quality of care, effectiveness of advocacy efforts, quality of strategic alliances and local partnerships, strength of linkages between grassroots projects and global surveillance systems, and financial efficiency.

Note

1. CARE has developed an instrument, the Management Capacity Assessment Tool, for assessing management systems. This instrument, which has been applied in countries such as Bangladesh and Haiti, is available upon request.

References

Murray, C.J.L., and Lopez, A. D. (eds.). *The Global Burden of Disease: A Comprehensive Assessment of Mortality and Disability from Diseases, Injuries, and Risk Factors in 1990 and Projected to 2020.* Cambridge, Mass.: Harvard School of Public Health, on behalf of World Health Organization and World Bank; distributed by Harvard University Press, 1996.

World Health Organization. *World Health Report.* Geneva, Switzerland: World Health Organization, 1997.

CHAPTER SIX

Public and Community Health

William H. Foege
Mark Rosenberg

Epidemiologist William H. Foege is widely recognized as a key member of the successful 1970s campaign to eradicate smallpox. Presently he is Presidential Distinguished Professor of International Health at the Rollins School of Public Health, Emory University. Foege is the author of more than 125 professional publications and the recipient of many awards, including the WHO Health for All Medal, the Healthtrac Prize, and the Calderone Prize. He holds honorary degrees from eleven institutions and was named a Fellow of the London School of Tropical Medicine and Hygiene in 1997.

Mark Rosenberg is director of the National Center for Injury Prevention and Control (NCIPC) at the Centers for Disease Control and Prevention (CDC). Board certified in both psychiatry and internal medicine, he has authored more than one hundred publications and has received the U.S. surgeon general's Exemplary Service Medal and also the Meritorious Service Medal and Outstanding Service Medals from the U.S. Public Health Service.

Successful public health leadership in the next millennium will require three abilities:

- *The ability to form effective coalitions.* Public health leaders will need to identify and work successfully with new partners. Coalition building will require not only interpersonal skills but also the ability to form an idea of a common goal or vision, share it, and develop support for it.

- *The ability to see the whole and its parts simultaneously.* Public health leaders will need to see what they are doing and how it fits in with the larger picture; to see what they are doing and how it fits in with what their partners are doing; to see what they are doing now and how it fits in with everything that will be done. They need to scan and to focus and to see relationships. And they need to do these all at the same time.

- *The ability to be tenacious.* Public health leaders need to persevere in each objective: to hold on and see it through. This ability comes from our having seen the success of public health efforts in the past and from the idea that our efforts to change the world will be successful.

In 1796, when Edward Jenner immunized James Phipps with cowpox material taken from the hand of Sarah Nelms, he began a chain of events that led to smallpox eradication, polio vaccine, and measles vaccine, a chain that will some day lead to vaccines for malaria and AIDS. The links in this chain include key elements of the public health approach developed as part of the response to these diseases: surveillance systems, a public health infrastructure, and the notion that a global response is appropriate for many of these health threats. As the science of public health has accumulated to include knowledge of sanitation, tuberculosis, and nutrition, it has culminated in the past third of a century in infant mortality rates that have dropped by half and life expectancy for the world's population that has increased by fifteen years. As the focus of public health has expanded from infectious diseases to chronic diseases to lifestyle factors, environmental health, occupational health, injury control, and now even to mental health, its tools have been refined. These tools are many, yet they all emanate from the following four concepts, which define the field of public health and the foundation of public health leadership:

- This is a cause-and-effect world, and public health takes responsibility for changing those causes that lead to bad effects.
- Public health takes responsibility for people in the aggregate.
- Public health takes responsibility for the future health of people living now and for the health of people who will live in the future.
- Public health problems constantly reemerge in new forms, and public health takes responsibility for keeping ahead of these changing problems in a changing world.

THE NEW WORK OF PUBLIC HEALTH

These four defining concepts of public health form a consistent and useful framework for approaching and leading the work of public health in a rapidly changing world. Leadership in public health demands the ability to chart a clear path through this changing environment, and this ability, in turn, requires the ability to see what is changing. Public health ideas about agent, host, and environment have changed tremendously over the past two hundred years. And much more than these notions has changed. Over the same period the world in which these factors operate and in which we do business has become much more complex in many ways. These changes and the increased scope of the public health task pose challenges for several leadership activities: using facts and data for rational decision making; appreciating human character and the psychological factors that affect individual behaviors, especially within the workforce; and understanding and predicting organizational behavior. An appreciation of the changes in each of these domains is necessary for leaders who want to move public health forward in the next millennium.

MAKING DECISIONS WITH MORE INFORMATION

To begin with, decision making is more complex. From its initial focus on only a few infectious diseases, public health grew to address a broad range of infectious diseases and then tackled noninfectious diseases such as reproductive health problems, cancer, and cardiovascular diseases. The issues then expanded again to include environmental problems, occupational health and safety, and injuries. And as the scope of public health attention expanded, the data available for analysis within each area increased rapidly.

Further, the potential for opposition also increased. Bacteria, viruses, and parasites have few advocates. But when prevention turned to cardiovascular diseases, smoking-related illnesses, and traumatic brain injuries following motorcycle accidents, the contributing causes of these problems—such as fatty foods, cigarettes, and motorcycles—also provided perceived benefits to large parts of the population. Supporters rallied to preserve these benefits and make public health policy development more challenging.

More data and more types of data are now available to public health leaders, and they are expected to use these data in ever more rapid decision making. In fact the whole public health infrastructure is more complex: data handling, proactive communications, and such new means of communication as the Internet offer new opportunities and demand more attention.

In addition to developing systems for collecting and handling these data, leaders will have to develop the capacity to change these systems as our understanding of particular problems grows. This is an iterative process: the better we understand a problem, the better we can specify exactly what information is needed to control it.

The sources for funding public health research and programs and the mechanisms of support have also changed. National, state, and local government funding has traditionally been a mainstay of support for public health programs, and the funding process used to be relatively straightforward: legislation was developed to authorize particular programs, and then governmental funds were appropriated for these programs. Today, many projects and ventures are supported through new mechanisms, including large entitlement programs, huge pots of money created by taxes on particular goods (like tobacco or alcohol), interagency and interdepartmental agreements, and public-private ventures. Some public health programs are initiated and supported not just in part but entirely by the private sector.

Public health has also become more politicized: the growth of managed care and the economic importance of health care has brought much greater interest in public health decisions, especially those affecting health care services. And as public health begin to address problems that involve behaviors and conflicting values, funders, including the federal and state governments, have begun to interject their own value systems, making the process of seeking program support yet more complicated.

LEADING A NEW WORKFORCE

In addition to changes in public health issues and information, changes in the individuals who make up the public health work force add to today's complexity. The increasing complexity of the public health tasks we face demands mastery of a greater range of skills, often requiring not only the traditional public health disciplines but collaboration with behavioral scientists, computer specialists, engineers, and communications specialists. Making this amalgam work requires the effective blending of many different technical specialists on projects that previously would have been unidisciplinary. Even more important, our workforces are becoming more ethnically and racially diverse. Greater racial and ethnic diversity brings strength but also increases the time and effort required to achieve true understanding and agreement. Unfortunately, more time is the one thing we no longer feel we have.

GUIDING ORGANIZATIONAL EVOLUTION

Organizations that affect public health have also become more complex, with cultures and standard operating procedures that can be difficult to understand and even more difficult to change. The public health enterprise itself is larger and more complex: more lives and people to be protected, larger budgets, more money flowing to more places, and more people employed (but now more separated from each other). To operate effectively, public health organizations need more rapid responses to get through more layers of bureaucracy. And each bureaucracy now covers a wider range of issues that have greater complexities and require greater depth of coverage.

The relationship of public health to the public and to the body politic has also changed. Public health issues are not just issues of science and medicine; they are now political issues, and public health leaders work in a highly politicized environment. In addition to the larger economic stakes now involved, several other factors are contributing to this politicization. First, people have much greater awareness of the potential of public health to contribute to their health and well-being in arenas far beyond contagious disease. At the same time, it has become clear that today's public health interventions involve more than simply providing antibiotics or vaccinations.

The traditional public health structure can no longer deliver public health alone. To do their jobs effectively, public health leaders must develop coalitions with groups outside the traditional public health domain. These new coalitions bring new problems as well as solutions, but we have no choice. Today, public health partnerships with outside groups are increasing in number and complexity. In part this reflects the need for public health to take on issues that are increasingly value and conflict laden. When these values bump up against individuals' personal belief systems, then individual change requires people and partners who are trusted by target audiences and who can convey credible messages to them. At the national level, for example, public health leaders must develop new constituencies, reaching beyond their traditional partners in state and local health departments to community groups. However these new coalitions also make communication more complex, difficult, and stressful.

This level of complexity has developed extraordinarily fast, and it is mirrored by similar levels of complexity in other areas of science, society, politics, and economics. Once public health was practiced on a local scale; this current complexity is global. Fifty years of global practice and use of global organizations are not enough to know what works best.

Ideas are the wealth of public health, and by cultivating ideas, public health has the potential to provide leadership on a far broader scale than has traditionally been considered its domain.

PART TWO

The New Health Care Organization

CHAPTER SEVEN

What Comes After Consolidation?

Jeffrey C. Barbakow

Jeffrey C. Barbakow is chairman and chief executive officer of Tenet Healthcare Corporation, one of the nation's leading health care services companies. Under his leadership Tenet's core revenues have grown from $2.5 billion to approximately $10 billion. He is a member of the CEO board of advisers of the University of Southern California School of Business Administration, the board of trustees of the UCLA Foundation, and the chancellor's council at the University of California at Santa Barbara.

⌐∽∾∾⌐

Fast forward with me, for a moment, to the not-too-distant future.

Consolidation—that rallying cry during the 1980s and 1990s for so many major U.S. industries seeking to improve their global competitiveness—has gone about as far it is going. For the hospital industry, this means that most inefficiencies have been squeezed out of what was once a highly fragmented, wasteful system. Purchasing leverage has been maximized. Administrative efficiencies have been captured. Capacity has been carefully rationalized. As a result the formerly loose-knit U.S. hospital industry has evolved into a somewhat smaller (but still substantial) number of fully integrated delivery systems, each offering a continuum of care—from inpatient acute care to outpatient surgery to home health services.

It does not take much of a crystal ball to see this far into the future. It is just about here. According to the American Hospital Association, about 50 percent of its 4,400 member hospitals now consider themselves part of a system, up from 11 percent in 1993. The number of integrated delivery systems nationwide stands at 280, of which 231 are not-for-profit, 44 are for-profit, and 5 are run by the government.

The real forecast has to look further out. What comes after consolidation?

I admit that my role as chairman and chief executive officer of an investor-owned hospital company in the process of building regional integrated networks across the country colors my view on that question. But because I wrestle every day with issues that affect the future of our business, I believe I have a pretty good vantage point.

And from all I can see, it is clear that the industry is about to undergo yet another significant transformation. I am also convinced that this will be a change for the better, because it will help preserve the best elements of U.S. health care today as it eliminates some of the less desirable aspects.

This transformation, I believe, will involve three major parts. First, today's emphasis on consolidation will be replaced by a new era of collaboration among hospital operators (with each organization's tax-paying status becoming increasingly irrelevant) and between the hospital operators and the insurance companies.

Second, health care providers will assume more of the risk for their patients' medical management. In their consolidations they have gained expertise in bearing risk. Now they will need to develop new, collaborative risk models with payers and other providers. Additionally, insurance will increasingly be about covering individuals, not just groups, as employees gain *portable* coverage that follows them from job to job. This off-loading of risk will create a market for new products designed collaboratively by insurers and providers.

Third, and perhaps most exciting, consumers will have much greater selection of and control over their own health care. Competition among providers in the future will focus increasingly on quality, and consumers will have the benefit of vastly more sophisticated information on outcomes as well as on perceived quality and service.

Now let's take a closer look at these major shifts that I see ahead. Clearly many new questions are raised. What will be the impact on services? How will success be measured? How will purchasing decisions be made? What new leadership skills will be required? Obviously I will be drawing from Tenet's experience in talking about these issues, but the application is universal.

As hospitals move into a new era of collaboration and risk sharing with payers and other providers, the nature of the services they offer will change dramatically. Increasingly, I believe, they will find it prudent to deal with two distinct at-risk populations in their service areas—people who have acute illnesses and require ongoing disease management and people who are generally healthy and need only episodic care.

In order to optimize the health of that segment of the population requiring extensive disease management, the newly consolidated health delivery systems will have to offer a full continuum of services at various points throughout their service areas. Take, for example, the case of a patient with coronary artery disease. In order for his health to be truly improved, this individual may require a broad range of services—everything from diagnostic procedures to open-heart surgery to rehabilitation. To effectively manage its entire population of individuals suffering from coronary artery disease, the health system of the future will have to offer this full continuum of services not just at one flagship hospital within the system but at various locations within its core service areas. Each location will have to demonstrate excellence in quality and efficiency in order to offer these services. Providing such depth of service also allows the hospital, as the bearer of an increased amount of risk, to match care intervention and setting to the patient's clinical requirements. This will ensure quality of care at an affordable cost.

For those generally healthy individuals who require only episodic care, hospitals will need to make a much more significant investment in preventive and wellness programs than they are currently doing. As they bear more risk for this population, their objective will be to help keep these individuals healthy so they do not need costly medical services. For example, Tenet's regional delivery network in South Florida has already seen the value of this approach. Tenet's mobile wellness program has performed more than sixteen thousand screenings—including mammograms and blood pressure, diabetes, cholesterol, and prostate exams—since its inception two years ago. That translates to sixteen thousand additional opportunities to identify and treat potentially life-threatening illnesses before they progress to the more expensive acute care stage.

The good news for individual hospitals in the future is that they will no longer need to be one-stop shops for health care consumers, as long as a broad range of services exists elsewhere in the system, preferably within easy reach of the population and taking into account the clinical needs of each service. For example, the logical location for a cardiac catheterization lab is close to a facility with an open-heart surgery program. Additionally, systems may choose to provide these services through various partnerships and alliances with other providers. Undoubtedly, hospital administrators of the future will be faced more and more frequently with deciding whether to make, buy, or contract for services—all the more reason for collaboration among payers and other providers.

Because it will be geared toward serving the particular health needs of the population for which it is at risk, the hospital system of the future must be on a solid financial footing. Collaboration among traditionally not-for-profit research and teaching organizations and financially strong system operations will grow. And as increasingly sophisticated consumers shop for quality in health care, connections between prestigious quaternary hospitals and larger regional systems will become an ever more important selling point.

This is particularly significant for academic medical centers and quaternary care hospitals that by their nature are expensive to operate. As Tenet's own experience operating teaching hospitals for premier academic medical centers shows, as long as these hospitals are part of larger networks and are sized appropriately to serve their particular population's needs, they should be able to prosper—even if as independents they would be on shaky financial ground. Through its affiliations with the University of Southern California (USC) School of Medicine at USC University Hospital in Los Angeles, Creighton University Medical Center at St. Joseph Medical Center in Omaha, and most recently, Saint Louis University School of Medicine at Saint Louis University Hospital in St. Louis, Tenet is able to offer these facilities all the advantages of being part of an integrated network.

For at least the past decade, hospitals have been implementing efficiency programs to reduce their costs. Much of the savings have come from the purchasing leverage offered by programs such as Tenet's group-purchasing organization, BuyPower. BuyPower, with annual purchasing volume of about $1.8 billion for more than 3,200 members, uses that leverage to obtain highly competitive prices from vendors for supplies and services. Other efficiencies have come from reengineering efforts at the individual hospital level and from spreading costs for systemwide maintenance or other functions across regional systems.

In the future, as more of the financial risk is borne by the provider instead of the insurer, the ability to optimize resource use will become even more central to the individual hospital's financial performance. But I must caution that *optimize* is the key word here, because quality of patient outcomes will be the most significant factor guiding tomorrow's consumer as she decides whether to entrust a particular hospital or provider with her health care needs.

Some patients may benefit from more expensive procedures that require longer stays in the hospital because the clinical outcome will be significantly better and their long-term health greatly improved. Others can be treated with less expensive procedures yet have the same outcome. In the future, clinicians and hospitals will still be grappling with tough utilization decisions as they do today, but consumers will play a much bigger role in that decision-making process.

Some of Tenet's clinical resource management programs are beginning to tackle this issue. Our hospitals have developed specific protocols for hip and knee replacement surgery that ensure patients are matched with the appropriate implant for their health, age, and lifestyle. And by placing a cap on the price they will pay vendors for any implant, they have been able to reduce their costs significantly. For example, Tenet's South Florida hospitals have cut costs by more than 30 percent. As hospitals and physicians join forces to share in risk management, the importance of these programs will be recognized. With that recognition, physicians, who control the resource utilization decision, will take greater personal responsibility for making sure that resources are used in the most appropriate and effective ways.

Under the current reimbursement system, payers who bear most of the risk have been responsible for bundling together provider networks to serve their customers' needs. As part of that process they have attempted to match provider geographies and services with the employee needs of the groups they represent. Their control over utilization has come through handling claims, referral requirements, and customer service. As a result, many consumers when surveyed include their payer's administrative efficiency and the geographical availability of care among the important criteria that influence their selection of a health plan.

These same surveys have found that consumers place little emphasis on the ability of providers to deliver quality clinical care and patient outcomes. Mostly likely that is because it has been difficult for consumers to measure success in health care. That, however, is about to change.

In the new era of collaboration, risk sharing, and vastly increased information available about outcomes and service, consumers are likely to make a major change in how they shop for health care. Purchasing decisions will increasingly focus on a provider's ability to manage the consumer's health and on its demonstrated success in outcomes.

At Tenet we recognize the need to measure quality of services and outcomes at our hospitals. And we know that these measurements will become essential to the success of the hospital of the future. For that reason the company has developed and continues to refine its own computerized outcomes management system that provides extensive patient care information in various different diagnostic categories, adjusted for severity of diagnosis. The system enables Tenet hospitals to compare medical costs and outcomes as reported by physicians and hospitals across the country. For example, the system can be used to compare the performance of individual physicians treating the same condition at the same facility or to contrast the overall performance of hospitals within the Tenet network.

Tenet's USC University Hospital is taking that system one step further. By adding a variety of other measures, such as clinical outcomes, patient satisfaction, and quality-of-life indicators, the hospital is working to gain a balanced view of patient outcomes. When combined with benchmark data from across the nation, this data will allow the hospital and its physicians to identify opportunities for improvement and to develop clinical initiatives for the future.

But even though I believe we at Tenet are moving in the right direction, it is also clear to me that our industry's newly expanded role in managing the health care risk of entire populations will require vision and leadership.

Tomorrow's hospital leaders must develop the ability to think strategically about their networks and plan accordingly. Key questions facing them will include where sites should be located, what services should be offered at each site, and how sites should be configured for maximum efficiency. These are quite different issues than those grappled with by the leaders of the past.

The make, buy, or contract out decision I mentioned earlier is one that administrators will have to address more and more frequently, and that will not be easy for an industry in which organizations are used to self-sufficiency and doing everything alone. Making the correct decision will require solid analytical and financial skills.

As they are today for insurance industry leaders, pricing and actuarial skills will be essential for tomorrow's hospital leaders. It has been said there is no such thing as a bad risk, only bad prices. This will be increasingly true in tomorrow's hospitals. At Tenet we have the advantage of having operated for many years in some of the most heavily penetrated managed care markets in the country (Southern California, for example). And our experience in New Orleans, where we were chosen by the Health Care Financing Administration to implement an innovative managed care plan offering Medicare recipients a greater range of health care choices, should stand us in good stead in the future. At least it has given us a window on the future.

In a nutshell, I believe that this industry has a number of brand-new challenges ahead, postconsolidation.

First, anticipating the clinical needs and utilization patterns for entire populations, and pricing them appropriately, will be central to the future economic viability of the hospital industry.

Second, the ability to measure and analyze outcomes and to communicate these measurements effectively will be critical to our future success. All of us—providers, payers, and consumers—will have to agree on a definition of *quality* in health care. And consumers will increasingly cite quality as their top priority in selecting a provider.

Third, to attract business in an industry that if anything will be even more competitive than today, the next generation of hospital leaders will need skills that combine clinical knowledge, epidemiological knowledge, and knowledge of customer expectations.

Fourth, the nature of our marketing will change. To effectively meet the needs of individuals, hospitals, as part of larger regional systems, will increasingly have to focus on the specific population segments for which the system has the right mix and location of services.

Some systems may be geographically driven; some may be demographically driven. The ability to understand market segmentation will be vital to success.

And finally, this fragmented business that served so well for so long as America's last great cottage industry will have to pull together collaboratively to share risk, increase efficiency, and respond to the needs of a much more sophisticated consumer who will know more and demand more of us.

From where I sit today, I believe we are up to the challenges.

CHAPTER EIGHT

Growing Effective Leadership in New Organizations

John D. Henry Sr.

Roderick W. Gilkey

John D. Henry Sr. is chief executive officer of Emory University Hospitals in Atlanta, Georgia. He serves on the boards of the University Hospital Consortium, Georgia Hospital Association, and the Atlanta Chamber of Commerce Quality Resource Center. A Fellow of the American College of Healthcare Executives, he is a member of the faculty of the Emory University School of Medicine and serves as associate professor in the Department of Community Health.

Roderick W. Gilkey is executive director of the Center for Healthcare Leadership at Emory University. He holds joint appointments in the School of Medicine, Department of Psychiatry, and the Goizueta School of Business and has received the university's highest teaching honor, the Emory Williams Award. The coauthor of Joining Forces *(with Joseph McCann, 1989) and a contributor to* Organizations on the Couch *(edited by Manfred Kets de Vries, 1991), he has also consulted to a number of global and Fortune 500 companies.*

The emergence of integrated health care delivery systems creates new opportunities and challenges for leaders. With the demands of increasing complexity, comes the need for ever higher levels of organizational and human performance. Leaders become more dependent on their people and on the capacity of those people to attain ever higher levels of achievement.

We have chosen to focus here on two major leadership strategies: developing and distributing the leadership to create change and aligning and coordinating leadership so that the organization's activities are strategically focused and its values are consistently applied. We call our approach *empowerment within boundaries*. It develops the organization's capacity for leadership and change while it creates an environment (structures and processes) where such leadership can be effective.

The term empowerment has come into fashion because it is an apparent solution to today's challenge to do more with less, or, in the vernacular of health care, to generate value by improving care and diminishing costs. The logic for a new leadership paradigm is compelling. The order once provided by chains of command, spans of control, and standards of protocol becomes an impediment to action in time-sensitive, competitive market environments. Power, authority, and decision making all must be dispersed before organizations can provide responsive point of service delivery. As a result, ponderous structures and systems, and the authoritarian personalities and leadership styles that they sometimes spawned, are now dysfunctional.

In the new health care environment, leadership and power will be dispersed as widely as possible so that everyone can be involved in providing services, as Stan Davis, author of *Future Perfect* (1997), puts it, "anytime, anyplace no-matter." This has prompted some experts, like Francis Hesselbein, president of the Drucker Foundation, to refer to leadership in the next millennium as *distributive leadership* (Hesselbein, 1996). In this context, leadership performance is best measured by its capacity to leverage human intellect and energy in the service of shared visions and collective aspirations. Leadership becomes similar to art as described by Degas: "with art it is not so much a matter of what *you* can see, it is a matter of what you can get *other* people to see." We are living at a time when a new form of leadership—leadership as the ability to inspire, empower, and exert broad influence—supplants leadership as the exercise of centralized power and control.

If empowering employees is a solution to the challenge of managing in a more competitive environment, it can also be a problem. For example, empowerment without the continued involvement of top management is abdication. In this instance, empowerment becomes giving employees enough rope to hang themselves. Leaders who empower in this manner, delegating and disappearing, are justifiably subject to criticism. They can inadvertently or unconsciously set people up to fail; their efforts are at best ineffective and potentially unethical. At the other end of the empowerment continuum we find leaders who delegate but then micromanage their people. Their actions reflect their ambivalence and anxiety about losing control. Their ineffectiveness easily contributes to underperformance and decline as they add to the numbers of overmanaged and underled organizations.

The key challenge is achieving the proper balance of empowerment and oversight, steering clear of indirection or micromanagement. This can be accomplished only with in-depth understanding of the competence and readiness of the employee to become empowered. The effective leader of today and tomorrow will need to have a more intimate and insightful understanding of people than her predecessor did.

Empowerment must be preceded by understanding. In a previous era it may have been possible for leaders to treat employees as cogs in a mechanistic organizational wheel. In such environments people are seen as replaceable if not incidental. That era is now followed by one that calls for growth fueled by innovation and ideas produced by effective management of human capital. In a knowledge and service economy, people are assets whose ideas generate products, services, and internal organizational improvements that increase revenues and decrease costs.

The transition from mechanistic to more humanistic models of labor was illustrated by items in two recent issues of *The New Yorker*. The first contained a cartoon of a classic tycoon rushing through a room of cubicles, hurriedly offering to one of the myriad anonymous employees, "Keep up the good work, whatever it is, whoever you are!" In contrast, in a second issue, an executive of one of America's premier financial services corporations repeats an oft-heard saying as he talks about his employees to a reporter: "You have to remember, in this business your most important assets go down the elevator and out the door every night; you hope to God they return the next day."

Dispersing power and responsibility can be relatively easy—the challenge is to distribute it and at the same time to define the boundaries and limits within which it should be exercised. This challenge can be met only when the leader understands how much can be dispersed, to whom, and when. Making such critical judgments requires a profound depth of relationship and understanding. It requires new or improved appraisal skills for assessing current and potential performance.

To address new challenges it is necessary to look for solutions in nontraditional knowledge bases, for example, our experience as parents and grandparents. First, we create highly protective environments for infants, then we gradually expand boundaries and limits and shift our focus from protection to exploration and learning. In time we support children's capacity for initiative and taking charge of their world. If we are successful in managing this unfolding process, mature, generative human beings result. Similarly, leaders need to sponsor others in a developmental process that generates high-performing individuals and regenerates the organizations where these individuals work. The good news is that as Erik Erikson stated in a personal interview in 1970, "the plan for growth is all there if we will but let it live." Like parenting, leadership has the major task of balancing empowerment and the boundaries that provide the definition and clarity necessary for focus and productivity. And also as in parenting, if this balancing is done with a reasonable amount of precision (not perfection), the inborn potential for growth and success will unfold.

The challenge is to create boundaries without installing barriers. A boundary should define a domain for acting and learning, practicing and reflecting, experimenting and learning. A fundamental task of leadership is to provide well-defined but permeable boundaries that afford practice fields for management and leadership development.

Although it is important to understand theories of empowerment boundary definition, leadership is ultimately a matter of practice. We have found that there are four areas of leadership practice crucial to developing organizational performance through empowerment within boundaries: engagement, attention, information, and individual and organizational development.

ENGAGEMENT

The leaders of health care organizations cannot be remote figures acting from afar. They need to be fully engaged, with an active presence that is accessible, responsive, and quick. In this sense leaders must be living examples of the system they wish to create. *Being the change you are trying to create,* to paraphrase one of Gandhi's favorite exhortations, is a challenge that must be taken very seriously. We have found that one way of achieving a higher level of engagement is to conduct *CEO rounds,* in which top management visits all the departments in the system in rotation. The meetings are led by the department directors, who oversee these scheduled rounds, and consist of a brief, formal presentation followed by a great deal of informal interaction and discussion. The agendas and topics in these discussions are orchestrated by the directors and their staffs; however, the topics that arise are often more emergent than planned. After initial moments of nervousness the conversations that follow tend to be open and spontaneous. Trust is a precondition for achieving the level of candor necessary to make these sessions worthwhile. In some sense the limits of candor and insight that can be achieved are set by the degree of openness of the leader.

These forums are an opportunity for leaders to ask questions, share stories, and develop relationships with people from all organizational areas and levels. The learning that transpires cuts across the organization. For example, in one large department having some serious difficulties, the CEO brought the entire senior management team to the rounds. As team members listened to the accounts of departmental problems, they were able to identify ways they could help. The discussion became a mutual problem-solving session in which top managers demonstrated that they were engaged and committed to helping their colleagues solve departmental problems by spending their own time and resources in doing so. In one of these sessions the senior management team caucused (with the department members present) and discussed how they could help—the CEO took his suggestions along with those of others and asked individual members of his team to assume specific responsibilities to help.

This kind of leadership engagement allows everyone to gain a deeper understanding of the organization's people and capacities, neither of which can be deployed or developed effectively without such understanding.

ATTENTION

One of an organization's most precious resources is its attention. A leader creates the dominant focus for an organization by directing that attention to the most value-added activities. As role models, empowering leaders manage their attention so that it is at once focused and flexible. This means paying attention to both strategic and tactical matters and inviting others to do the same. In one of the most effective strategic practices we have developed at Emory Hospitals, we distribute quarterly strategic updates at department directors' retreats, attended by over 140 hospital managers. Moving strategy from the drawing board to the departments has been greatly facilitated by these sessions, which feature presentations by hospital leaders, followed by vigorous discussions. A key part of these sessions is offering encouragement and counsel for communicating the strategy throughout the system. The goal is to make certain that everyone from top to bottom has as much understanding as possible of the organization's strategic direction and focus. The retreats, informal briefings, and ongoing communication are an attempt to make strategy a participative living process rather than an abstract set of ideas articulated from above. This practice makes it possible for employees to focus their attention and link their day-to-day activities to evolving strategies.

Attention is also focused on the operational details that allow strategy implementation. In one CEO round a worker showed the senior management team a machine that was not working well. One of the executives noticed that the safety switch had been installed improperly. The machine was immediately put out of service until repairs were made. By correcting a previously undetected problem, team members demonstrated the importance of the smallest detail. They also displayed their commitment to the safety and well-being of the workers.

INFORMATION

Leaders determine the level of candor in their organizations—what is permissible to discuss and what is not. The ability of health care organizations to meet the imperative to innovate and create new, responsive systems of care is profoundly influenced by the extent to which information and ideas can be exchanged freely and openly. The need for candor and dissent is clear, and though this need must be communicated, it is better demonstrated than discussed. New norms for candor and improved communication require leaders to develop and use mechanisms to share information. It was not enough for us to create quarterly management retreats, for example; they had to become vital forums for sharing new information. Similarly, when the CEO of a new hospital system received a difficult mandate from the board that would place heavier demands on everyone, the CEO chose to stand before the management and read the letter. In this way everyone received the same message, the same way at the same time. Although the mandate (which defined exactly what the board did and did not want) was not particularly welcomed, it defined the reality and brought everyone together with a common goal and clear boundaries. The CEO took a substantial risk in sharing this information so directly. Fortunately, employees rose to the occasion and justified the CEO's confidence. The information was used constructively and ultimately elevated morale and commitment to the objectives of the mandate.

INDIVIDUAL DEVELOPMENT

In management, sponsoring or developing others, parenting them in a sense, is described as mentoring. Mentoring may be one of the highest forms of leadership. It requires maturity and integrity to mentor effectively and unselfishly. Psychologist Helene Deutsch once observed (1973) that maturity meant achieving the proper balance of narcissism and altruism. Narcissism in this context meaning healthy self-esteem and self-respect, the kind that gives us the confidence necessary to be leaders and to contribute to the lives of those around us. Altruism means having the capacity to be enhanced by the growth and success of others. Leadership in this context means achieving success through commitment to the success of others.

Because traditional leadership in formal, centralized organizations emphasized command-and-control tactics, it reinforced the narcissistic characteristics of managers at the top. In contrast, as we in health care move toward more decentralized and informal (or even virtual) organizations, our facilitating and empowering approaches will depend on top management's altruistic capacities. It will be interesting to see if it becomes increasingly difficult for individuals to reach the top through self-promoting and self-aggrandizing maneuvers when success in the top job increasingly requires creating an environment in which others can succeed.

Leadership by coaching and mentoring is neither an abstract idea nor a lofty sentiment. It is a way of managing that makes a difference. For example, one of the most valuable questions that a leader can ask during coaching sessions is, What can I do to help you? It is also helpful for the leader to reinforce the idea that the new health care organization is a collaborative, cross-functional network acting in the service of shared aspirations. In this context the vital concept is one of servant leadership—that is, leadership based on exercising power and gaining efficacy by helping others exercise their skills.

In the new paradigm, leaders not only seek their fulfillment in the success of others, they also create environments where people can perform real work—work that is a form of self-expression, work that reflects the inner hopes, aspirations, and ideals of the people who perform it. Such work is described by Abraham Zaleznik in his article "Real Work" (1997), where he argues that the majority of individuals' energy in most corporations is in fact spent on psycho-politics, that is, constant maneuvering to create personal and political gain.

If success in tomorrow's health care environment means drawing on the best performance from everyone, then the commitment to development must be broad and offer opportunity for the many, not just the few. Therefore managing diversity will become a means rather than an end. The ability to manage diversity well is a good measure of an organization's performance, of its excellence; it is not simply a legislated goal or fashionable outcome.

The practice of empowerment is based in part on the theory that people with a sense of strategic direction can assume responsibility for implementation. This theory places yet another demand on emerging leaders, the need to communicate a compelling vision and a clear strategy. Without a vision and strategy, employees cannot be expected to move beyond the ordinary to achieve the extraordinary; unempowered people can repeat conventions but they cannot create them. In more severe cases they cannot create new strategies or imagine a new future. The resulting paucity of internal talent and impoverishment of available resources leads the organization to excessive dependence on the outside world. It quickly becomes reliant on external resources such as consultants or outside managers to develop the new strategies it needs to meet changing demands. It begins to outsource management thinking. The unempowered organization loses increasing amounts of control over its destiny—in effect, the organization's autobiographical narrative is written by ghost writers.

We have addressed the increasing importance to leaders of understanding their associates—both their strengths and developmental needs. In addition, leaders must gain increasing depths of self-knowledge. This means they must understand their motivation. Unless a leader understands his need for power, for example, he may exercise power largely to overcome a sense of personnel inadequacy. His leadership will be more a compensatory attempt to achieve personal restoration than a wholehearted effort to achieve organizational excellence.

Despite all these challenges, there are reasons to be hopeful about the evolving paradigm of leadership. For example, as we move away from command-and-control leadership, the opportunity for people to misuse leadership positions for their own narcissistic ends diminishes. In the new vocabulary of empowering leadership, leaders are described as sponsors, facilitators, enablers, coaches, catalyzers, and even midwives. We can and should expect new kinds of individuals—healthier and more mature people—to emerge in positions of leadership in the future.

Once the empowerment process is under way, looking for small successes to celebrate becomes especially important. People's need for affirmation is particularly strong during times of major organizational change, such as mergers. Typically there are outstanding performers and great organizational strengths on both sides of the merger. This needs to be communicated and acknowledged quickly in order to help overcome people's fear factor, which can become the greatest demotivator of all.

The starting point for dealing with the potentially adverse effects of large-scale change is the individual—all of us want to know that we have worth and value. Once leaders confirm that worth, they start empowering people and building a new organization. Thus self-development at all levels is a precondition for organizational development. This means investing in people, even in difficult economic times. It is preferable to manage expenditures so that educational efforts can be increased and that greater education can then help management deal more effectively with the economic challenges.

—*∿*—

Empowerment is not a technique, it is a process, and as such it requires a profound and enduring commitment from the top. It is relatively easy to talk of empowerment, but what kind of power is it that is being transferred? Empowering others means being committed to giving them the coaching opportunities to acquire a range of power and expertise sufficient to succeed.

Although empowerment can be a difficult challenge for leaders, creating boundaries can be even more difficult. First, as stated previously, boundaries must be based on a thorough knowledge of people's emerging competencies. Once established, the boundaries must be both definitive and permeable. They must allow the individual to advance into new areas and the different parts of the organization to cross-pollinate, acquiring new insights and practices from each other. Like empowerment, boundary management is an ongoing task. The leader must continually monitor the progress of those empowered, making sure boundaries offer both adequate definition and sufficient latitude.

Leadership is now more than ever a matter of the heart as well as the head. It requires both knowledge and wisdom to orchestrate the human and technical assets of an organization. Leadership is a science and an art, best practiced with an attitude of humility—and of gratitude for the immense potential presented by individuals who are willing to commit themselves to the pursuit of organizational excellence.

References

Davis, S. *Future Perfect.* (2nd ed.). White Plains, N.Y.: Addison Wesley Longman, 1997.

Deutsch, H. *Confrontations with Myself: An Epilogue.* New York: Norton, 1973.

Hesselbein, F., Goldsmith, M., and Beckhard, R. (eds.). *The Leader of the Future: New Visions, Strategies, and Practices for the Next Era.* Drucker Foundation Future Series. San Francisco: Jossey-Bass, 1996.

Zaleznik, A. "Real Work." *Harvard Business Review,* 1997, *75*(6), 53–63.

CHAPTER NINE

Reinventing the Academy

Darrell G. Kirch

Darrell G. Kirch is dean of the School of Medicine at the Medical College of Georgia and dean of the School of Graduate Studies. A graduate of the University of Colorado School of Medicine, he completed his residency training in psychiatry in 1982. From 1982 to 1993, he served in various capacities at the National Institutes of Health, and in 1993, he served as acting scientific director of the National Institute of Mental Health.

━∾∾━

Although many features of modern universities date back to the schools' medieval roots, university academic health centers are relatively recent creations that are unique and exceedingly complex enterprises. At the core of an academic health center is the medical school, a graduate-level professional component of the university, dedicated to educating future physicians. The medical school often is joined in the academic health center by several other health-related professional schools, ranging from nursing to pharmacy. Like their parent universities, medical schools have developed research programs that represent major sources of biomedical innovation and in many cases generate millions of dollars in sponsored support for the campus.

What makes an academic health center unique is that in the majority of cases, the university also has developed its own health care delivery enterprise centered around one or more teaching hospitals and their associated clinics. These hospitals and clinics serve as teaching venues for faculty members in their interactions with students and resident physicians in training. Typically they are wholly owned and managed by the university. At this writing, there are 125 accredited medical schools in the United States, and roughly 100 of them are part of larger academic health centers, including some form of clinical care delivery system. When examined as an overall financial entity, the teaching hospital and its affiliated clinical programs often represent the largest single source of revenue in the budget of the academic health center and its medical school. As a corollary, the academic health center's budget may also be the largest single component of the parent university's budget.

As the health care industry expanded in the latter half of the twentieth century, so did these university-affiliated clinical enterprises. Most observers would agree that their considerable growth yielded great benefits for their associated medical schools and universities. It is clear that the expanding income of academic health centers, fueled by the unprecedented growth of fee-for-service medicine after World War II, in turn allowed them to cross-subsidize faculty academic and research endeavors. An index of this expansion is the fact that U.S. schools of medicine demonstrated ninefold growth in their budgets (in constant dollars) from 1960 to 1993, when the gross domestic product increased less than threefold. Similarly, during the same period, the number of practicing physicians who served as full-time faculty in medical schools increased elevenfold (Cohen, 1995). Not all these physicians, however, were reimbursed for the care they provided. An additional important financial feature of academic health centers is that as a function of their service mission and often of their urban location, they provide nonreimbursed health care services to relatively high proportions of indigent patients.

THE NEW ECONOMIC REALITY

Other chapters in this volume paint a vivid picture of recent turmoil in the overall organization and financing of U. S. health care delivery. As I have described, the growth of academic health centers in recent decades was supported by their expanding role as direct providers of services. As a result they have become exceptionally dependent upon clinical income. Now they find that their special status as components of the university in no way protects them from the turmoil currently dominating the larger health care marketplace. In this context their commitment to indigent care may become especially burdensome. In the current climate the ivory tower simply does not offer a refuge for the clinical enterprise of the academic health center.

Strong programs in tertiary medical care, subspecialty training, and technological innovation for many years characterized the academic health center. These strengths have become significant liabilities in a world emphasizing community-based primary care, the key role of generalists, and cost containment. In a highly competitive, cost-conscious marketplace, many academic health centers have found themselves to be poorly positioned. In addition, universities have long struggled with town-versus-gown tensions as they sought to define their place in the community. For the academic health center these tensions are reaching new heights as many physicians in private practice perceive their former teachers at the local medical school as competing providers who threaten private physicians' financial well-being.

THE ORGANIZATIONAL CHALLENGE

The sources of current tensions within academic medicine go far beyond competition with other local health care providers. Until recently the economic structure of medicine in the United States was dominated by not-for-profit hospitals, solo practitioners, and indemnity insurance products with cost-plus reimbursements. That cultural pattern now is shifting dramatically to *corporate configurations*, such as for-profit hospital chains and large physician-managed corporations, with payers shifting financial risk downstream to providers.

The traditional culture of universities and their academic health centers is far from corporate. It is highly individualistic, with a strong emphasis on the independence of each faculty member, a highly prized autonomy deriving from the principles of academic freedom. The net result is that many academic physicians hold tenure. This lifetime employment commitment, which frequently includes significant compensation guarantees, may be a potential obstacle to organizational renewal in universities. With the demise of mandatory retirement, tenure looms even larger as a possible barrier to change. Another feature of the academic culture is a system of shared governance that relies heavily upon faculty input. The resulting system is often exceedingly laborious and oriented toward vigorous debate, peer review, and due process rather than rapid, decisive action.

Another reality is that universities and their medical schools tend to be hierarchical, almost feudal, in their emphasis upon departmental structures representing specific specialties. Individual academic departments in the medical school of an academic health center are led by department chairs wielding considerable authority, and these departments often operate essentially as independent financial entities. Most academic health centers have faculty practice plans that at best function as loose confederations with common billing and collection rather than as tightly integrated, operationally efficient multispecialty group medical practices.

To further complicate this organizational culture, academic health centers are accountable to (and often under great pressure from) multiple constituencies, including legislators; regents or trustees; the leadership of multicampus university systems; alumni; donors; and internal stakeholders including faculty, students, resident physicians, and support staff. Although each group may justifiably claim only partial interest in the academic health center, it may often act more like a majority shareholder.

The challenge for academic health centers is clear. How can this traditional academic culture, made up of highly independent faculty members operating within autonomous academic departments and responding to diverse sources of external and internal influence, be reconciled with the marketplace pressure to attain high levels of corporate integration and efficiency in the clinical enterprise?

NEW LEADERS FOR ACADEMIC MEDICINE

The challenge for the academic health center is daunting. As arms of the university, medical schools and academic health centers have been led by individuals holding such titles as dean, provost, and chancellor.

Traditionally these individuals presided over scholarly activities and maintained the academic culture. The new economic reality facing faculty physicians and teaching hospitals, however, calls for decisive, action-oriented leadership akin to that of a chief executive officer. This new reality also demands cohesive strategic planning, exceptional organizational flexibility, and a willingness to take risks.

The leadership style of a contemporary chief executive officer and the flexible, systems-oriented structures emerging in the corporate world are not easily brought to the academic health center. For example, much of the current literature on leadership and organizational change emphasizes the importance of building nonhierarchical, functionally focused teams. Thus some health care organizations are creating interdisciplinary teams focused on providing longitudinal, cost-efficient, outcome-oriented management of chronic diseases such as diabetes or asthma. To achieve this level of patient care, team members must exercise a high degree of cooperation. Such teams may significantly empower professionals not traditionally given leading roles, such as nurses serving as case managers. To be cost effective, instead of emphasizing episodic delivery of subspecialty services in a tertiary care hospital, the teams often deploy the majority of their resources to primary care providers based in the community. However, the creation of such teams in an academic culture (with long-standing barriers between professional disciplines and even between medical subspecialties, with a relative shortage of primary care physicians and physician extenders, and with such barriers reinforced by independent financial structures) may be difficult indeed.

To create effective teams the new leaders of academic health centers must shift from their historical role of presiding over a loose confederation of independent faculty members and autonomous departments to the role of creating a culture that acknowledges the exquisite interdependence of diverse units. Deans and other academic leaders in the past often spent much of their time mediating disputes and resolving conflicts of interest, but their work now is to clearly identify a confluence of interests in the form of a common vision in order to bring disciplines together across traditional barriers. The task is to lead the academic health center to become corporate in the literal sense of the word, that is, to become *a single body*.

Just as those who lead medical schools and academic health centers, and the parent universities, face the same forces of change and the same challenges as leaders in the corporate world do, they have the same fundamental opportunity to reinvent their organizations. Those leaders who can embrace change and stimulate reinvention, as they assure an often reticent faculty that core academic values and competencies will be preserved, will be positioning their schools to be the models of the twenty-first century.

Reference

Cohen, J. J. "Finding the Silver Lining Without the Golden Eggs." *Academic Medicine,* 1995, *70,* 98–103.

CHAPTER TEN

Leading Academic Health Centers

Michael Johns
Thomas J. Lawley

*Michael Johns leads Emory University's widespread
academic and clinical institutions and programs in the
health sciences as executive vice president for health affairs,
director of the Robert W. Woodruff Health Sciences Center,
and chairman of the board and chief executive officer of
Emory Healthcare. He oversees the Emory University
schools of medicine, nursing, and public health; the Yerkes
Primate Research Center; the Emory Clinic (a nonprofit
group practice); more than a dozen primary care centers;
and Emory University, Crawford Long, and Emory-
Adventist Hospitals. Editor of the* Archives of Otolaryn-
gology *and a specialist in management of head and neck
tumors, Johns is an internationally recognized cancer
surgeon and researcher on outcomes of treatment.*

*Thomas J. Lawley is dean and William P. Timmie Professor
of Dermatology at the Emory University School of Medicine
(and former chair of the Department of Dermatology), vice
president of Emory Healthcare, and president of Emory*

Medical Care Foundation. His research addresses auto-immune skin diseases, the cell biology of endothelial cells, and regulation of cell adhesion molecules. He has served on many boards and committees, including an NIH study section, and currently serves on the National Advisory Allergy and Infectious Diseases Council for the National Institute of Allergy and Infectious Diseases of the National Institutes of Health.

T he decade of the 1990s has been a time of unprece-dented challenges for leaders of medical schools and academic health centers (AHCs). The threefold mission of the AHC is to pioneer new discoveries, educate and train the health professional workforce, and develop better health care. Over the course of more than five decades, AHCs became the world's leading centers of biomedical discovery and health care, spurred by this nation's unparalleled commitment to bio-medical and behavioral research and by a health insurance system that reimbursed liberally for modern, procedure-based medicine.

However, by the late 1980s a significant backlash was building against the ever increasing share of national income going to medical care. At its peak just a few years ago, health care's share of the GDP was 13.9 percent and projected to reach 16 percent or higher by the year 2000 (Levit and others, 1994). Ingrained in all these policy issues was a challenge to the dominant role of the academic health center. Some policy leaders felt the AHCs had spawned much of what needed to be reformed. Some saw the AHC as a dinosaur that would, or should, quickly die as national priorities and the health care system changed dramatically.

The role of leadership in today's academic health center must be addressed in the context of both the development of a new, increas-ingly consolidated, and highly competitive health care industry and the implicit challenge to the AHCs' traditionally dominant role. The unprecedented challenge for AHC leadership is this: to supply the

The authors wish to acknowledge the contributions of Jonathan F. Saxton to the preparation of this chapter.

vision and direction necessary to catalyze the appropriate reengineering and reinvigoration of the AHC so that its extraordinary talents, resources, and services can best be realized in the pursuit of new discoveries, improved health professions training, and better health care services and policy.

A UNIQUE LEADERSHIP CHALLENGE

What is unique about this leadership challenge is that both organizational and cultural changes are required. AHCs have functioned in relative isolation from many traditional market forces. For faculty and staff of these centers, it can be difficult to change traditional behaviors and practices, to adjust to the fact that price can count as much as or more than quality in people's choice of health care services, and to reconcile the expansive and often expensive ambitions of modern medicine with the economic forces now driving health services consolidation and cost containment. And unlike the case in many private sector organizations, it is neither possible nor desirable for significant change to be imposed from above.

The AHC is a complex organization, normally consisting of a university medical school, an owned or affiliated teaching hospital, and one or more other health professions schools (for example, nursing, public health, or dentistry). In most cases, the academic health center designation is simply a convenient shorthand designation for a collection of institutions focusing on health and biomedical science and contained within a university's purview rather than a description of a functional organizational entity. The first order of business for most AHC leaders is to organize these health services for a competitive marketplace. The budgets of virtually all AHCs, and to some extent the budgets of their parent universities, rely heavily upon faculty practice and teaching hospital revenues. Ensuring the viability and competitiveness of these revenue sources is critical in the short run. The leadership challenge here is to create consensus across the AHC. This consensus will be the foundation for the most efficient and effective service organization possible.

Embedded within this challenge, however, are issues that go to the heart of the functions of a traditional academic institution. Medical faculty often choose academic careers in order to pursue more than clinical care, which they could do in private practice, or more than straight bench research, which they could do in a corporate setting.

The academic setting allows, and in fact demands, more. Most often the faculty member has more than one major role: clinician and scientist; scientist and teacher; clinician, scientist, and mentor; teacher and administrator. These bi- and tripartite roles are inherent in the very idea of an academic institution and an expert faculty. However, clinicians who are also research scientists may not be as clinically productive as clinicians in private practice. Research scientists who are also teachers and who must regularly compete for grant support may not be as prolific as their full-salaried counterparts in private industry. Until recently such comparisons between academic and nonacademic life were seen as comparisons between apples and oranges, made mostly for the purpose of choosing career paths. With the rise of large and vigorous competitive industries in health services and key areas of biomedical research, suddenly the comparison is no longer like that between apples and oranges, but like that between different processes for making the same widgets. Now faculty practice groups and teaching hospitals must compete directly for access to patients within an aggressively price-competitive marketplace, where productivity often is paramount.

The advent of a dynamic, competitive managed care marketplace means that AHC leaders must be capable of successfully leading the change to a new form of organization. They must be able to provide not just vision and direction but also confidence, and they must manage sometimes high levels of turbulence and anxiety throughout a set of diverse and complex organizations. It will be immensely helpful to them to have leadership experience beyond the academic environment and familiarity, if not experience, with marketplace economics and dynamics. They also must have or develop personal and professional relationships with key marketplace leaders and players. And perhaps more than ever before, AHC leaders must have a deep and abiding appreciation for the overarching academic missions of academic health centers and a vision for preserving and strengthening those missions. If all we AHC leaders had to do was take care of patients, we could organize to do it as efficiently as anyone. Our real challenge is to maintain our academic and educational functions—our core leadership missions—in the face of changes wrought by the emergence of a new health care industry. In short the real challenge for AHC leadership is to reinvent the AHC for the twenty-first century.

ORGANIZATIONAL IMPERATIVES

In the current and foreseeable environment the entire AHC enterprise is at risk unless the parts and parcels of the AHC can work as a team, as an integrated practice in a patient-centered organization.

Through capitation contracting and other mechanisms, provider organizations, including academic health centers, are being forced to assume more and more of the financial risks of managing the health care of populations. The ingredients for success in this evolving arena are not yet fully defined. But at a minimum we know this much:

- Managing risk requires size—a relatively large population of covered lives over which to spread risk.

- Managing risk requires integrated and coordinated management of patient-centered health care services.

- Managing risk requires an organization that has the flexibility and responsiveness to anticipate and adapt to new market realities.

- Managing risk requires a real presence in the marketplace: brand-name equity; product and service differentiation; local, regional, or national influence; and a sophisticated business, marketing, and public relations operation.

THE KEY: CREATING CHANGE AGENTS

Achieving the organizational and cultural change required in this environment means instituting and leading a systemwide, personnel-engaging, change-engendering process. The key is to engage a critical mass of faculty and staff in planning for the future. The goal is not simply to create a viable plan but to create a process in which as many individuals as possible become participatory change agents. Absolutely critical to success is a broad and open strategic planning process that creates a shared vision built upon expert analysis of internal AHC and external market conditions and university priorities. These steps must be coupled with strong and ongoing organization-wide communication, to ensure that accurate information is always on hand to counter the inevitable flow of rumor and uncertainty that will emerge in a changing environment.

MEDICAL SCHOOL LEADERSHIP

Because of the medical school's central role in the AHC, leadership in the medical school will be critical in this environment. This leadership must focus on the important not just the urgent. Academic values must not be simply protected but also championed, especially as specific values are reevaluated in the light of evolving social and professional norms.

The medical school dean, department chairs, and senior faculty all face a phalanx of new and emerging issues and responsibilities. Not only must they offer overall vision and direction to the organization but they must continue to perform professional mentoring and to manage the day-to-day operations of faculty and staff, including the transition to new forms of faculty practice and new institutional and professional expectations. Department chairs will continue to have primary responsibility for the performance, reputation, and success of the academic and clinical programs. They are likely to feel a great deal of pressure to enhance departmental revenues and may feel they are being pushed toward lessening the importance of academic missions. Given the three missions (in research, patient care, and professional education) that the AHC must fulfill, even the most sophisticated transition planning can seem like a zero-sum game when it comes to the intellectual and physical energy available to department chairs to meet the multiple mission responsibilities.

Chairs face new challenges in managing their faculties. Faculty, whether junior or senior, clinicians or scientists, feel strongly the impact of the new competitive environment. Many are not sanguine about the changes in their academic and professional endeavors. Clinicians see managed care hurting the physician-patient relationship, and clinician scientists see the increased demands to see patients impinging on their research time. Nonclinicians see the new emphasis on protecting and increasing revenues as potentially or actually distorting departmental priorities. Deans and chairs must work closely together to ensure that chairs have the information, mandates, and resources to meet these responsibilities. Chairs then need to work equally closely with their faculty to ensure that each person can make the necessary adjustments in his or her work and professional goals in order to succeed and contribute within the overall departmental and institutional framework.

For some department chairs, managing in this new environment will be particularly difficult. Some will lack a complete set of the new skills necessary to manage all aspects of a demanding clinical enterprise. Some may have professional priorities that run to other core missions in research or education. Others may lead departments with particularly serious problems to manage in the newly competitive environment. In these cases sometimes the best solution is simply to replace the leader, but more often, with proper guidance and resources, existing leaders can succeed in creating the necessary organizational capabilities within their departments. Many chairs will need to appoint people to handle the clinical enterprise as a distinct operating unit within the department. Others may require the expert assistance of outside consultants as they reorganize the department for maximal effectiveness across all mission areas. Each situation will be different, and a dean must have the ability to help each department address its needs.

Chairs must take primary responsibility for leading departmental and professional discussion about the ways in which the imperatives of the new environment affect traditional models of academic and professional values, recognition, reward, and promotion. In an era requiring more functional specialization among faculty, the traditional triple-threat mission needs to be revisited. There must continue to be a place for the triple threat, but it can no longer serve as the only paradigm for highest academic honors and accomplishment.

Reconciling the need for more functional specialization with the AHC's triple mission must be an ongoing priority. The key to resolution at the institutional and departmental levels will require developing more-sophisticated teamwork models, including new forms of clinical practice, across specialties, functions, and departments. The alternative is a further balkanization of departments into specialized groups that do not communicate well and have different interests. New avenues will be needed to mainstream, or integrate, the more specialized person. Across the board in AHC leadership, there is significant room for innovative solutions.

Reference

Levit, K. R., and others. "National Health Spending Trends, 1960–1993." *Health Affairs*, 1994, *13*, 16–17.

CHAPTER ELEVEN

Decisions for Insurers

Patrick G. Hays

*Patrick G. Hays is president and CEO of the Blue Cross and
Blue Shield Association, a confederation of fifty-five inde-
pendent Blue companies—collectively the nation's largest
insurer. Previously, he was president and CEO of Sutter
Health, a Sacramento-based integrated delivery system.
He also held leadership positions at Kaiser Permanente,
Methodist Medical Center, and Henry Ford Hospital.
He is a Fellow of the American College of Healthcare
Executives and past chairman of the California Association
of Hospitals and Health Systems.*

The author is indebted to Tracey Noe of the Blue Cross and Blue Shield Association's Washington, D.C., office for her key assistance in developing this
chapter.

Health care leaders—indeed, all citizens—are involved in one of the great social experiments in U.S. history. The ongoing revolution in the U.S. health care system is probably the most profound social redesign this country has undertaken since it became an industrialized nation. With our votes and our dollars we Americans have demonstrated our desire for a competitive, market-based health care system instead of a federalized approach. We seek an environment in which health plans compete not just on price but on quality of outcomes. We want to preserve our country's long-standing tradition of clinical excellence as we continuously improve the process of care, fostering innovation, promoting consumer choice, and providing top-notch customer service.

This uniquely U.S. perspective has fueled profound change in the health care marketplace. Like the auto, defense, and banking industries in the 1980s—and like today's telecommunications and energy providers—today's health care system bears the brunt of massive transformation. Insurers face growing price pressure from purchasers, combined with quantum changes in technological capabilities and rising consumer expectations. (It has been observed that in most other Western societies, death is considered inevitable, but for Americans, it's optional.) Seemingly overnight, the definition of *value* has shifted focus: from high-cost, inpatient, procedure-oriented care to an increasingly patient-centered system of wellness, prevention, and improved health outcomes. The revolution is complicated, however, by the lack of a national, ethical consensus about the appropriate level of health care spending in both the public and private sectors.

Faced with a volatile marketplace, insurers carefully evaluate their market positions. Many reorganize to leverage core strengths, achieve greater economies of scale, and promote continuous quality improvement. Others reengineer their operations to improve efficiency. Still others acquire their competitors or physician practices. Each of these decisions is a local one based on how the insurer believes it can most effectively provide its existing and future customers with high-quality, affordable health care services.

This health care revolution fascinates those of us who are part of it; we are witnessing a turning point in U.S. social history. For patients, however, the revolution is confusing, often frightening. Cartoons, editorials, and news articles treat the phrase *managed care* as an epithet. It conjures up visions of faceless bureaucrats denying needed services, imposing long waits for treatment, and putting profits ahead of patients. These concerns are sometimes well founded; massive change frequently is accompanied by a period of chaos. Moreover, on the path toward effective competition, we have done a good job of managing costs, but we have not always done an equally effective job of managing quality.

The good news is that the much maligned system known as managed care is evolving into the management *of* care—a concept that focuses on maintaining health for all instead of merely restoring it for the sick. In recent years insurers have expanded their role from mere claims payers; they are building comprehensive, integrated health management systems that provide physicians and other health care professionals the data, technology, and back-office support they need to keep pace with the rapidly changing environment and the increase in scientific discoveries. Effective health plans serve as partners in care management by encouraging patients to receive important screenings and tests; developing innovative, customized programs for those with chronic illnesses; and helping physicians learn about new treatments. Health plan expertise in information analysis, financial management, and benefits administration makes it possible for physicians, hospitals, and other health professionals to manage the growing need for information and better understand the appropriateness of the care they provide.

The shift in focus from fragmented, unmonitored fee-for-service and passive indemnity insurance holds the promise of dramatic improvements in the U.S. population's health status and productivity as it approaches the new millennium. If we are to fully realize this vision, four steps are key. We must promote teamwork among *all* players in the health care system. We must provide physicians the tools they need to make effective clinical decisions. We must develop a flexible regulatory climate that preserves competition and rewards innovation. Finally—and perhaps most important—we must develop a more effective approach to educating consumers about how organized systems of care work, why they are beneficial, and where the health care field is headed. No market functions effectively if participants lack information they need to make educated choices.

If we are to achieve meaningful teamwork in a competitive health care environment, the needs and interests of physicians, hospitals, purchasers, and health plans must be aligned toward the common goal of patient wellness or preservation of quality of life. All too frequently, players in the health care system gang up on each other—a destructive approach for all, especially those we serve. Instead we need to share power and respect the resident expertise and needs within each discipline. Managed care, if implemented as its designers and visionaries intended, can align clinical and financial incentives for the first time in U.S. medical history.

With such alignment, successful health plans of the future will reward clinician partners for providing the right *kind of care,* at the right *time,* in the right *setting.* These performance-based incentives can be developed only through investment in outcomes research. Evaluation of clinical outcomes helps physicians choose among different approaches and protocols to customize their services to meet patients' individual needs. Health plans can make these decisions easier by summarizing reams of data into clinical practice guideline information; physicians then can use the scientific method in which they were educated. Conversely, alignment of clinical and financial incentives is impossible when health care professionals feel disempowered.

Health plans should also use their advanced computer systems to track specific patients' health status and treatment outcomes over time. Insurers can provide such information to physicians and assist them in educating patients about the importance of early detection, for example. Even today many health plans send letters to their female subscribers urging them to obtain annual mammograms and perform monthly breast self-examinations. Similar reminder campaigns encourage subscribers to receive Pap smears, cholesterol tests, prostate cancer screenings, and various immunizations.

Insurers are also increasingly using their information systems to launch population-based approaches to managing chronic illnesses. The large panels of patients enrolled in managed care plans are ideal databases to use in research studies that identify best practices. By analyzing clinical data from thousands of real cases, we can predict which patients with chronic conditions like asthma and diabetes will eventually develop complications and which will likely respond to various treatment approaches. Physicians can use this evidence in their future decision making.

Enhancing database management is just one step toward achieving a truly patient-focused health care system. Next we must develop a more effective division of labor among physicians themselves. The limitations of the gatekeeper approach devised in the 1990s are becoming evident, with the turf battles it fostered between generalists and specialists, or *proceduralists* and *cognitives*. A Northern California physician once told me of a different way to conceptualize care management: recognize that more and more of the illnesses Americans face are chronic rather than acute. In fact, chronic conditions now account for 80 percent of all health care expenditures, a trend that will intensify as the population ages. To care for these patients appropriately, my physician colleague suggested, the choice of clinician—generalist or specialist—to serve in a *principal* role or a *consulting* role ought to depend on the patient's condition at various points along the care needs spectrum. In today's postacute environment, rigid definitions of generalists and specialists are useless. Innovative managed care plans are already empowering pulmonologists and endocrinologists to be the principal physicians for patients with the appropriate chronic illnesses; the family doctors take the consulting role for these patients. This kind of approach is proving more clinically and cost effective. Other insurance plans are convening *care clinics,* where patients with similar diseases share experiences with their peers, family members, and doctors. These settings allow health care professionals to *integrate* acute treatment, follow-up care, health education, and psychosocial support.

Insurers can provide expertise in coordination of care processes and quality improvement techniques to help make this integration reality. For example, many health plans employ nurses specially trained as *care managers* to conduct baseline health screenings for new members. These nurses interview patients by telephone to identify immediate and potential health needs. Care managers' assessments help physicians understand health histories, determine the risk of serious complications, and distinguish relatively simple health care needs from more complex problems. By sharing results of these health surveys with primary care physicians, care managers assist in developing treatment programs uniquely suited to each patient. Here is an example. Once a person is identified as having congestive heart failure (CHF), the care manager visits the patient at home to explain the disease's symptoms, causes, and treatments. The care manager also teaches the patient the importance of tracking his or her weight in a daily log, because weight gain is an important indicator of CHF complications. The care manager then calls the patient daily or weekly to monitor eating habits and weight fluctuations. By keeping such detailed records, the care manager can often detect complications that might require a visit to the emergency department or a hospital stay if left untreated. This constant support not only improves the quality of care for patients, but also helps physicians get the information they need to adjust treatment protocols.

Insurers can also assist physicians in treating the new, complex problems facing our aging population. For example, the Blue Cross and Blue Shield Association, the nation's largest confederation of health benefits companies, recently joined forces with the American Geriatrics Society to offer primary care physicians education about the unique health care needs of older adults. Through this alliance, known as the National Blue Initiative for Quality Senior Care, the two organizations are helping health professionals learn to identify and manage geriatric health problems, promote geriatric wellness, and assist their older patients in living more comfortably and independently. By working together toward the common goal of improving elder care, physicians and health plans can develop strong partnerships to benefit people of all ages.

Such new partnerships cannot work effectively unless they occur in a flexible regulatory structure. To ensure a vibrant health care marketplace that can rapidly respond to new demographics, and even new diseases, government officials will need to develop rules and regulations that protect consumers without micromanaging health care. Recent years have seen a troubling state and federal trend of passing piecemeal laws and regulations mandating that health plans cover specific treatments for specific medical conditions—or even prescribing certain modes of medical treatment. Although these laws are well meaning, they often produce unintended consequences, freezing medical science in place and protecting the status quo. My experience suggests that managed care, properly implemented, actually fosters clinical innovation. Moreover, governmental restrictions usually cause premiums to rise, because health plans are required to absorb the costs of compliance. As the marketplace matures the government's role should be to create more effective, enlightened regulatory structures that encourage *evidence-based* treatment decisions and stimulate more consumer-friendly competition, instead of protecting myriad special interests in health care or yielding prematurely to alleged situations. Facts, evidence, and cool heads are called for.

Finally, perhaps most critically, we must educate our fellow Americans about how health care is evolving and how they can take part. I have no doubt that tomorrow's treatment and financing environment will result in better health care, but there has been no meaningful public policy debate about how the changing marketplace affects *people.* As health care leaders it is our responsibility to lead that debate.

We owe it to those we serve to guide them through the confusing maze of mergers, benefit changes, and marketing claims. We must create a forum for explaining the different models of health care delivery and the fundamental trade-offs involved in an environment of scarce resources. We must encourage our schools to emphasize the importance of rationality, critical thinking, and the scientific method, not just in classes like biology or mathematics or economics but in all disciplines. Above all we must strengthen our efforts to capture valid data comparing clinical outcomes of competing health plans and providers and to explain these comparisons in language consumers can understand.

Despite the current chaos of change the twenty-first century is poised to become a most exciting era in U.S. health care. Already we have witnessed remarkable improvements in caring for—and preventing—some of nature's greatest threats. The emergence of hormone replacement therapy offers a potent new weapon against heart disease and osteoporosis. Other new drugs offer renewed hope for patients with cardiovascular problems, Alzheimer's disease, and AIDS. By the turn of the century, scientists are expected to finish mapping the entire human genome—opening the door to new treatments for hundreds of inherited illnesses. At the same time, we are exploring some of the most challenging public policy questions this country has ever faced: How can we address the need for improved health care access, quality, and affordability in the United States without breaking the federal bank? How can we expand the ranks of the insured without forcing businesses to assume an undue portion of the burden? How can we prepare our clinical systems for the shift toward chronic illness and long-term care as our population ages?

Such questions do not exist in some parallel universe full of policy wonks. On the contrary, in health care, the most intimate of human services, these questions have a profound impact on all people. In the health care marketplace we must remember that we are not manufacturing widgets. Health care is *not* a commodity. Those who serve in this arena carry special ethical, moral, and compassionate obligations.

The rapid state of change in health care is painful, both for those inside it and for many who need it. But I believe today's evolving marketplace is setting the stage for a new era of competition in health care: competition among organized delivery systems, involving informed consumers making educated choices, with physicians fully engaged, and with health plans competing to provide superior patient outcomes and demonstrated customer value. For the first time in medical history, doctors, nurses, hospitals, and health plans have an opportunity to align clinical and financial incentives. These aligned incentives will restore public trust in our delivery system—and will benefit those who need care the most.

Over the years colleagues have heard me say, "If the future cannot be predicted, it can be invented." I believe we can reinvent our health care system so the *care* in managed care is meaningful. How many kids get immunized in Health Plan X? What are the return-to-work statistics for injured employees who choose Health Plan Y? What percentage of people with catastrophic illnesses in Health Plan Z regain normal, active lives? These are the questions customers are asking. As we face the new millennium, we are developing a health care system that can answer them.

CHAPTER TWELVE

Seeing Insurance Through the Customer's Eyes

Leonard D. Schaeffer
L. Carl Volpe

Leonard D. Schaeffer is chairman and chief executive officer of WellPoint Health Networks, one of the nation's largest publicly traded managed care companies, operating Blue Cross of California and UNICARE. Previously he served in Minnesota as president of Group Health and as adminis-trator of the Health Care Financing Administration, over-seeing federal Medicare and Medicaid programs. He serves on the boards of numerous organizations, including the Blue Cross and Blue Shield Association, the National Institute for Health Care Management, and Allergan, and is a member of the Institute of Medicine, National Academy of Sciences.

L. Carl Volpe is director of health policy and analysis at WellPoint Health Networks, overseeing development of public policies and positions. Previously he directed health legislation for the National Governors' Association. His interests include health care financing, market-based systems of care, and state and federal relationships in health care industry regulation. Representing the nation's governors, he was a consultant to President Clinton's Health Care Task Force.

—◦◦◦—

In the U.S. culture very little is more personal to us than our health. When sick, we Americans are quite demanding. We want it all—a health care system that assures coverage, provides immediate access to the most qualified health professionals and facilities, and ensures superlative quality of care. Moreover, we expect to be cured of almost every ailment and want care regardless of the cost and irrespective of our relative health status. Problems and limitations of the system are neither well understood nor tolerated. Unfortunately, as our population ages over the next two decades, health care utilization and costs will increase, and the pressures on the system will increase.

Americans' demands as health care consumers are part of a reality that, at some level, must be accommodated by insurers and health plans.[1] The late Speaker of the U.S. House of Representatives, Thomas P. O'Neill, claimed that "all politics is local" (Matthews, 1988, p. 10). That is to say, politicians are successful when they understand and address the unique needs of their constituents. The same can be said for health care insurers. The challenge for insurers in the next millennium is to recognize that all health care is local. To be successful, insurers must address the perspectives of the individual customer.

UNDERSTANDING THE CUSTOMER THROUGH PRODUCT CHOICE

Employers are the primary source of health care financing for nonelderly Americans. As a strategy to attract and retain employees, companies offer benefits that pay all or part of the employee's health care premium and frequently offer coverage for dependents as well. In 1996, it is estimated that employers provided health coverage for 72.3 percent of nonelderly employees and 49.6 percent of their nonemployed, nonelderly dependents (Fronstin, 1997).

The authors wish to acknowledge Mourn O'Haren, Steven Wojcik, and David van der Griff for their critical reviews and advice during the preparation of this chapter.

As the primary payer the employer has primary responsibility for selecting the type and extent of coverage. Until recently that choice most likely was indemnity coverage. With indemnity products the employee chooses a provider, pays the claim, and seeks reimbursement from the insurer. Aside from benefit limitations, there are few, if any, meaningful cost-control mechanisms on care. This unfettered access to health care services generated high satisfaction among employees and, for many years, correspondingly strong support on the part of employers. But as health care costs increased at an accelerated pace through the 1980s, so did employers' interest in cost-efficient alternatives to indemnity coverage, and health maintenance organizations (HMOs) emerged as a formidable, more affordable coverage alternative. In 1985, about 18.9 million Americans were enrolled in HMOs. By 1996, there were an estimated 67.5 million HMO enrollees (American Association of Health Plans, 1998).

HMOs remain appealing to employers. Through defined provider networks, HMOs have reduced the rate of growth in health care premiums. Figure 12.1., however, shows the relationship between cost and member choice on the product continuum. Indemnity products offer maximum provider choice without meaningful cost controls, and HMOs offer significant cost controls but with limited provider choice. Figure 12.2 shows the employer-employee dilemma created by the continuum. Employers want to maximize cost efficiency, but employees want maximum provider choice and control over health care services for themselves and their families. As employers moved to HMOs, employees have become less satisfied with their health plans because of the constraints placed on health benefits in the HMO model.

In response to employee dissatisfaction, employers have begun to seek out innovative *hybrid products* that provide some level of cost control as they also offer greater provider choice (Figure 12.3). A market response to changing customer demands, hybrid products take on many forms. Some are HMOs that offer some limited out-of-network coverage (for example, point of service [POS] products). Also popular are preferred provider organization (PPO) products, which allow consumers to choose between visiting a provider who is part of a designated network and visiting an out-of-network provider, if preferred. The PPO encourages enrollees to remain within the cost-effective network by establishing higher copayments or coinsurance for out-of-network care.

Less	Cost Control	More
Indemnity		HMO
More	Member Choice	Less

Figure 12.1.   Cost and Member Choice Continuum.

Employer Preference

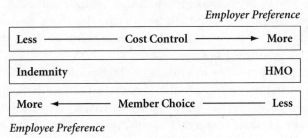

Figure 12.2.   Employer-Employee Dilemma.

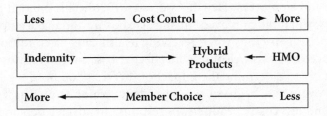

Figure 12.3.   Emergence of Hybrid Products.

The trend toward hybrid products is well documented. In 1988, 89 percent of employers with over two hundred employees offered indemnity products, 12 percent offered PPOs, and 72 percent offered HMOs. In 1997, indemnity dropped to 51 percent, PPOs increased to 58 percent, and HMOs remained the same at about 70 percent. Like PPOs, POS plans have experienced growth, with 42 percent of large employers offering them in 1997, compared to 23 percent four years earlier (KPMG Peat Marwick, 1997). Employees took advantage of these new options. Between 1992 and 1996, more than half of all employees using indemnity products moved to managed care. In firms with over five hundred employees the proportion of employees in PPO, POS, and HMO products increased from 48 percent in 1992 to 77 percent in 1996 (Foster Higgins, 1997). For health plans and insurers to survive into the future, they will have to continue to be responsive to market demands for affordable coverage that offers choice.

Research conducted at our own company shows that employers want a greater choice of cost-efficient plans for their employees. They prefer more direct access to certain providers and greater management of high-cost individuals. Employees that we have surveyed indicate that they want to share in their health care decisions, to have more flexibility in their health plans, and to have access to the best professionals when they get sick.

The development of hybrids is not static, and changes in health care financing may affect product design. Data show that employers, although continuing to offer a health benefit, are requiring employees to take a greater financial responsibility for premiums and cost sharing. Between 1990 and 1997, the percentage of employees whose health benefits were fully paid by their employers declined from 30 to 11 percent for PPO coverage offered by firms with more than one thousand employees (Hewitt Associates, 1996). This trend, if it continues, will limit employers' financial exposure and make employees more cost conscious when receiving health care—a condition that health economists welcome as an effective cost-control measure.[2] It is too early to determine the impact of this trend on product design. Employees may begin to act as prudent economic purchasers and demand less costly products. In response to adverse personal economic realities, this country is also seeing a call for greater governmental regulation of the health care industry. The full impact of this trend also has yet to be seen.

Health plan choice is influenced by the employer. Provider choice reflects the interests of the consumer. As voluntary or required participation in network-based care grows, customers are focusing their attention on the availability of providers and the quality of care they receive.

UNDERSTANDING THE CONSUMER THROUGH NETWORKS AND QUALITY OF CARE

Until recently the relationship between a consumer and his health care provider was considered sacrosanct. The family physician was a known and respected member of the community. The typical hospital was a community institution with local management. Moreover, the relationship between the provider and the family was stable, lifelong, and in many cases transgenerational. For most Americans the hospital and doctor were familiar and were always there when people needed them.

Whether this depiction is real or an exaggeration of a more limited reality, it represents people's perception that the relationship between consumers and providers offered security. That relationship is now perceived to be threatened. Now consumers must be cost conscious about their care and provider choice is limited, yet conventional wisdom still says that specialists and subspecialists are needed to treat even basic health problems. If market-based health care is to remain viable, health plans must respond to the threat in that view. The challenge is to construct networks so that market forces continue to operate yet beneficiaries can be given some sense of security about their care. Key to this balance is an understanding of quality in patient care.

UNDERSTANDING QUALITY IN CONSUMER CHOICE

Public discussions of quality are relatively new to the calculus that defines U.S. health care. The perception of choice eclipsed the importance of quality in the heyday of indemnity products. Consumers asked friends about providers and moved to another doctor when unhappy. Moreover, the doctor or hospital, when faced with a significant challenge, could enhance the perceived *quality* of care by increasing the *quantity* of care. Because indemnity products reimburse more comprehensively and operate without significant utilization controls, both the provider and consumer were satisfied.

To the benefit of all Americans, today's health plan incentive structures have precipitated a serious and public discussion of quality. With limited access to providers, who are in addition often unfamiliar to the patient, consumers have begun to question the quality of their care. Moreover, health plans market their products mostly as cost-efficient care. In response to initial criticisms of their efficiency, they have argued that within the coverage limitations of the policy, they provide all *medically necessary* care. Because that argument implies that *medically unnecessary* care is not provided, it begs some questions: What care is medically necessary? What care is not? And who decides?

More than most other issues, these questions and the ways health plans have handled the answers to them have challenged consumers' security. Unlike some other questions of health coverage, these questions are understood by the typical consumer. Although there are no easy answers, the success of health plans, in part, depends on acceptable responses.

Questions of health plan quality come from two health plan practices. First, prior authorization and utilization review protocols have been imposed that assess physician decision making in the context of the health plan contract. Second, financial incentives for individual providers and provider groups have been designed to increase the probability that only medically necessary care will be given. In each of these practices an incentive exists to limit care. Fueled by the concerns of providers, Americans are beginning to equate limited care with substandard care. Americans are worried. In a recent study, 45 percent of Americans expressed concern that the quality of health care has deteriorated under managed care (Henry J. Kaiser Family Foundation and Harvard University, 1997).

But what is quality care and how do we measure it? In health care and health care coverage, quality definition and assessment have taken three general approaches. In the first two, quality is founded on expert medical opinion. In the third, it is empirically based. Thus credentialing of providers, at a minimum, is one approach. It begins to ensure that a provider has had the training and experience thought to lead to good outcomes. Utilization review and prior authorization of treatment protocols by experts, though controversial, is another approach. The least biased approach and potentially the most durable is the identification of empirical linkages between treatment protocols and specific health outcomes. Unfortunately, many more years of basic biomedical and clinical research are needed before such standards will be reliable and predictive of quality care. The extent to which any of these three approaches will give the consumer comfort about the quality of her care remains to be seen. However, all quantify quality assessment, and quantification is an essential element in addressing consumer concerns.

Of the three approaches, consumers appear most concerned about health plans' utilization review and prior authorization methods. Some consumers believe that health plans deny necessary care, that health plan decisions interfere with the physician-patient relationship. Although health plans vehemently deny this assertion, utilization review and prior authorization techniques lend themselves conveniently to litigation, and consumers have found that a viable recourse. Ironically, the real and perceived threat of litigation can increase costs directly, through the cost of settlements and through increased utilization in the form of defensive medicine. Litigation is not the only result of this consumer concern, legislative remedies are emerging as well. Recently enacted state legislation in Texas makes health plans, like physicians, liable for the practice of medicine and therefore makes utilization review and prior authorization decisions subject to malpractice claims. As an alternative to health plan liability, some legislative proposals have called for an independent process for grievances and appeals, to give consumers a recourse outside of or prior to a judicial review of plan behavior.

Although the crisis of confidence in health plans may be fueled more by an active advocate community, disgruntled providers, and the press than directly by consumers; health plans can neither ignore nor deny the consumer concerns. With indemnity products, insurers served an administrative and risk-spreading function. Now, by virtue of the products they sell and the tools of cost control, health plans are partners in patient care. In response to consumer concerns, health plans must take action to restore consumers' sense of security. If they do not, the industry is likely to continue to see legal and legislative challenges until the public is satisfied.

What can be done? The industry must assure consumers and purchasers that consumer satisfaction and quality are important to health plans. Stronger industry self-policing is needed. Cooperative efforts between health plans and purchasers to enhance customer satisfaction and quality of care would also help. Concurrently, the industry must be clear with providers and consumers about the guidelines used to determine necessary care. Together, these steps should significantly improve the current situation, but to truly rebuild consumers' trust in the quality of their health care, a longer-range solution is needed.

That more comprehensive answer probably lies in the complex nexus between network and product offerings. The strength of hybrid products, previously mentioned, offers part of the solution, greater consumer choice. The remainder of the answer probably lies in health care network design.

Health plans will continue to compete for excellent providers whether those providers are individual physicians, medical groups, hospitals, or centers of excellence specializing in treatment of certain classes of disease. Once appropriate specialty referral mechanisms are in place, there is limited utility in careful cost management of basic primary and preventive health care needs. This care is given relatively infrequently and is typically not costly. Consumers view aggressive cost management of basic primary and preventive care as unnecessary and inconvenient. Unfortunately, existing cost management approaches do not distinguish easily between basic and specialty care. It might be better for health plans to direct aggressive cost management activities toward serious illness and disease.

When seriously ill, consumers are most concerned about who takes care of them and where that care is provided. They want to be assured of getting the very best treatment available. Seriously ill cases need medical management, and when these consumers are assured of high-quality care, they are likely to accept strong medical management. As health plans, we can meet this challenge. By employing the best available providers practicing the best medical techniques currently known and applying the most effective medical management techniques, we can achieve the best possible outcome for the seriously ill consumer as we meet the economic interests of both health plans and purchasers.

In the future, successful health plans will design products and assemble networks that assure consumers some freedom in their selection of providers for their basic care, ideally providers who are known in the community. Moreover, consumers will be assured that if they get sick, their cases will be well managed and that they will have access to and treatment by well-known and respected specialty providers. Accomplishing this goal will not be easy and may call for a rethinking of product and network design. However, achieving this goal is necessary if health plans are to begin to contribute to the sense of security that consumers need.

Health plans and insurers are faced with some of the most significant challenges in recent history. Ignoring individual and family needs in the name of shaping national health policy can no longer be tolerated. The current health care debate has evolved from a focus on broad issues of cost control to a focus on more complex issues of quality and choice and flexibility. Only those health plans that make a similar transition will survive.

Notes

1. In the remainder of this chapter the terms *insurer* and *health plan* are used interchangeably. Although a historical distinction exists between the insurer that offers indemnity coverage and a health plan that offers a managed care product, that distinction has blurred considerably in recent years. When relevant, product types will be discussed directly.
2. A by-product of this change has been a decline in employer-based dependent coverage, which could exacerbate the problem this country faces of uninsured children and adults.

References

American Association of Health Plans. "Number of People Enrolled in HMOs, 1976–96." [http://www.aahp.org/menus/index.cfm]. Jan. 1998.

Foster Higgins. *National Survey of Employer-Sponsored Health Plans: 1996.* New York: Foster Higgins, 1997.

Fronstin, P. *Sources of Health Insurance and Characteristics of the Uninsured: Analysis of March 1997 Current Population Survey.* Issue brief. Washington, D.C.: Employee Benefit Research Institute, Dec. 1997.

Henry J. Kaiser Family Foundation and Harvard University. *National Survey of Americans' View on Managed Care.* Menlo Park, Calif.: Henry J. Kaiser Family Foundation; Cambridge, Mass.: Harvard University, Nov. 5, 1997.

Hewitt Associates. *Salaried Employee Benefits Provided by Major U.S. Employers in 1990 and 1995: A Comparison Study.* Lincolnshire, Ill.: Hewitt Associates, 1996.

KPMG Peat Marwick. *Health Benefits in 1997.* New York: KPMG Peat Marwick, June 1997.

Matthews, C. *Hardball: How Politics Is Played—Told by One Who Knows the Game.* New York, Summit Books, 1988.

CHAPTER THIRTEEN

Leadership Skills and Strategies for the Integrated Community Health System

Paul K. Halverson

Paul K. Halverson, faculty member of the Department of Health Policy and Administration at the University of North Carolina School of Public Health, is currently on assignment as director of the National Public Health Performance Standards Program at the Centers for Disease Control and Prevention (CDC), Public Health Practice Program Office. He is a Fellow of the American College of Healthcare Executives, and his research interests center on performance measurement in public health and the interaction between public health and hospitals and managed care.

Health care leaders within the community, especially leaders of hospitals, are faced with an important opportunity: to design and make real a health system that enables people to work and live in an environment that protects and promotes the health of the community. Accomplishing this goal requires us to use the painter's brush of leadership, to use our experience, knowledge, and influence to organize the community to focus on improving the health status of its members.

BACKGROUND

The craze among provider organizations of developing *integrated delivery systems* was an attempt to retain patients newly aligned with managed care organizations. We in nonprofit health systems bought and sold physician practices, developed marketing efforts to declare our virtues, and emphasized the *comprehensive* nature of our systems. However, most efforts toward improving the health of the community were superficial and generally insufficient to make a significant impact. Although most of us proudly felt identification with our service area, we really wondered how much the institution of the hospital should focus on what some regarded as the social ills of the society. We saw the impact of teenage pregnancy and failure to seek sufficient prenatal care, for example. But somehow we missed the biggest opportunity—to mitigate the causes of this and other problems. It was easy to feel good about providing a needed service even when ignoring the cause of the problem. We were not being paid to deal with the causes, only the consequences.

As our financial incentives changed to fixed-fee payments, we increasingly emphasized providing services as efficiently as possible. Competition to retain and grow patient volumes often focused our attention on building an integrated delivery system that combined hospital resources with physicians who were responsible for keeping the hospitals occupied. Coterminous with the integration movement was the increased attention paid to the tax-exempt status of most hospitals and the presumed *community benefit* derived from these hospitals' contributions of service to the community in lieu of corporate income tax. This attention generally resulted in fairly complex calculations to determine the amount of free service provided and the number of activities involving the hospital that somehow might be said to provide a *community good*.

For many leaders this reflection on the community was an important reminder of the strength of the community they served. For some hospital CEOs it was a turning point, a realization that if the hospital were to continue to provide real value to the people who created the institution it must return to the primacy of its origin as a health resource for the community (Shortell and others, 1996).

Moreover, as health plans increasingly made hospital prepayments on a per-member, per-month basis, hospitals began to realize that the key to their long-term survival was keeping community members healthy. It is not until hospitals understand that being the lowest-cost, highest-technology provider is insufficient to accomplish this community health goal that they seriously consider forming an integrated community health system.

THE INTEGRATED COMMUNITY HEALTH SYSTEM

An integrated community health system is not owned by the hospital, nor does the government regulate it. An integrated community health system is made up of a multitude of health providers, community agencies, public health organizations, and community advocates that coordinate their efforts in support of improving the health of their community. The real value of a community health system lies in the collective energies and synergistic outputs that come only from organizations working together to accomplish great things (Baker and others, 1994). Public health departments can talk all day about the virtues of population-based strategies to improve health, hospitals can build and staff clinics in every neighborhood and shopping mall, and community advocacy groups can unendingly complain about specific issues and organize campaigns for change—and yet they will all individually fail if their underlying goal is to significantly improve the health of the community. Health is a complex issue, one not easily surmounted by the creation of a new program, the purchase of a facility, or the training of staff. Health is changed when health care leaders collectively harness the talents of multiple organizations and individuals to earnestly persevere in creating the conditions under which individuals can live healthy lives (Centers for Disease Control and Prevention, and Agency for Toxic Substance and Disease Registry, 1997).

Leadership of an integrated community health system has many dimensions. The leadership experience and managerial acumen of the professional health care executive is critically important in the development of the system. There are important differences, however, between managing a medical care delivery system and leading an integrated community health system. First, a community health system belongs to the community, not the hospital, the public health department, or any other organization or agency. Second, the creation of a multiorganizational alliance will take more time, energy, and perseverance than most people anticipate. It is therefore critical that the lead organizations in the system consider their participation as a high-priority, strategic, long-term investment and not as a short-term, peripheral project. Third, community health organizations are most successful when the senior management of participating organizations takes a serious personal interest. If the participating CEOs are unwilling to make the system a top priority, the likelihood of success is doubtful.

PAINTING THE PICTURE

Given the history and purposes of the integrated community health system as defined here, there are three primary characteristics leaders must consider if they are to operate successfully within that system: inclusiveness, innovation, and integrity.

Inclusiveness

Inclusiveness means that once you believe you have all the people necessary at the table to solve a problem, look again. In most cases you will discover several more who can claim a part of the problem or who should be part of the solution. Inclusiveness means that you need to have more people involved than may technically be necessary. Be aware also that in most cases in which problems are left unresolved, it is not because there is no technical solution but because the political will does not exist to implement the solution. Consider the following additional points about leading with an inclusive style:

• *Learn to lead by giving up control.* Community health systems generally do not have one single executive leader to whom everyone reports, but several organizational leaders who coach the organization through consensus building. Within the community health system, leadership means getting the right people to the table and supporting their ability to arrive at solutions. Many organizations may lend staff to support community health system projects, and the job of defining strategic and operational goals must be accomplished by partners who consider themselves equal. The role of the leader, therefore, is to bring the parties to the table, provide them with the tools, and respect the process. The work of people involved in solving community problems takes time and generally cannot be short-circuited. That does not mean, however, that work within the community health system can be done without a strategic plan, specific goals, or timelines. What it means is that the new organization must set these plans, goals, and timelines.

•   *Seek out new and different people to join the team.* If improving the health of the community were easy, it would be done by now. Reach out to include people who may bring unusual points of view or offer perspectives not represented by the original group. Realize that involvement of certain groups of people may require you to adjust the normal meeting place or time. For example, if you are trying to include nonworking single mothers, recognize that transportation, child care, and time of day can be barriers to participation.

•   *Open your ears and close your mouth.* Usually we think we have a better handle on a problem than we really do. Remember that facts about community health are only as strong as the community perception of them. For bringing about change, what the people think is important is generally more critical than what the statistics demonstrate.

•   *Gain common vision and agreement on goals.* Unlike lack of objection in the boardroom, lack of objection in community health system meetings does not necessarily equal consent. Most governmental and volunteer organizations require a very open and deliberate process to obligate the organization to a specific action or participation in a joint program.

•   *Take your estimate of the time required to accomplish the task and double it; also learn to be happy with half a loaf.* Unlike most hospitals or business organizations, many of the organizations in a community health system have very complex governance systems that frequently try the patience of even the most committed corporate leaders. Early in the life cycle of a new community health system, it is especially important to celebrate forward movement and be grateful for progress on objectives even though not all the program goals will have been met.

Innovation

The second major theme to consider in leading a community health system is innovation. The process of building community health systems lacks a familiar and well-developed pattern, and the constituent organizations may be steeped in their own traditions. However, just coming together as organizations interested in improving health is not enough to solve the tough issues that pervade sustainable improvement in community health. To succeed, the organizations in the new community health system must harness their collective ingenuity to arrive at new and innovative approaches. Consider the following suggestions on developing organizational innovation:

- *Develop an atmosphere conducive to innovation.* It is hard to be innovative in an organization where never making a mistake is the order of the day. Explicit conversations among the leadership and with staff about the value of innovation and the need to try new things are important. An atmosphere conducive to innovation generally does not arise out of one cataclysmic event but out of repeated successful and valued innovations on a small scale.
- *Create an innovations fund.* Some innovative ideas may not pass the same financial hurdles that mainstream traditional activities are expected to pass. An innovations fund with separate criteria can be established for funding pilot projects and experimental programs that offer new approaches to important problems but lack proven evidence of success.
- *Create structured ways to learn from failure.* Each new program or initiative should have an agreed reasonable trial period followed by honest evaluation. Ideas that do not meet their objectives should be modified or terminated. Gaining new insight and building team cohesion can be important benefits even from projects judged ultimately to have failed in their original design.
- *Do not bureaucratize good ideas.* Resist the temptation to overmanage the innovation process, with complex approval mechanisms, for example. Create an organizational process that encourages new ideas by staff throughout the organization.
- *Give credit where credit is due.* The old adage of accepting blame and passing out praise seems to fit here.
- *Celebrate success!* Health care organizations do not celebrate enough. For the community health alliance, just maintaining a joint work focus for a year may be enough to celebrate.

Integrity

There is no agreement that can be written that eliminates all risk. A baseline requirement for leaders working to build a community health system is integrity. The community may not understand every aspect of how and why the system is being developed, but if people believe that the leaders are honest and have their best interests at heart, they will generally be willing to support change. Conversely even the most brilliant scientific proposal will fall flat if led by an individual who is not regarded as having the highest integrity.

• *Recognize that success is based on trust.* The new community health system structures generally are built upon new organizational structures that in turn are based on the contributions of teams. People must learn to trust these new organizational systems, which are generally untried and may not be comfortable initially. Leaders must work hard to make them functional for both the teams and the individuals. Team members must be able to trust that individual success that they may sacrifice will be offset by team benefits and recognition.

• *Tell the truth.* People know that the leaders do not know everything. Tell them the truth; insist that everyone subscribe to a policy of full disclosure.

• *Walk the talk.* It is not as much about what you say as what you do. Being consistent in words and deeds will do a great deal to bolster your credibility.

• *Communicate.* When you are sure that everyone has heard you, say it again. But listen twice as much as you talk. The listening part is far more important.

• *Own up to vulnerability.* Leadership is an art, and designing health systems with the community comes with risk. Be confident about plans, but do not pretend the future is certain.

• *Follow the Golden Rule.* "Do unto others as you would have others do unto you." It works—try it.

References

Baker, E. L., and others. "Health Reform and the Health of the Public." *JAMA,* 1994, *272,* 1276–1282.

Centers for Disease Control and Agency for Toxic Substance and Disease Registry (CDC/ATSDR). Committee on Community Engagement. *Principles of Community Engagement.* Atlanta, Ga.: Centers for Disease Control, Public Health Practice Program Office, 1997.

Shortell, S. M., and others. *Remaking Health Care in America: Building Organized Delivery Systems.* San Francisco: Jossey-Bass, 1996.

CHAPTER FOURTEEN

Alliances in a Changing Industry

Arnold D. Kaluzny
Howard S. Zuckerman

Arnold D. Kaluzny is professor of health policy and administration at the School of Public Health and director of the school's Leadership Program, senior research fellow in the Cecil G. Sheps Center for Health Services Research, and a member of the Lineberger Comprehensive Cancer Center at the University of North Carolina at Chapel Hill. A consultant to private and public research organizations, he recently served as chairman of the board of scientific counselors for the National Cancer Institute's Division of Prevention and Control. He published extensively on the areas of organizational innovation and change and the role of alliances in health services.

Howard S. Zuckerman is professor of the Department of Health Services at the School of Public Health and Community Medicine, University of Washington. He is also director of the Center for Health Management Research, serves on the board of stewardship trustees of

*Catholic Health Initiatives, and is a member of the govern-
ing council of the American Hospital Association's Section
on Health Care Systems. He consults to a number of
health care systems and alliances, is a frequent lecturer
to health care groups, and is the author of* Multi-
Institutional Hospital Systems *(1979).*

———————

P erhaps the most dramatic change in health services is
the configuration of organizations and the development of alliances
to achieve strategic purposes that cannot be achieved by any single
organization (Zuckerman, Kaluzny, and Ricketts, 1995). Such alliances
are designed as cooperative, interorganizational mechanisms for adaptation to a changing environment—built on the basis of commitment
not control and emphasizing interdependency and sharing of knowledge, capabilities, resources, and risks. In this chapter we examine the
roles of alliances in a changing health care system, identify the opportunities for different alliance functions, and outline challenges and
managerial guidelines for health care leaders working in a changing
industry.

Consider just a few of the different alliance arrangements health care
organizations have made in recent years and their varied functions.

•   *1997.* The creation of the Coalition of Not-for-Profit Health
Care, composed of hospitals, health systems, health maintenance organizations, and other not-for-profit provider organizations. The coalition is designed to ensure the survival of nonprofit, tax-exempt
providers in the nation's health care delivery system. It monitors and
seeks to influence with legislative advocacy, research, and public education federal legislation and regulatory policies affecting the interests of nonprofit providers.

•   *1995.* The merger of three large hospital and hospital system
alliances—American Healthcare Systems, Premier Health Alliance,
and SunHealth—to form Premier, Inc. This new alliance of not-for-
profit health care organizations includes some 1,700 hospitals, fully
one-third of the community hospitals in this country, and represents
over $8 billion in annual purchases. It exemplifies collaboration to

achieve economies of scale, enhanced access to needed resources, and greater collective power.

•   *1994.* The creation of Community Care Networks as a collaborative effort of the American Hospital Association (AHA), Hospital Research and Educational Trust, Catholic Health Association, and Voluntary Hospitals of America, with support from the W. K. Kellogg Foundation, the Robert Wood Johnson Foundation, and the Duke Endowment, in conjunction with the American College of Healthcare Executives and the Coalition for Healthier Cities and Communities. These networks were designed to test the AHA vision for locally reformed health care delivery and financing involving a community focus, management within fixed resources, and a seamless continuum of care and community accountability.

•   *1991.* The creation of the Center for Health Management Research, designated by the National Science Foundation as an Industry/University Cooperative Research Center. Bringing together fourteen integrated health care systems and fifteen universities, the center undertakes research projects and commissions papers of importance to the practice community and also of interest to the academic community.

FUNCTIONS AND OPPORTUNITIES

The initial focus of many early alliance arrangements was to enhance purchasing power, but in the future they will place less emphasis on delivering the absolute lowest price. Instead they will be strategic, emphasizing long-term relationships with key stakeholders (for example, suppliers) to provide value to both parties and to develop services and activities designed to help service delivery organizations become more efficient, cost effective, and competitive. These emerging alliances will seek to secure a broader array of benefits, including enhanced capability to learn and adapt new competencies; to share development costs of new products, services, and technology; to manage uncertainty and solve complex problems; and to respond rapidly to market demands and technological opportunities. Consider some of the opportunities that collaboration affords service providers.

• Service-directed activities: the provision of integrated care to populations in local communities through a full range of service providers, such as long-term care and public health agencies and physicians. Although each provider group presents unique challenges, it is perhaps the latter that is most difficult and demanding yet central to any collaboration (Zuckerman and others, 1998).

• Supportive activities: the infrastructure to support low-risk and high-value collaborative activities. For example, a collaboration can support the development of clinical and financial indicators, benchmarking, physician support services, and human resource management services such as interchangeable benefit packages.

• Research: the evaluation of evolving collaborative service and support activities. Some collaborative activities will succeed and others will fail, but regardless of the outcome, all will be learning opportunities. If leaders are to make effective decisions, they must understand the relevance of the activity and its relative efficiency, effectiveness, and sustainability. Although organizations are likely to have greater in-house evaluation capability in the future, the resolution of evaluation questions will require collaboration with research organizations.

CHALLENGES

The development of an alliance requires a new way of thinking about the management and leadership processes. Rosabeth Moss Kanter's analysis of industrial organizations (1989) applies equally well to the challenges facing health service organizations: "In the future, if an increasing amount of economic activity continues to occur across, rather than within the boundaries defined by the formal ownership of one firm, managers will have to understand how to work with partners rather than subordinates. And that alone promises a revolutionary change in the way America does business" (p. 192).

What are the challenges and opportunities that managers and leaders face as they attempt to transcend their respective organizations and collaborate with others to provide efficient quality care to populations within the communities they serve?

• *Culture.* Each organization participating in any alliance activity presents a different culture, that is, a pattern of fundamental assumptions developed by the organization for dealing with problems of internal and external adaptation (Schein, 1985, 1996). For example,

in health care the general transition from a predominantly professional culture with emphasis on technical quality and physician autonomy to a predominantly business culture with emphasis on cost
containment and accountability means that different organizations
may be at different points in their efforts to accommodate these two
perspectives (McLaughlin and Kaluzny, 1990). Therefore the ability to
accommodate both perspectives is critical to collaborative success.

• *Trust*. Trust is the underlying glue of any collaborative activity.
It involves mutual respect and confidence and requires open and frequent communication, congruent goals and objectives, and joint problem solving. One manager embarking on a collaborative arrangement
stated that "if you don't have trust, you must build it," and it is important to recognize that trust is gained and retained the old-fashioned
way—by earning it (Zuckerman and others, 1998, p. 17). Building
trust within an organization is particularly challenging because
encounters occur across operational levels, and thus trust must be
demonstrated at all levels. Particularly critical is the cooperation of
middle managers, who often perceive any collaborative activity as a
threat to their positions.

• *Commitment*. To achieve the commitment that sustains an
alliance over time, leaders and managers must rethink management
fundamentals. Specifically, the command-and-control orientation,
with emphasis on power and individual accountability, needs to be
replaced with a participative orientation, with emphasis on developing commitment, learning, and teamwork. As Ohmae (1989) has
observed: "good partnerships, like good marriages, don't work on the
basis of ownership or control. It takes effort and commitment and
enthusiasm from both sides if either is to realize the hope for benefits.
You cannot own a successful partner any more than you can own a
husband or a wife" (p. 148).

MANAGEMENT GUIDELINES

The management of an alliance of any sort is a very complex business.
Walter McNerney (1985) described the situation well some years ago:
"There is more to management than crisp efficiency. In the health
field, perhaps more than any other, management involves moral issues
and ethical choices. It involves a deep commitment and personal
courage. It involves a resolve to be just and right, not only a resolve to
win" (p. 339).

Kanter (1989, 1994), observing alliances in many industries, suggests that these crucial factors characterize successful partnerships:

The partnership must be perceived as strategically *important* by all parties.

The partnership must be viewed as a serious *investment,* requiring time and resources.

The partnership must be based on an acknowledgment and acceptance of mutual *interdependence.*

Each partner must display *individual excellence* and bring added value.

There must be effective *integration* of purpose and activity.

Exchange of *information* must be open and frequent.

The partnership must be *institutionalized* or formalized.

Relationships must be based on *integrity* and trust.

Health care organization experience so far suggests some practical approaches and guidelines to developing and managing an alliance.

• *Select the right partners.* Not all organizations are equal candidates for collaboration. For an alliance to succeed, organizations must seek partners with complementary service functions and cultures. For example, a hospital-dominated system might do better collaborating with a system or organization containing primary care physicians and long-term care facilities than it would collaborating with a system or organization based as it is on hospital service activities.

• *Think in terms of sequential implementation, or small wins.* The development of an alliance is a process, and although many activities are possible, leaders and managers should initially seek collaborative activities that have a reasonable chance to succeed. Based on the *theory of small wins* (Weick, 1984), this strategy offers the chance of a visible and therefore encouraging success within the larger ongoing process. It also gives the alliance organizations practice in the required interpersonal relationships, builds trust, and establishes a basis for more complex collaborative activities (Kaluzny, Warnecke, and Associates, 1996).

• *Align incentives.* Any alliance involves risk, and it is critical that this risk be shared among the participants because risk is an important incentive for organizations to change behavior. However, it is not the only incentive. Others that need to be taken into consideration are gaining the capacities to do the right thing (Cohen and Bradford, 1990) and to share a common vision, gain expertise and resources from partner organization, and achieve a degree of security. As Ohmae (1989) puts it, health care organizations "are beginning to learn what nations have always known—in a complex uncertain world, filled with dangerous opponents, it is best not to go it alone" (p. 143).

• *Establish procedures.* The development of a collaborative relationship will undoubtedly involve conflict and negotiation. Thus, at the onset, participants should agree on the domain in which the alliance will operate and on the operational procedures that will be used to resolve conflict in a systematic and nondestructive manner.

• *Look for and encourage boundary spanners and idea champions.* Alliances do not emerge from the ocean fully clothed. They emerge because an individual or small group of individuals with vision is committed to the success of the activity. These individuals have the respect of all parties and are able to move back and forth among them, clarifying issues, facilitating communication, managing conflict, articulating the vision, and unrelentingly building consensus and energizing the process (McKinney, Warnecke, and Kaluzny, 1992).

• *Set realistic time frames.* Alliances are not necessarily short-term arrangements but rather may be seen as a journey for the participants. Not to be underestimated is the substantial time investment required of the participants.

• *Establish performance expectations.* Alliance members should have mutually agreed-upon performance expectations, which can ultimately also be the basis for judging alliance efficacy. Such expectations should be coupled with explicit performance measures and realistic time frames. A significant problem for many alliances is the temptation to judge success by short-term financial results rather than by long-term strategic objectives. It is essential that partners learn from and be strengthened by the alliance and gain a clear sense of added value from participation. As Jordan Lewis (1990) observed, "If the partners do not benefit, there is no reason to collaborate." ·

Alliances offer health care organizations the opportunity to significantly improve their ability to provide quality care in their communities. Alliances can be developed to conduct both direct service and support activities, including research and evaluation. The leadership challenge is to recognize that each partnership is really an innovation within the context of care and carries with it a range of profound social and economic consequences for not only the organizations in the alliance but also the larger community served by the alliance. The study of innovations has clearly shown that any innovation needs careful monitoring and requires a great deal of effort to be fully and effectively implemented and institutionalized. The simple presence of an innovative activity will not necessary result in its acceptance by all the various service delivery program members and participants. Health care organizations are full of the debris of good ideas; clearly one role of leaders and managers is to ensure idea implementation and institutionalization, thereby also ensuring that intended effects are achieved.

Achieving the intended effects will require organizational learning by all parties at all levels. In the terminology of the day, successful alliances must become *learning organizations* (Senge, 1990). Historically, to the extent that organizational learning occurred it occurred through benchmarking, that is, comparing organizations with each other. Though benchmarking will undoubtedly continue, it a defining characteristic of alliances that they require learning from within. Leadership must set the tone, provide the perspective, and define the challenges required for alliance members to learn from each other and for the alliance as a whole to learn from itself and from the experiences it encounters within a changing industry.

Finally, it is important to recognize the limitations and potential negative consequences of health care alliance arrangements. For example, despite substantial benefits, alliances remain complex and often ambiguous arrangements, sometimes requiring organizations to simultaneously cooperate and compete. Once we acknowledge that not all innovations are good, it becomes the role of leadership to assess both positive and negative consequences of alliance arrangements. As described by Bennis and Nanus (1985), the difference between management and leadership is that "management is doing things right while leadership is doing the right thing." During the changes ahead, as various alliances are developed to pull together an increasingly complex industry, the challenge will require both management and leadership and thus the opportunity to not only do the right thing, but through an understanding of alliances' various functions and challenges, the opportunity to do things right.

References

Bennis, W., and Nanus, B. *Leaders: The Strategies for Taking Charge.* New York: HarperCollins, 1985.

Cohen, A. R., and Bradford, D. R. *Influence Without Authority.* New York: Wiley, 1990.

Kaluzny, A. D., Warnecke, R. B., and Associates. *Managing a Health Care Alliance: Improving Community Cancer Care.* San Francisco: Jossey-Bass, 1996.

Kanter, R. M. "Becoming PALS: Pooling, Allying and Linking Across Companies." *Academy of Management Executive,* 1989, *3*(3), 183–193.

Kanter, R. M. "Collaborative Advantage: The Art of Alliances." *Harvard Business Review,* July–Aug. 1994, pp. 96–108.

Lewis, J. *Partnerships for Profit: Structuring and Managing Strategic Alliances.* New York: Free Press, 1990.

McKinney, M., Warnecke R., and Kaluzny, A. "Strategic Approaches to Cancer Control Research in NCI-Funded Research Bases." *Cancer Detection and Prevention,* 1992, *16*(5–6), 329–335.

McLaughlin, C. P., and Kaluzny, A. D. "Total Quality Management in Health: Making It Work." *Health Care Management Review,* 1990, *15*(3), 7–14.

McNerney, W. J. "Managing Ethical Dilemmas." *Journal of Health Administration Education,* Summer 1985, *3,* 331–340.

Ohmae, K. "The Global Logic of Strategic Alliances." *Harvard Business Review,* Mar.–Apr. 1989, pp. 143–154.

Schein, E. H. *Organizational Culture and Leadership.* San Francisco: Jossey-Bass, 1985.

Schein, E. H. "Culture: The Missing Concept in Organizational Studies." *Administrative Science Quarterly,* 1996, *41*(2), 229–240.

Senge, P. *The Fifth Discipline: The Art and Practice of the Learning Organization.* New York: Doubleday, Currency, 1990.

Weick, K. F. "Small Wins: Redefining the Scale of Social Problems." *American Psychologist,* 1984, *39,* 40–49.

Zuckerman, H., Kaluzny, A., and Ricketts, T., "Alliances in Health Care: What We Know, What We Think We Know and What We Should Know." *Health Care Management Review,* 1995, *20*(1), 54–64.

Zuckerman, H., and others. "Physicians and Organizations: Strange Bedfellows or a Marriage Made in Heaven?" *Frontiers of Health Services Management,* 1998, *14*(3), 3–34.

PART THREE

Serving Special Populations

CHAPTER FIFTEEN

Challenges for Women's Health

Gloria Feldt

*Gloria Feldt is president of Planned Parenthood Federation
of America (PPFA), the nation's oldest and largest reproductive health care organization, and president of the
Planned Parenthood Action Fund, PPFA's political arm.
Previously she served as executive director of two regional
Planned Parenthood organizations. She has received many
awards for her work and has published articles on abortion
rights, sex education, clinic violence, and reproductive
health in major newspapers and national magazines,
appeared on network news and talk shows, and testified
before Congress on women's reproductive health issues.*

*No woman can call herself free who does not own and
control her own body.*

*Margaret Sanger, Planned Parenthood founder
(1920, p. 94)*

M argaret Sanger launched the American birth control movement in 1916 with an extraordinary vision: to give women the opportunity to shape the course and quality of their lives by choosing when and if they would become parents. That vision once sent shock waves reverberating throughout this country. Nearly a century later it has become one of our most cherished and supported ideals.

Women's leadership has fueled this enormous transformation in Americans' understanding of the link between access to family planning and the ability of individuals to achieve their fullest potential in life. Now women's leadership is needed to increase awareness that *reproductive health* is absolutely fundamental to *women's health* and that *reproductive health care* is an essential component of *primary health care.*

For too long, women have been either disregarded or viewed as a special population by mainstream medicine, even though they comprise more than half the population, they are the nation's largest consumers of health care, and they spend 68 percent more in out-of-pocket expenses for their health care than men, primarily for reproductive health care (Women's Research and Education Institute, 1994). Nevertheless, women have traditionally been excluded from clinical research trials. Women's health issues, including breast, ovarian, and cervical cancers, have been woefully underfunded. Women's reproductive health is often discussed as a political or moral, rather than a medical, issue.

Compartmentalizing or neglecting women's health poses significant health risks to women—and by extension to millions of children and families who rely on women as primary caregivers. Comprehensive approaches to health care are needed to enhance women's health and ultimately the health of all Americans.

Planned Parenthood Federation of America (PPFA) has used a comprehensive approach for more than eighty years. The world's largest and oldest voluntary family planning organization, PPFA has 133 affiliates that operate nearly nine hundred reproductive health centers located in forty-seven states and the District of Columbia, part of a network of seven thousand family planning clinics in the United States. An estimated 6.6 million women—and men—rely on these facilities for a wide range of reproductive health care services, primarily birth control, gynecological services, breast and cervical cancer screenings, prenatal care, abortions, testing for sexually transmitted infections (STIs), sex education, and counseling. Growing numbers of these clients use reproductive health centers as their sole source of health care, despite the array of choices managed care has allowed them.

Why do family planning clinics inspire such fierce loyalty? The answer is simple: their top priority is people, not profits. As mission-driven institutions, they recognize that the *way* in which health care is provided is as important as the actual care provided. Family planning clinics not only offer a wide range of high-quality services, they offer these services in a way that conveys that they see clients as diverse and valued individuals who have families; a place in the community; and their own traditions, beliefs, and value systems. These clinics give information to women and explicitly encourage women's participation in reproductive health care decision making. By empowering women to take charge of their reproductive lives, the clinics help them control other areas of their lives.

Our practice at PPFA is guided by the belief that women's health is determined by the social, political, and economic context in which women live, not just by their unique biology. This is a distinct departure from mainstream medicine, which continues to focus on treating the physical symptoms of acute illness or disease with little attention to the socioeconomic, political, or environmental factors that contribute to those symptoms. We know that the best medical treatments in the world mean nothing to a poor single mother who cannot afford to pay for them. We know that a birth control prescription is useless to a woman whose religion prohibits contraception. We know that bandages and painkillers will not assuage the fear of a battered woman.

This comprehensive, contextual, and patient-centered approach not only makes sense but costs less and produces better health outcomes, including a dramatic improvement in maternal and child health in this country. In fact, the vision of managed care as a system that provides coordinated care and emphasizes prevention, self-care, education, and knowledge *is the reality reproductive health centers have been practicing since their inception.*

That is why the search for new cost-effective health care models must include the lessons learned from reproductive health centers and the women who have served as the guiding force behind their successful development. The same prescience and vision women used to launch a domestic and international family planning movement—probably the single most important factor in improving maternal and child health during this century—can now be used to identify and address the women's health care challenges of the future.

CHALLENGE ONE: UNDERSTAND THE RELATIONSHIP BETWEEN POLITICS AND WOMEN'S HEALTH

Women's health cannot be separated from the political context in which it is defined and addressed. Despite the existence of a legal right to make childbearing choices, women continue to confront formidable barriers in exercising that right. The more autonomy women gain over their reproductive lives, the more threatening they become to those determined to turn back the clock on women's progress. Legislative and legal attempts to roll back access to choice have been increasing both in number and intensity. Clinics that offer abortions and, increasingly, those that offer only family planning services have been the targets of violence in recent years. These actions are having the most devastating effects on those least able to fight back—the young, the poor, the geographically isolated, and those uneducated about family planning.

If health care leaders are serious about improving women's health, they must become more united and more public in their support of reproductive freedom. First, health care organizations must recognize the importance of family planning, sex education, and reproductive choice in their mission statements, policies, and procedures. Second, they must understand that any attempt to chip away at women's access to reproductive health care threatens women's overall health and well-being and also the health and well-being of children and families. Third, they must speak out against efforts to promote *abstinence-only* sex education, to force minors seeking birth control to acquire parental consent, and to thwart access to contraception and safe legal abortion.

At the practice level, health care providers must provide reproductive health care services in a way that acknowledges that for women the personal *is* political. It is not enough to write a prescription for contraception or to test for STIs. Providers must back these services up with information, education, and support that will help empower women to become actors in their own lives.

CHALLENGE TWO: BREAK THE CENSORSHIP BARRIERS

Censorship comes from both internal and external forces. Today we all are bombarded with sex and sexual images in our culture—on television, in movies, and in advertising. Rarely, however, are public portrayals of sex accompanied by parallel messages about responsibility or the consequences of irresponsible sexual behavior. Sex is easier to find on television than the weather report, yet most television stations refuse to air contraceptive advertisements. Legislators would rather champion abstinence-only programs than provide adequate funding for responsible, age-appropriate sex education. Some health care providers are reluctant to openly discuss sexual health issues with their patients.

Young people, especially, suffer the most dramatic consequences of these mixed messages. As they learn from popular culture that it is glamorous to have sex, young people are also learning that it is not OK to talk about or plan for sex. It is no surprise, therefore, that the same country that censors open and honest discussions about sex—discussions essential to helping young people grow into healthy adults capable of making responsible decisions—has teen pregnancies and STIs that are among the highest rates in the developed world. These are enormous public health problems that ultimately we *all* pay for in the long term.

Those who are concerned about reproductive health care need to take a leadership role in promoting more open and honest discussions about sexual issues. We must stop censoring ourselves from fear of controversy. We must remind the American public that censoring information that can help *prevent* unintended pregnancies, HIV/AIDS, and STIs is irresponsible and dangerous. And we must support the development of realistic and responsible educational tools, information, and programs about sexuality and sexual behavior, programs that resonate with diverse constituencies, their experiences, and the way they see the world.

At the community level, health care providers must ally themselves with educators to guarantee that balanced and age-appropriate sex education—which American voters preponderantly support—is part of every school's curriculum. This school-based sex education, which has been proven to increase the likelihood of teens using birth control and acting responsibly about sex, must complement parents' efforts to serve as the primary sex educators for their children. To that end we must train parents and teachers so they are better able to talk openly about sex and sexual decision making with children and teens.

At the practice level, providers need to offer guidance and ask questions about their clients' sexual practices, risk factors, behavior, and beliefs at every appropriate opportunity. Practitioners must be comfortable in discussing these issues openly, using correct terminology, and communicating in ways that are jargon free and nonjudgmental. Clients of all ages should be encouraged to ask questions and be given honest answers. Clients' diversity, whether of race, religion, geographical location, sexual orientation, or age, must also be respected and acknowledged as an important factor in the process of providing more responsive and effective reproductive health care.

CHALLENGE THREE: PROVIDE, PROTECT, AND EXPAND CHOICES FOR BOTH WOMEN AND MEN

Even though women and men currently have more reproductive health options than ever before, these options are still not yet a reality for many people, especially the poor and powerless. We need to work harder to ensure greater access to all *available* reproductive health options and also to create and promote *new and expanded* options that will improve the health and well-being of women, men, and their families.

First, the health care community must demonstrate its unified support for the family planning program provided by Title X of the Public Health Service Act. Signed into law by President Richard Nixon in 1970, it provides low-cost birth control and reproductive health services to millions of low-income women. Each year, Title X funding helps women avoid 1.3 million pregnancies and more than 600,000 abortions. Every Title X dollar spent to provide family planning services saves an estimated three dollars that would otherwise be spent in Medicaid costs for pregnancy-related care. Nevertheless Title X continues to be a favorite target of anti-choice forces, who relentlessly advocate to eliminate it.

Second, we must promote emergency contraception as a viable and effective contraceptive option. Often erroneously referred to as the morning after pill, emergency contraception uses ordinary oral contraceptives or an intrauterine device to prevent pregnancy soon after unprotected intercourse. This regimen has been found to be 75 percent effective in preventing pregnancy; its widespread use could prevent up to 2.3 million unintended pregnancies and 1 million abortions each year (Stewart, 1996). Few women, however, know enough about emergency contraception to request it, and many practitioners, unfamiliar with prescribing the regimen themselves, do not discuss this option with their patients.

Third, we need to advocate for increased funding for reproductive health-related research and clinical trials, including those for new methods of contraception. Research funding for women's health is generally inadequate, but funding for reproductive health is even more abysmal. According to Planned Parenthood, a recent study revealed that less than 1 percent of the federal health budget is devoted to contraceptive research and evaluation.

Fourth, we must educate health care providers about early medical and early surgical abortion procedures and encourage greater use of them. These procedures can be performed quickly and in the confines of the provider's office, giving women more privacy and control over their decision. These procedures can also be administered during the first days of a suspected pregnancy, making them a safer and less stressful experience for women.

Fifth, we must agree on a standard, comprehensive definition of *quality reproductive health care* that includes contraceptive services, supplies, and outpatient care; abortion services and voluntary sterilization services; infertility services; screenings for STIs, HIV, and breast and cervical cancers; sexuality education and counseling; preconception risk assessment and care; and all stages of maternity care—prenatal, delivery, and postnatal. We must then advocate for expanded insurance coverage that recognizes and includes these services as essential to quality reproductive health care.

CHALLENGE FOUR: HELP WOMEN AND MEN USE CHOICES WISELY

Choices, applied wisely, lead to knowledge and fulfillment. That is why it is critical that health care providers better enable their clients to decide *which* choice is best for them and their circumstances. Many family practice physicians, the primary caregivers often called upon to address a range of reproductive health care needs, are still not receiving adequate training in the prevention or management of unintended pregnancies. Today, only 12 percent of all OB-GYN residency programs require abortion training, and 84 percent of U.S. counties have no abortion services at all ("Training Family Practice Residents . . .," 1997). As a result, as older abortion providers retire, the pool of younger physicians willing to replace them becomes increasingly smaller.

This information and training gap extends to patient education services. A recent national survey of women of reproductive age found that nearly half of them assumed that they are screened for STIs when they visit their OB-GYN for annual checkups. In reality, however, STI testing is optional, and women must request it. One-third of women at risk for an unplanned pregnancy said that neither they nor their doctors mentioned birth control during their most recent visit.

To ensure women's access to a full range of health care services and options, better training programs and curricula emphasizing all facets of reproductive health care need to be instituted in medical and professional schools. Health care providers already practicing must also have opportunities to update their skills through specialized workshops and other educational programs. All health care providers should be required to learn counseling and communication techniques that will improve their ability to convey information and options in a way that is *heard* and *understood* by clients. It is also important that providers listen to women and use what *women* say they need to make more informed reproductive health decisions as the basis for designing more responsive programs and services.

Health care providers must also be aware of and sensitive to the special needs of underserved constituencies such as immigrant populations, low-income people, the uninsured, the homeless, battered women, and others who may need services above and beyond reproductive health care. To meet these complex needs, health care providers can develop stronger links and partnerships among a wide range of community-based agencies to provide a more coordinated and responsive system of care for underserved constituencies.

CHALLENGE FIVE: RECOGNIZE THAT WOMEN ARE MORE THAN A SPECIAL POPULATION

If we are to improve women's health and the health of their families, we must abandon the distinction of women as a special population, a practice that contributes to their segregation and diminishment. Ultimately this will require a major attitude shift in the way we as a nation think about, treat, and value women.

The health care community can facilitate this attitude shift by acknowledging that women's leadership can improve the way we provide health care in this country. A first step would be appointing more women to positions of authority. Today, although women constitute more than 40 percent of all medical school students, less than 5 percent of academic chairs and only a quarter of all medical school faculty are women (American Academy of Medical Colleges, 1996).

Health care practitioners can bolster women's empowerment by encouraging their full participation in decisions about their reproductive health. Practitioners should work *with* women, view them as experts on their needs, and value their strengths and experiences as resources that can help meet these needs.

Another important way the health care community can contribute to women's equality is to include men and boys in discussions about reproductive health. Male responsibility must be encouraged in preventing pregnancy and STIs and in developing cultural messages that promote sex as more than "scoring" and as a responsible and mutually loving and caring act.

Health care providers must also speak out against rape, domestic violence, and sexual harassment and frame them as public health problems that have devastating effects on women's health and their lives. We can help prevent these problems by easing societal pressures on girls to please everyone but themselves and also the pressures from and on boys to be sexually active too soon. Providing girls with the information they need to make their own decisions, live their own lives, and determine the course of their futures will contribute to the development of the next generation of women leaders.

—◆◆◆—

Working together, reproductive health care providers and the rest of the health care community can meet these leadership challenges *and* use them as opportunities for building a world in which *all* women and men are acknowledged as moral decision makers; in which *all* women and men have access to the reproductive health care they need to make healthy, responsible choices; and in which all children are welcomed joyfully by parents prepared to care for them. This is the vision that women's leadership has created. Transforming that vision into reality is our challenge and our mission.

References

American Academy of Medical Colleges. "Increasing Women's Leadership in Academic Medicine." *Academic Medicine,* 1996, *71*(7), 799–811.

Sanger, M. *Women and the New Race.* New York: Brentano's, 1920.

Stewart, F. "The Effectiveness of the Yuzpe Regimen of Emergency Contraception." *Family Planning Perspectives,* 1996, *28*, 58–64, 87.

"Training Family Practice Residents in Abortion and Other Reproductive Health Care: A Nationwide Survey." Family Planning Perspectives, 1997, *29*(5).

Women's Research and Education Institute. *Women's Health Care Costs and Experiences.* Washington, D.C.: Women's Research and Education Institute, 1994.

CHAPTER SIXTEEN

Fulfilling a Women's Health Agenda

Wanda K. Jones

Wanda K. Jones is deputy assistant secretary for health (women's health) of the U.S. Department of Health and Human Services. Previously she was associate director for women's health at the Centers for Disease Control and Prevention (CDC) in Atlanta. She is recognized for her leadership on women's health issues in the federal and state public health communities. She prepared this chapter as part of her official duties at the CDC.

In the past decade the rising costs of health care have forced society to reevaluate how health care is delivered in this country, with a focus on managed care as a way of controlling costs. Interest in women's health as a social, medical, and public health issue has accompanied the changes in health care delivery. Publication of *Our Bodies, Our Selves* by the Boston Women's Health Book Collective in

1973 was the first concrete step in a movement that has invited us to look at women's health as more than just women's reproductive organs. In the mid-1980s, a task force of the U.S. Department of Health and Human Services reported that women and minorities were underrepresented in health research, prompting legislative action. And by 1994, all agencies of the U.S. Public Health Service had established offices or designated a lead official for women's health. These events and countless others have led to a broad research agenda that is beginning to yield insights into the similarities and differences between men and women: they learn in different ways, possess different biologies, may react to illness and drug therapy differently, and largely maintain different societal roles and responsibilities.

CURRENT ISSUES IN WOMEN'S HEALTH

Women often still live their lives in the context of others—their parents, siblings, spouses, or children. Unfortunately the U.S. health care system too often fails to recognize this. When a woman misses her health care appointment, she may be labeled noncompliant, hard to reach, even irresponsible. In fact she may have missed her appointment because her child care arrangements fell through, she lacked bus fare, or her car just wouldn't make the forty-mile journey that day. Conventional approaches to the delivery of health care rarely are able to accommodate these difficulties. Some enlightened clinics provide on-site drop-in child care for parents with appointments, Medicaid covers some transportation costs, and community volunteers (mobilized through faith communities or grassroots or service organizations) transport or accompany clients to their appointments.

Properly addressing women's health issues requires a contextual evaluation of individual women, their medical problems, and their health risks. National, state, and local data on major causes of illness and death among women can be useful in targeting efforts to particular demographic groups of women, but they are no substitute for understanding the health risks of an individual woman. For example, national data suggest that heart disease in postmenopausal women; sexually transmitted diseases in young, sexually active women; and pneumonia and influenza in the elderly are areas for appropriate intervention. However, national data may not provide a *complete* picture of the health status of some population groups and subgroups. Two examples are the near-poor who are uninsured (who do not use health services until an emergency arises) and immigrants who speak English poorly or not at all (who do not use health services because they do not understand what is being done and why). Data sets derived from health care visits likely would overrepresent severe illness or injury among these population groups. Further, in an assessment of an individual woman's risks, too great a focus on the national data picture could result in overlooking serious health problems for that woman. Younger women can develop heart disease even if it is quite rare, sexually transmitted diseases can be acquired by any sexually active woman at any age, and pneumonia and influenza can be very serious for any woman with a chronic medical condition such as diabetes, autoimmune disease, or HIV/AIDS. Therefore a complete medical and family history can help fill out the risk picture for an individual and shorten the diagnostic path. Not every set of hoofbeats is a herd of zebras, but one might think differently hearing hoofbeats in the Serengeti.

Until recently, health care has focused on the treatment of disease as it occurred, and an entire structure of hospitals and medical research institutions has evolved to deliver what Americans have come to expect in high-technology, high-quality health care. But it is expensive health care. Some are wondering how much more expensive it can get. Some are postponing preventive screenings such as mammograms and Pap smears because they cannot afford to pay what their insurance no longer covers (or perhaps never did). Some are trying to reduce those costs by acting sooner along the continuum from health to disease, focusing on ways to maintain health, postpone disease onset, or optimize outcomes for the individual. For this particular purpose, unconventional medicine (dietary supplements, chiropractic, acupuncture, ayurveda, imagery, hypnosis, homeopathy, folk remedies, and other practices not commonly taught in U.S. medical schools) has become enormously popular. Although one extensive survey of the use of unconventional medical practices in 1990 found no significant differences between men and women (Eisenberg and others, 1993), about a third of respondents with at least one principal medical condition saw neither a medical doctor nor a provider of unconventional therapy. It is not clear from this study how many of these individuals used unconventional therapies; overall about a third of the respondents reported some use of them. However, for five of the ten most frequently cited principal medical conditions (back problems, insomnia, headache, anxiety, and depression), more respondents reported use of unconventional therapies with or without consulting a medical doctor. One may infer from this list of conditions, at least three of which (headache, anxiety, and depression) are reported more frequently by women, that women indeed are major users of unconventional therapies. And given that women also report that these three conditions are not adequately treated or not taken seriously by some health care providers, their pursuit of relief through other means would not be surprising. Burg (1996) suggests that providers may not routinely ask patients about their use of these therapies, and that doing so may help improve communication between patient and provider. Clearly this is an area that needs to be explored.

Despite the increased awareness of women's health issues, the way in which those issues are addressed is often narrow. For example, breast cancer is one of the most highly publicized women's health issues. Some efforts to promote women's health services focus only on breasts, although some also address the reproductive tract. But women are not well served by these efforts when other health risks are ignored—poor diet, physical inactivity, and violence and also alcohol, tobacco, and other drug use. Women can expect to spend half of their adult lives beyond their reproductive years. With that longer life span, women face more chronic illnesses than men, including cardiovascular disease and stroke, cancer, osteoporosis, diabetes, osteoarthritis, and Alzheimer's disease. What we know and learn about the causes, prevention, diagnosis, and treatment of these diseases will not only help women *and* men, it will drive the health care industry toward improvement in both academic research and in clinical care.

DISEASE PREVENTION AND HEALTH PROMOTION FOR WOMEN

Where and how should we focus our efforts on women's health then? Disease prevention and health promotion are powerful partners to the diagnosis and treatment of disease. Their combination draws on the strengths of public health and health care, presenting a unique opportunity to improve health and quality of life for all. A balanced approach that recognizes women can control major determinants of their health status is a good place to start. Second, positive, practical steps that are age and culturally appropriate can help women make changes to improve their own health status and also that of their families. For women of any age, nutrition and physical activity are major topics to address for disease prevention and health promotion. For teenaged women, specific issues to target include avoidance of tobacco and drug use, postponement of sexual activity, and avoidance of violence and injury. Sexually active women need to know how to reduce their risks of unintended pregnancy and sexually transmitted diseases. For women at midlife and through the elder years, the issues shift toward prevention and early detection of chronic disease.

Health care providers can work with women to pinpoint lifestyle factors key to women's health risks and then can identify modification strategies. Behavioral change is difficult; considerable evidence suggests that recognizing several stages of behavioral change and delivering the health message that targets an individual's stage is more likely to be effective than delivering a general health message. Even then change may come slowly, with intervening relapses to the old behavior. Peer educators, role models, telephone support networks, and support groups of women for women can reinforce health messages. Community resources have been mobilized around many women's health issues including physical activity, breast cancer, osteoporosis, and family violence. These and other approaches have been evaluated for their efficacy in promoting and sustaining behavioral change among women. Many have been incorporated into routine services by innovative providers who serve women.

Some managed care organizations are leading the research and implementation of these innovations. They see the benefit to their enrollees in improved utilization patterns and customer satisfaction. Innovation can also be a marketing tool, complementing consumer education in health promotion and disease prevention. Readily available health information supports women in becoming more informed consumers and in turn should result in improvements in health care as women become full partners with their providers. This outcome is characteristic of the more successful initiatives that address disease management for women. The challenge, however, is to ensure that the full spectrum of a woman's health needs are met no matter who her provider is; and if those needs cannot be met by a single provider, a combined practice is the most practical way to address them. This latter approach is the strength of comprehensive women's health centers and managed care organizations that have integrated their systems of care.

LEADERSHIP IN WOMEN'S HEALTH

Many of today's popular leadership models build on women's traditional strengths of communication, collaboration and cooperation, empowerment, and inclusion. Women have practiced these skills since time immemorial as they faced the complexities of managing the home and family with limited resources. As leaders for the health and welfare of their families, women have educated and communicated with those around them and then have done what was necessary to ensure the family's survival.

Health care leaders should recognize that women are considerably more informed than ever about health issues and that their interest in health issues is extremely high. However, although more health information is available in lay magazines and the electronic media (including the Internet) than ever before, that information is of varying quality, and women may not understand all of it. They may not be able to apply it to their own situations, or they may misinterpret it and conclude that a health risk is far greater or less than it actually is. Women need to know where to find in-depth and accurate information about their own or their families' health problems when they need it. Information about a particular health problem may not be salient for a woman until she or someone close to her develops that problem.

It is critical to gain a better understanding of how specific diseases affect women by studying them in women, not by extrapolating from knowledge of those same disorders in men. The numbers of women in clinical trials and studies of disease conditions has increased over the past ten years, but many disorders that affect women disproportionately (such as autoimmune disease, osteoporosis, and arthritis) have not been studied adequately in women. Further, women can contribute information to study design and enrollment issues, increasing the likelihood of successful study recruitment. And even where no study is involved, providers can consult women as consumers to inform clinic services, design, and other features and make the health care setting woman friendly.

Health care leaders should have a broad systems perspective on women's health issues, taking steps to understand and then to address their complexity and interconnections. Despite women's increasing access to economic resources, many continue to work in jobs that offer no or minimal health coverage. Connections between health care services and community and social services that can address the gaps some women face are critical. Also, preventive services and activities offered in the workplace can go far in improving women's health. Evidence suggests that employees who participate in physical activity, injury reduction, and other lifestyle programs have lower rates of illness and absenteeism than other employees do and also tend to be happier in their work. These benefits will add to the bottom line of any business, not just that of health care organizations.

Developing a *total* focus in delivering care, as opposed to the piecemeal or body-part-specific focus of the past, and striking a balance between individual and societal needs, cost, and quality when shaping care and policy are key elements of a women's health agenda. But more than that, these steps represent a tremendous opportunity for improving the health of women *and* men. The willingness to take risks, to learn from mistakes and move on, seeds the success of much of business and industry. The business of health care and women's health should be no exception as it strives to attain a system of services across the spectrum of life needs, services that complement but do not compete against each other, services informed by and responsive to the women who use them.

References

Burg, M. A. "Women's Use of Complementary Medicine. Combining Mainstream Medicine with Alternative Practices." *Journal of the Florida Medical Association,* 1996, *83,* 482–488.

Eisenberg, D. M., and others. "Unconventional Medicine in the United States. Prevalence, Costs, and Patterns of Use." *New England Journal of Medicine,* 1993, *328,* 246–252.

CHAPTER SEVENTEEN

Caring for an Aging Population

Martha A. McSteen

Martha A. McSteen is president of the National Committee to Preserve Social Security and Medicare. In the 1980s, she was acting commissioner of the Social Security Administration for three years. The recipient of numerous awards, including the Presidential Distinguished Executive Award, the Presidential Meritorious Executive Award, the HEW Distinguished Service Award, and the Commissioner's Citation, the Social Security Administration's highest award, she serves on the board of directors of the Alliance for Research in Aging, the International Federation on Aging, and the Setting Priorities for Retirement Years Foundation.

For much of the past half century, the United States has embraced and been enlivened by the energy and vigor of the post–World War II generation of baby boomers. From art and academics to advertising and politics, a youth culture pervaded and infused virtually every sector and sanctuary of our modern society. And indeed, with their unprecedented numbers, the baby boomers gave the United States a demographically and demonstrably youthful profile.

The emerging face of the United States in the twenty-first century, however, will be much more mature—increasingly retired and considerably older. The numbers of citizens we will call seniors will be truly historic. Call it what you will—the graying of America or the aging of the baby boomers—the transformation we now are about will pose national challenges unlike any we have confronted before.

The opportunities to broaden and deepen our culture and public dialogues with the experience, reflection, and wisdom that age can provide are full of promise and should be welcomed. At the same time the sheer scope of reordering society and all of its support structures to encompass the largest retirement population in U.S. history will be daunting. Nor will the attention required come and go with the baby boomers. The startling gains of recent years in longevity and the advances in nutrition and medicine and in safer and healthier workplaces are combining to virtually guarantee a significant and long-living population of seniors for decades after the baby boomers.

Can the United States marshal the national leadership that will be crucial for caring for an aging population? We certainly have the national can-do spirit it will take; the United States often has met challenges head-on, with an eagerness to lift anchor and set sail. In fact, I perceive an excitement today within the medical and scientific communities and among many in the social services about preparing for and addressing the dramatic generational changes of the next century.

Make no mistake, however. The dimensions of the leadership and resources required will be extraordinary. Anything less than full and total commitment at all levels and from all parts of society will fall tragically short of the effort it will take to greet and care for the population of U.S. seniors that is just over the horizon—and to do so with the dignity and respect they have earned.

UNDERSTANDING THE
DIMENSIONS OF CHANGE

That population will expand to an astonishing size. In the near term the number of Americans aged sixty-five or older will climb moderately from thirty-four million today to nearly forty million by the year

2010, according to the U.S. Bureau of the Census. But in just the following two decades, the population of seniors will explode in number, leaping by 75 percent and reaching more than 69 million by the year 2030. Two out of every ten Americans by that year will be sixty-five or older (U.S. Bureau of the Census, 1996)!

In the years between 2030 and 2050, according to the best projections of demographers, the population growth of older Americans will subside but still continue at a 14 percent rate. After the midpoint of the twenty-first century, the age segments of the nation's overall population will grow at fairly even rates. Of particularly great concern, however, is the expected swelling of the ranks of Americans aged eighty-five or older. As the baby boom generation retires and ages, the eighty-five-and-older group is estimated to vault from 5.9 million in 2010 to 8.8 million in 2030 and to 18.9 million in 2050. Over the next half century this population of the oldest seniors is expected to grow by more than 400 percent (U.S. Bureau of the Census, 1996).

We will have to learn how to manage our new aging population, especially its oldest members. In the past "the aged" were a small percentage of the nation's population, and the tender loving care of families was often the traditional and primary source of their emotional and financial well-being. For medical professionals, treating seniors was generally perceived to be a responsibility but often not a challenging one because there were few major health breakthroughs to enhance senior citizens' well-being.

Now, profound changes in U.S. society and lifestyles and striking advances in the medical sciences guarantee that our approach to the coming generation of seniors will be different.

Today's families, despite what wishes they may have, confront factors not faced by families of the past in providing for their older members. Our modern and highly mobile lifestyles and the employment demands of the new economy routinely separate by hundreds, even thousands, of miles members of the once-cohesive nuclear family. The unparalleled growth of single-parent and two-wage-earner households and the marked prevalence of both divorce and remarriage add to the difficulties and emphasize the challenge ahead for those inventing and providing housing and living arrangements for seniors in the new century.

Thankfully, a lack of meaningful breakthroughs in medicine for the senior population no longer is the problem. It is finding the funds for the sometimes complex treatments and cures of modern medicine and finding enough physicians and other health professionals to cope with the surging and increasingly older population that will be tomorrow's dilemma.

MEETING RESOURCE
AND RESEARCH NEEDS

Adequate resources to meet the medical and health needs of older Americans will be undeniably costly, but not providing adequate care and not investing in the research for new treatments and cures will be even more costly. Today Alzheimer's disease costs the nation an estimated $100 billion a year. Cardiovascular diseases and stroke cost an estimated $100 billion a year. Treating and caring for seniors afflicted by osteoporosis costs some $14 billion every year, and the costs of urinary incontinence are another $16 billion (Task Force for Aging Research Funding, 1998).

The United States now spends about $350 billion a year on health care for our population age sixty-five and older (Task Force for Aging Research Funding, 1998). We know from solid studies, however, that medical research for ways to slow the progression or delay the onset of these and other age-related diseases may significantly reduce the costs that the nation otherwise will somehow have to shoulder. According to some estimates, 50 percent of cataract operations could be avoided and $2.5 billion a year saved if the rate of cataract development were delayed; a five-year postponement in the onset of Alzheimer's could provide savings of as much as $50 billion a year; and delaying by five years the beginnings of hearing loss among older citizens could save $28 billion a year (Task Force for Aging Research Funding, 1998).

Those and other savings will become increasingly crucial as the eighty-five-and-older population of seniors continues its rapid growth. The oldest of the old traditionally have had the highest rates of disability, nursing home use, and multiple chronic conditions, and they incur health expenditures at a significantly higher rate than either the general population or younger seniors.

As our population ages, age-related research then becomes not just useful but invaluable. To better understand diseases and disabilities prevalent among seniors, long-term studies of normal aging in healthy adults are vital and already have shown that growing older does not automatically mean becoming sick and dependent. Research in the building-block sciences, such as cell biology and neuroscience, holds the potential for truly breakthrough cures and treatments. Finding how, for just one example, to remineralize human bones could prevent the bone thinning of osteoporosis and the 237,000 costly and painful hip fractures it causes in senior citizens each year.

Research on functional disabilities in older persons has been designated a top priority by the National Academy of Sciences' affiliate, the Institute of Medicine, and the reason is altogether understandable. Incontinence, impaired muscle strength, and diminished mobility are especially costly and devastating for the senior citizens who suffer from these and other functional conditions.

MEETING NEEDS FOR GERIATRICIANS

Just as critically, the United States confronts a dramatic and alarming shortage. According to the Alliance for Aging Research (1996), the nation faces a shortfall of more than 13,000 doctors in geriatrics, the area of medicine that addresses the sometimes complex health care needs of older patients. In fact less than 1 percent of the 685,000 doctors in the United States are certified in this field. Yet groups like the Alliance for Aging Research estimate that by the year 2030, the nation will need at least 37,000 geriatricians—a sixfold increase over the number working in the field today—in order to care for aging baby boomers (Alliance for Aging Research, 1996).

Moreover, the nation's medical schools are unprepared to educate and graduate these doctors. The alliance points out that students entering medical school today can anticipate that by the time they begin practicing at least half of their patients will be over the age of sixty-five. Yet, only 14 of the 126 U.S. medical schools require a course in geriatrics of their graduates, and according to the latest survey of just a few years ago, just 3 percent of medical school graduates had taken even an elective course in geriatrics (Institute of Medicine, 1993).

In many regions and at many schools, there is a serious shortage of teachers and medical researchers in the field of geriatrics. Although some medical specialty fields are chronically oversupplied with teachers, organizations that advocate for seniors conclude that more than four times the present number of teachers in geriatrics is needed to address the shortage in geriatrics (Institute of Medicine, 1987).

Of course not all older patients, by any stretch, require geriatric specialists for their health care. Indeed most medical experts agree that primary care physicians should continue to be the backbone of care for seniors. Primary care doctors, particularly those with some training in geriatric medicine, will be critical in addressing the looming shortage of specialists.

ENCOURAGING LEADERSHIP AT MANY LEVELS

We have the advantage at this point of a growing awareness and knowledge of these and other challenges the United States faces with its increasingly aging population. The issues of senior citizens' retirement, expanded longevity, and health needs and care are moving to the foreground of public debate.

Caring for an aging population is in fact an all-generation issue. We will fall short if the challenges ahead are perceived as merely today's aging problem. We will succeed, however, if younger generations recognize that their futures hold greater promise if thoughtful, committed action is taken now.

Surely government at all levels from the federal on down will play a pivotal role in gathering the resources and designing the strategy for adjusting to an older population. But we will fail if the problems are left only to government; the scale of the undertaking is too massive and the need for personal, grassroots, local approaches is too great to expect government either in Washington or in the state capitals to respond adequately on its own.

Churches and civic associations, the business community from Main Street to Wall Street, our foundations and nonprofit organizations, all will have to offer their attention and cooperation and leadership to create an enduring strategy that will see the United States through this demographic transformation and see to it that the aging population is not abandoned or ignored.

A lasting and practical solution that organizations such as the Washington, D.C.–based Setting Priorities for Retirement Years (SPRY) Foundation are pursuing approaches aging and the retirement as events requiring a lifelong personal strategy. SPRY envisions a social environment in the United States that encourages individuals throughout their lives to establish long-term goals for their personal health, financial security, and overall well-being.

The national leadership for an aging population also will have to keep a wary and watchful eye out for swindlers and sharks and their money-making schemes. They already prey upon seniors and almost inevitably will multiply as the number of seniors skyrockets. The fraud that has plagued the Medicare system is a clear indication of the troubles with scams that lie ahead.

Some of the work ahead can and should be undertaken now, without delay. The Department of Health and Human Services has laid out a number of important steps in its white papers on geriatric education. For example, to begin easing the shortage of medical practitioners for a growing senior population, the steps are straightforward: provide ongoing federal funding for the training of professionals and paraprofessionals to work in the long-term care system, develop strategies for enhancing the attractiveness of faculty careers in geriatrics, increase financial support for recruiting students into geriatrics and long-term care programs, stress interdisciplinary team training for health professionals who care for senior patients, and implement a major consumer education program in long-term care, with an emphasis on home and community-based services.

The U.S. medical community must be at the forefront of efforts to meet the needs of the aging population, and I call on the American Medical Association in particular to take the lead. The increased participation and continuing interest of the medical profession is essential; it is the medical practitioners and health professionals, more than the members of almost any other occupation, who deal with the elderly and who possess the special knowledge and experience that communities and the country will be relying upon.

The national leadership that will be successful and effective will also find the forum and invent the means to reach out and involve each citizen in the solution. Each citizen is intimately and irrevocably bound up in this transformation of our population. This year or next year it may be our grandparents or our parents who reach their senior years; shortly after them, it will be ourselves and then our children. What kind of health care do you want in years to come? How do we as a nation address that issue? Each citizen must be to asked to answer these and other questions.

Ultimately the challenge of leadership belongs to health care professionals; history will not judge us kindly if we tarry or shirk our obligation. Millions of our fellow citizens, many now and many more in the next few decades, are depending on us to do well. We cannot afford to let them and ourselves down.

References

Alliance for Aging Research. *Will You Still Treat Me When I'm 65?* Washington, D.C.: Alliance for Aging Research, May 1996.

Institute of Medicine. Committee on Leadership for Academic Geriatric Medicine. "Academic Geriatrics for the Year 2000." *New England Journal of Medicine,* 1987, *316,* 1425–1428.

Institute of Medicine. Committee on Strengthening Training in Geriatrics for Physicians. (Report.) Washington, D.C.: National Academy Press, 1993.

Task Force for Aging Research Funding. *A Call for Action.* Washington, D.C.: Alliance for Aging Research, Jan. 1998.

U.S. Bureau of the Census. *65+ in the United States.* (Current Population Reports, Special Studies.) Washington, D.C.: U.S. Bureau of the Census, Apr. 1996.

CHAPTER EIGHTEEN

Geriatric Care

William L. Minnix Jr.

*William L. Minnix Jr. is president and CEO of the
Wesley Woods Center on Aging, a comprehensive long-
term care, housing, outpatient, and acute care program
that is part of the Emory University system of health care.
Active on the boards of the National Chronic Care Consortium and the American Association of Homes and Services
for the Aging, he is also a frequent lecturer at professional
meetings on the topics of long-term care, integrated health
systems, ethics, and public policy.*

Health care leaders must remember this truth
about geriatrics: aging creates complexity—physical, emotional,
social, family, economic, and spiritual complexity. Geriatric care
requires highly flexible, sensitive, tailored, subtle, competent, interdisciplinary, and ethical responses to need. Geriatric care is therefore
highly individualized.

Leaders must also remember this prediction: geriatric programs will become the centerpiece of health care. Improvement in quality of life at a reduced cost for an aging population is a demographic and an economic imperative. Two provocative perspectives support this conclusion, one from a geriatrician, the other from an economist.

Geriatrician Christine Cassel (1990) tells us that "it's important to distinguish between the diseases that cause death—such as cancer, heart disease and stroke—and those age-related diseases that . . . cause significant disability. This latter group of diseases includes most predominantly osteoarthritis, osteoporosis and resultant fractures, and degenerative neurological conditions such as Alzheimer's disease, Parkinson's disease and visual or hearing loss. . . . If nothing is done to better understand the causes and treatment of disabling, non-lethal diseases, the epidemic of dependency and disability will be truly awesome."

And economist Peter Peterson (1996) reports that "when we consider the great demographic drift that will shape our national future over the next fifty years, we are speaking . . . of a genuine transformation. . . . What concerns me most about America's coming demographic transformation is simply this: on our present course, we won't be able to afford it" (p. 56).

This chapter begins with a few stories illustrating axioms about geriatric care and ends with a discussion of management and leadership strategies fundamental to success.

SOME STORIES

Each of the following stories is a composite of actual situations we have encountered at Wesley Woods. Each story concludes with a few axioms, which are then woven into the strategies for success.

The Woman with Fifty-Six Medicines

A frail, mildly demented woman was referred to the Wesley Woods SOURCE program. SOURCE (Senior Options Utilizing the Community Environs) is a Georgia Medicaid demonstration project designed to support nursing home eligible elderly clients at home. The woman lived alone in her modest home, had multiple diseases, had not had a shampoo in two years, and was taking fifty-six medicines, including twelve inhalers. SOURCE established her with one physician (a geriatrician), brokered services, and transportation; eliminated most of the medicines (the twelve inhalers were replaced by one daily pill); and averted emergency room, hospital, and nursing home admissions.

Axioms

- Recruit a core geriatric team: a well-trained geriatrician, a nurse practitioner, and a social worker.
- Be prepared to help people in spite of fragmented and bureaucratic delivery systems.
- Understand that geriatric care involves a great deal more than medical care.

The Woman Who Wanted to Face Her Maker Unencumbered

An elderly woman living at home invited Wesley Woods staff for a visit to talk about her future. Assuming she wanted to move into one of our facilities, we were prepared with brochures and applications. Her conversation meandered through her concerns about finances, her mentally ill adult daughter, and zoning changes in her neighborhood. She also wanted a good doctor. She declared she did not want to be kept alive by artificial means. She politely asserted she had no interest in living anywhere but home. When asked how we could help, she replied crisply, "Good question! I want you to help me live my final years—and face my Maker—unencumbered by tubes and gadgets. I want to stay at home as long as possible. I want to plan responsibly for my daughter and I want to rest in peace. Can you help me put that plan together?" We referred her to a geriatrician, a lawyer specializing in elder law, and home support services. She lived the rest of her life—and died—as she wished.

Axioms

- Consider that what you currently offer may not necessarily be what the geriatric market needs or wants.
- Be prepared to orchestrate an array of trusted professionals and services.
- Position your organization as the place to turn when the public faces geriatric problems.

The Child Who Wanted to
Study Alzheimer's Disease

Wesley Woods conducted a workshop series titled "You and Your Aging Parent" for a large church. Typically attendees at such workshops are caregivers, usually women. However, a twelve-year-old attended this particular series, requesting information that would help him write a term paper on aging. By the fourth week of the course, the lad revealed his real need: "My grandma lives with us. She's acting weird—like pulling drapes off the wall and taking off her clothes. My mom and dad fight about her. My sister and I are scared of my grandma, and we're afraid Mom and Dad will get a divorce." We met with his parents and clergy. The boy's father was in denial about his mother's Alzheimer's disease and felt trapped by a "promise" made to his mother that he would never put her in a nursing home. He was avoiding the situation through business travel. With support, the family was able to place grandma in a long-term care facility and grew closer together.

Axioms

- Include the entire family in the plan of care and be prepared to address powerful family dynamics.
- Be present in places where the family market gathers; do not expect the market to come to you.

The Daughter Who Wanted to Be Responsible

A daughter brought her mother to Wesley Woods Hospital for acute psychiatric care. The mother had multiple diseases and was addicted to medications. In addition, the mother and daughter had long-standing relationship problems. At a care conference the daughter lashed out at staff, "Why can't you people make my mother well and happy? That's what I brought her here for!" When asked how long the mother had been unhappy, the daughter's husband replied, "Come to think of it, as long as *I've* known her." The daughter paused, then conceded, "You know, I believe you're right." Asked to reflect now on realistic treatment goals for her mother's care, she said, "My goal is not happiness for her at this point. I know she can't be cured, so I want you to make her as comfortable as possible. And for me, I want to be able to look myself in the mirror the day of her funeral and be able to honestly say I've done the best job as a daughter that I was able to do. I want the satisfaction of feeling I've been responsible." The mother was placed in long-term care and the daughter sought counseling. After her mother died the daughter could honestly say she had behaved responsibly.

Axioms

- Understand that family goals are often as important as patient goals.

- Understand that comfort and responsibility are fundamental goals because cures and happiness are often unattainable.

THE STRATEGIES

Four strategies can help health care providers put the axioms listed here into practice and provide high-quality care to the nation's aging population.

Strategy 1: Invest in a Competent Geriatric Team

The medical cornerstones of geriatrics are geriatric medicine, geriatric psychiatry, neurology, and rehabilitation medicine. The delicate ecology of the aging body is subject to imbalances precipitated by myriad internal and external variables. Therefore it is essential that a person from one of these disciplines be the primary care leader, with people representing the others close at hand for consultation. Hospitals and physician groups are typically in the best financial position to attract and support such medical teams. However, long-term and home care organizations can collaborate with hospitals and doctors to form the necessary core medical competence through collaborative program planning, joint recruitment, and partial salary support.

The demand for certified geriatricians is growing faster than medical schools can produce them—a trend not likely to change soon. Therefore the training of existing practitioners is a paramount professional development objective for health systems.

Geriatric psychiatrists are an equally important part of the geriatric care team. In addition to the growing problem of dementia, depression may well be the biggest undiagnosed and untreated disease in the elderly. A substantial number of people receiving geriatric medical care have untreated depression. The good news is that depression can often be treated successfully if recognized and treated appropriately. However, geriatric psychiatric programs are underdeveloped compared to need. Inpatient, partial hospitalization, and outpatient services can be economically attractive when structured properly and integrated as part of the geriatric service spectrum.

Geriatric medical services can be marketed to the public, other health care providers, and managed care organizations as comprehensive specialty services. Geriatric consultation, memory assessment, depression screening, and other services can be linked to comprehensive case management services. In fee-for-service arrangements, geriatricians are marginally viable financially through fee reimbursement but typically require financial support through medical administrative activities. However, in the managed care arena these physicians, along with geriatric nurse practitioners and case managers, are cost beneficial. Effective geriatric programs reduce unnecessary emergency room visits, hospitalizations, nursing home admissions, and physician office visits.

To offer leadership in geriatric care, providers must have interdisciplinary care competencies available. The interdisciplinary team can be recruited or trained from within, but without it there is no program. The investment is worth it.

Strategy 2: Infect Organizational Culture with a Healthy Philosophy of Aging

Ours is still an ageist society. We value youth, strength, independence, and physical beauty. Aging leads to vulnerability and dependence, conditions we fear. Too few people have discovered the unique satisfactions of age: the wisdom, the different pace of activities, the spiritual reflection, the sense of history, and the pathos and humor that inevitably accompany the indignities of health problems.

My in-laws are in their mid-eighties, with multiple health problems. During an extended holiday visit my father-in-law and my fifteen-year-old son discussed aging. My son, observing that older folks are often an object of humorous ridicule, made a poignant observation, "I think most people think a frail body means a frail mind." To which my father-in-law responded, "That's right! I remember my grandfather around our farm. I never talked to him much. I thought he was an old fool. I'd give anything to talk with him now."

My father-in-law then reflected on his recent stroke, which landed him in a hospital emergency room. He remembers how frustrating it was not being able to communicate and being treated as if he were "crazy." He felt avoided, that he "wasn't a priority." He remembers hospital staff talking about him "as if there wasn't a person inside me anymore." A few days later in the intensive care unit, he had a spiritual epiphany in which an inner voice told him to keep fighting—that he must grow from this experience.

This interchange between grandfather and grandson expanded during the rest of the holidays. There were discoveries of common interests, reflections about religion and philosophy, and disagreements about politics.

Leadership in geriatrics requires a respect for elders based on a healthy corporate philosophy of aging. This philosophy must be reinforced through staff development, elder-friendly systems, and treatment protocols that assume "there is still a person in there somewhere."

Erik Erikson (1963) observed that the personal psychospiritual conflict to be addressed in late life is "ego integrity versus despair" (p. 268). Has the past been fulfilling? Is the future one of hope or fear? Elders have a great need to reflect and talk, especially with the younger generations, and these issues often surface in the midst of health crises. Therefore behind every care plan should be the goal of helping elderly patients value what is good in their lives, come to terms with regrets, and openly explore hopes and fears about the unknown. Erikson (1963) believes healthy life cycles depend on it: "healthy children will not fear life if their elders have integrity enough not to fear death" (p. 269).

Strategy 3: Create a Learning Organization with a Therapeutic Oasis and an Ethical Mirror

The knowledge and demographic explosions are combining with the economic pressures in health care to create exponentially rapid change. Research about aging is proliferating. Health care is being reengineered by managed care. New procedural techniques are advanced daily. Information systems, telemedicine, and health informatics will soon create hospitals and nursing homes without walls.

In the eye of this hurricane of change is the impaired older person who must cope with frailty at one level and work through the Eriksonian late life conflict at another and whose care is being delivered by human beings with their own personal complexities. Therefore it is essential to create a work environment with therapeutic underpinnings, one that helps employees learn and grow.

Three interrelated human resource management concepts are important to geriatrics programs: the learning organization, the therapeutic oasis, and the ethical mirror.

The *learning organization* was introduced by Peter Senge (1990). The theory behind it assumes that employees can rekindle childlike curiosity in the workplace, that rapid change calls for lifelong learning and innovation, and that applied learning through work practice within the context of a team produces satisfied employees and extraordinary results. Senge describes five disciplines important to the learning organization and corporate health, the most important of which is *systems thinking*. Systems thinking solves and prevents major work problems through a holistic view of the enterprise and the use of analytical methodologies.

Consider this example. Several years ago, as our executive staff prepared for our annual planning retreat to define goals and objectives, it became painfully apparent that our goals and objectives were recycled. We concluded we had "multiple chronic management diseases." We identified twenty-three nagging symptoms of organizational ill health, such as employee turnover and grievances, periodic occupancy problems, recurring patient complaints, inadequate financial resources, professional staff tensions, problems in our relationship with the Emory University School of Medicine, and insufficient tools to help staff do their work.

Using Senge's systems thinking, we diagnosed seven root causes of organizational ill health from the twenty-three symptoms and developed a multiyear strategic plan to not only become healthy but chart a visionary future course. We clarified mission, vision, and values. We developed a plan to formalize our relationship with Emory Healthcare. We transformed a traditional personnel department into a contemporary human resource function. We created a marketing function. We defined short- and long-term financial standards. And we reengineered our corporate infrastructure to produce improved business planning, stronger governance, and more investment in technology support.

The holistic, analytical mind-set that Senge encourages also led us to the conclusion that many of the problems we encountered in geriatric care delivery were caused by antiquated and ill-conceived public policy. So, as a not-for-profit, university-affiliated organization, we set out to position ourselves to innovate a new model of care and educate policymakers about needed changes in state and national systems.

Learning organization principles have a special harmony with geriatric care programs.

The second component important to a geriatric care program is a therapeutic oasis. Geriatric care brings to the surface raw feelings of fear, loss, regret, frustration, and unresolved conflict in all parties involved. Staff have to be trained to respond therapeutically and not react defensively or ignore the patient. At the same time, staff have personal problems that they bring to work every day. A therapeutic oasis that can help staff manage their feelings and reactions can take many forms: pastoral care programs, psychiatric consultation for individuals and teams, employee support groups, employee assistance, and mental health benefits.

The third component of a healthy human resource environment for geriatrics is an ethical mirror. Geriatrics presents personal, professional, and organizational ethical dilemmas. The people involved want to believe they are doing the right thing. Therefore it is important to have an ethics process that helps them reflect on their options. Ethics committees can automatically review some decisions, such as a termination of care for someone with no family. They can serve as an open resource to help any family member, patient, or staff member think through his or her ambivalence over a key decision. Educational programs can use case examples to help people reflect before they face an actual dilemma. Testing dilemmas against ethical principles within the safe context of caring people can be enormously helpful to those who genuinely seek to be responsible.

A learning organization with therapeutic and ethical components is essential to support the people who work in geriatric programs.

Strategy 4: Develop Enduring Community Partnerships with a Chronic Care Perspective

Successful geriatric care depends on a continuum of services developed from a chronic care perspective. According to *Chronic Care in America*, a report prepared for the Robert Wood Johnson Foundation, "chronic care is an unfamiliar term because the health care system in the United States is geared first and foremost to acute medical care" (1996, p. 11). Moreover, "in comparison with acute conditions, chronic conditions call for a different kind of care: an integrated network of professional expertise, and a far greater reliance on nonprofessional and informal caregiving—that is, on family, friends, and community level organizations" (p. 13).

It is unlikely that any one health organization has the expertise or wherewithal to offer the complete continuum of geriatric care. Therefore partnerships are essential. They can be defined as formalized long-term relationships of providers and payers, which collectively offer geriatric services, based on need, for an indefinite period of time. It is essential that these partnerships be strong and enduring to eliminate the possibility of discontinuity of care.

An enduring partnership is based on four constructs: the healthy marriage, relationship marketing, the merger of systems and expertise, and leadership relying on orchestration not control.

The relationship between Wesley Woods, historically a long-term care organization, and Emory Healthcare, a specialty academic medical center, has taken several years to develop. Wesley Woods is now part of Emory Healthcare as its geriatric and chronic care arm. The key elements of the Emory–Wesley Woods relationship are commitment to a common vision that includes service, research, and education; agreement on common planning, management, and clinical processes; overlapping governance participation; the positioning of geriatrics at the same corporate level as Emory's other major service arm; joint recruitment and appointment of key administrative and professional leaders; and agreement on the major geriatric programs to be based at Wesley Woods.

I have referred to the relationship on occasion as a Catholic marriage with a hyphenated last name and separate checkbooks. Wesley Woods and Emory Healthcare are committed to each other with little or no possibility of divorce. Our names are joined in the title Wesley Woods Center on Aging of Emory University, and Wesley Woods remains responsible for its own finances and liabilities.

In effect Wesley Woods has linked long-term care together with a prestigious acute care and specialty physician care for the benefit of its market area. This linkage has been the major nucleus needed to begin care integration across time, place, and provider. Due in large measure to the Emory–Wesley Woods ties, Wesley Woods has been able to develop a network of other providers who want to be affiliated with Wesley Woods at Emory for all the benefits that can accrue to them over time. These organizations are well respected in their own fields and collectively represent the full continuum of care from home health care to community-based services, assisted living, day care, nursing home care, and hospice care. These relationships have been formalized around the same principles and commitments that characterize the Emory–Wesley Woods relationship. Together Wesley Woods and these partners have created a new organization called Atlanta Senior Care, in which each organization has a stake. A chronic care infrastructure is now in place that links acute, physician, and long-term care for the benefit of frail, vulnerable elderly people. Wesley Woods brought the parties together and is the manager of the new entity.

The marketing construct that permeates this chronic care infrastructure is relationship marketing. I define relationship marketing as the joining of two or more complementary businesses that together create more value for their markets than any of them can do separately, with special attention given to ongoing personal relationships with the customers served and among the partners.

Atlanta Senior Care offers services as if it were one organization so that corporate boundaries are virtually invisible to the people served. The partners work together as a team for a common purpose, regardless of individual corporate identity.

Wesley Woods and Emory Healthcare have assigned nursing and social work liaison staff to contact partners regularly and, in some cases, to be a standing member of a partner's clinical or management structures. Atlanta Senior Care also has a clinical management team that meets at least weekly to discuss individual patient needs.

Effective relationship marketing management in geriatrics requires integration of three important systems: case management, information, and financial. Case management is the *key* system that must be integrated if care is to be managed responsibly and efficiently. All parties involved *must* agree to a common approach, and all patients and families need to know about it and have access to it. Without this commitment, geriatric care disintegrates.

To support clinical care and case management, an integrated information system (IS) is important. The technology is available to achieve this objective, but health care organizations are often stuck with existing systems or bogged down in consultant processes. In addition many organizations have dozens of individualized subsystems that are difficult to change. IS planning and management is the toughest operations challenge facing health care, and lack of it is a classic (and ironic) demonstration of non-systems thinking.

Integrated financing is crucial to geriatric care. Whether fee-for-service or managed care, and regardless of payer source and number of partners involved, all parties need to know where costs are incurred and how revenues are distributed.

Case management, information systems, and integrated financing are the cardiovascular system of geriatric care. If there are flaws in any of these three components—or in their relationship—problems will inevitably arise with care delivery.

The final construct that must be addressed to ensure enduring partnerships is leadership. It should be obvious that effective and efficient geriatric care is not likely to be lodged in one organization. Geriatric care is a function of a number of organizations, which have multiple agendas. Therefore leadership based on formal authority is almost impossible. Leaders in geriatrics have to learn that their power comes from the vision painted, the commitment of stakeholders to a common mission and plan, the satisfaction derived from improved care delivery, and the integrity earned in fulfilling responsibilities.

Geriatric care requires an orchestra leader, not a field commander. Orchestra leaders are responsible for a symphony played by instrumental groups and soloists. Orchestra leaders coach, blend variety, direct tempo, and modulate intensity, though neither playing an instrument nor owning the symphony hall. And if the audiences are not satisfied, the orchestra leader is accountable.

Health care leaders must remember this challenge and opportunity: there is an urgent need for leadership in the development of geriatric programs that are healthy, affordable, ethical, and fulfilling. The aged are the fastest-growing segment of the population and have the highest utilization of current and future health services. Those who develop reverence for the complexities of aging and talent as orchestrators will lead the health care industry in the next century.

References

Cassel, C. K. "Growing Old in America." *Atlanta Journal and Constitution,* Jan. 1, 1990.

Erikson, E. H. *Childhood and Society.* (2nd ed.) New York: Norton, 1963.

Peterson, P. G. "Will America Grow Up Before It Grows Old?" *Atlantic Monthly,* May 1996, p. 56.

Robert Wood Johnson Foundation. *Chronic Care in America: A 21st Century Challenge.* San Francisco: Institute for Health and Aging, University of California, San Francisco, for the Robert Wood Johnson Foundation, Aug. 1996.

Senge, P. *The Fifth Discipline: The Art and Practice of the Learning Organization.* New York: Doubleday, Currency, 1990.

CHAPTER NINETEEN

New Perspectives for Long-Term Care

Lorraine Tarnove

Lorraine Tarnove is executive director of the American Medical Directors Association, a national professional association representing long-term care physicians. Under her leadership the association has grown from a membership of six hundred to over eight thousand. Tarnove has written health education and policy materials for major national organizations, including the American Association of Retired Persons, American Heart Association, American Cancer Society, and National Osteoporosis Foundation.

—∿∿—

Long-term care is a part of the U.S. health care system that is little understood, reviled by the public and media, and defined by onerous regulations. It stands challenged by the biggest changes facing our society—the aging of the U.S. population and the reform of the U.S. health care system. "You are heading for a demographic tsunami," warned Senator Wyden (D-OR) at the 1997

National Investment Conference for Senior Living and Long Term Care Industries, "and there is a need for particularly innovative solutions." Wyden and others speakers, including former administrator of the Health Care Financing Administration Bruce Vladeck, condemned the current leadership of the long-term care industry. This is a wake-up call for those leaders who have not as yet realized that they will determine the future viability of their industry.

One cannot discuss the topic of future leadership in any arena without discussing change, and discussions of the enormity and speed of change facing every aspect of our society dare banality with their frequency. Surely the health care leaders of the future must understand the changes facing our society and be able to interpret and overcome them with out-of-the-box vision and strategic thinking. No industry faces change more momentous than health care does, yet few leaders in the field seem aware of the changes in thinking and philosophy about effective leadership.

Regulations may have designed this industry, but they will not provide it with a vision and a way to survive change and succeed in the future world of health care.

The long-term care industry in this country evolved from the poor houses and group homes that arose in the mid-nineteenth century to care for the growing number of abandoned elderly who were poor and ill. By the late nineteenth and early twentieth centuries, the beginnings of institutional care emerged with board and care homes established by religious and charitable organizations. The nursing home as a free-standing care site emerged fully after World War II, taking on more patients and professional caregiving staff. In 1946, the Hill-Burton Act responded to such societal changes as longer lives, working mothers, and more mobile families with funding for construction of nursing facilities. It was the genesis of the current seventeen thousand nursing facilities and the regulations that govern them.

Today the industry has grown to over seventeen thousand nursing facilities and 1.5 million beds (FIND/SVP, 1993). Keith Krein (1995) has identified three key trends that will shape the future of long-term care: cost controls, niche strategies, and an emphasis on primary care physicians. In addition, increased competition and managed care penetration will shape the future of the industry. The remainder of this chapter offers further perspectives on the potential for change in long-term care and the potential role of industry leaders.

ACKNOWLEDGING THE
REGULATORY BARRIER

Clearly there is an opportunity for long-term care industry leaders to focus on quality, innovation, and customer needs at national, community, and facility levels. However, just as the established and fragmented structure of health care is not adequate to meet future demand, hierarchical leadership within the long-term care facility is not enough to succeed in the future environment of competition and consumer demand. Long-term care leaders must create an atmosphere that allows and encourages creativity and innovation. Even though the existing regulatory environment may seem to preclude such innovation, a true fundamental change in the nature of leadership can and should overcome this barrier. Certainly, at the individual facility level, there are enormous opportunities for empowering staff to solve problems and respond to customer needs and expectations creatively.

The regulatory environment presents a unique barrier to innovative change in the industry. As the second most regulated industry in the United States (nuclear energy is first), long-term care facilities have virtually every operation and aspect of care regulated by hundreds of pages of regulatory doublespeak and an army of national and state watchdogs who reach into facilities with yearly surveys that can result in criminal charges and financial fines of major proportions. These regulations define the structure and management of these facilities. There is a national trend toward deregulation, but given the public's enduring negative image of the nursing home industry and vigorous consumer advocacy at the national level, it is not likely that long-term care regulations will go away. Therefore leaders will have to adopt new ways of thinking, reaching beyond facility walls to networks.

PREPARING FOR THE
DEMOGRAPHIC TSUNAMI

Preparing for the inevitable demographic tsunami is more complicated than simply addressing the daunting number of older adults who will need medical care and social support. The fastest growing segment of the over-sixty-five population comprises those who are over eighty-five. These individuals will be medically complex. They will need many types of services and professional caregivers to coordinate these services and ensure patient needs are met.

Then there is the boomer factor. As consumers, the baby boomers are educated and demanding and need a high level and variety of services. The industry will have to respond with a more customer-driven approach.

The industry has already begun to diversify and offer alternatives to traditional custodial nursing home care in two main directions. Subacute care and rehabilitation facilities, with more staff and the capability to offer more medical services and procedures than nursing homes, are proliferating. On the other end of the spectrum, assisted living is the fastest-growing segment of the industry, boasting independence for patients with behind-the-scenes support services on an as-needed basis. It is not difficult to predict a collision between the needs of these patients and society's need to limit health care expenditure.

CHANGING A FRAGMENTED STRUCTURE TO A CONTINUUM OF CARE

The health care system cannot address the number and needs of expected patients with the current structure of health care organizations and payment systems. Vertical hierarchies are silos that impede delivery of integrated care and simply reinforce the fragmentation of our current long-term care system. This system is not even universally defined—types of long-term care emerge based on payers' payment policies. Assisted living responds to customer demands but may end up evolving into simply another name, more politically correct and less pejorative, for the custodial care nursing home.

The future leaders of long-term care need some notion of what the future holds. Long-term care has some immutable truths, such as the number of older adults who are likely to need long-term care services. The rest is guesswork.

One thing is certain, however. Long-term care must evolve into a virtual continuum so patients can receive services they need regardless of site or payment policy and under the supervision and care of a physician case manager. Sites like subacute care units, rehabilitation facilities, and home health agencies will form networks that make it easy for patients to move around and receive the care they need from the most-appropriate, cost-efficient provider.

MAKING END-OF-LIFE DECISIONS

A national debate is needed on the ethical issues surrounding the role of technology in end-of-life care. The public needs information and education for making these difficult decisions and for understanding the realities of death and dying. Patients and families are not prepared to face extended life spans and the near-infinite technical capacity to support life through resuscitation, tube feeding, and ventilators. In spite of the 1990 law that requires discussion of advance directives on admission to health care facilities including nursing homes, the rate of use among those over sixty-five is disappointing. Because we in this society have avoided the topic, individually and collectively, the debate continues to rage, somewhat hysterically and with an appalling lack of factual or logical information.

There is a significant opportunity for leadership to frame and propel this national debate, bring it to consensus, and then provide the communication, information, and education needed by the community, by the family, and by those at the bedside. Such an action would be the essence of leadership. The call from Congress for long-term care leaders to solve fiscal and service delivery issues creatively rings hollow when the ethical framework is missing and leads to confusion, misuse of resources, and pain and disillusionment for the dying, their families, and their professional caregivers.

USING A NEW DATA SOURCE FOR DECISION MAKING

Leaders in the field of long-term care have suffered a paucity of data about their patients, the care delivered, and the outcomes achieved. The big news in this connection is the establishment of the Resident Assessment Minimum Data Set (MDS) in the Nursing Home Reform Act of 1987. Every patient admitted to a Medicare certified long-term care facility must complete a comprehensive resident assessment by filling out a twelve-page MDS that covers every area of function and disease. By July of 1998, all these facilities are required to send this data to the Health Care Financing Administration electronically, in effect, creating the largest database of information on long-term care patients and facility practices ever collected. The potential for application to patient care is enormous; through the MDS, the documentation of clinical outcomes can be rationally applied to cost management. Leaders of the future may finally have the hard data to show what can be accomplished and to weigh care decisions and their outcomes rationally with cost concerns. This will be the key to an affordable system that is acceptable to the consumer.

References

FIND/SVP. *The Long-Term Care Market: A Market Intelligence Report.* New York: FIND/SVP, 1993.

Krein, K. "The Corporate Medical Director." *Clinics in Geriatric Medicine: Medical Direction in Long Term Care,* 1995, *11*(3), 403–417.

Wyden, R. Speech to National Investment Conference for Senior Living and Long Term Care Industries, 1997.

CHAPTER TWENTY

Rural Health Systems

Jon B. Christianson
Anthony L. Wellever

Jon B. Christianson is a professor at the Institute for Health Services Research at the University of Minnesota School of Public Health. An economist who teaches, researches, and writes about medical care financing and evaluation, he has collaborated with health care providers to evaluate new treatments. He is a member of the editorial boards of Health Affairs *and* Medical Care Research and Review *and the coauthor of a paper that won the 1995 Health Care Research Award of the National Institute for Health Care Management.*

Anthony L. Wellever is a research fellow and deputy director of the Rural Health Research Center at the University of Minnesota. He is the author or coauthor of a number of articles about his research interests: rural health networks, managed care in rural areas, and alternative models for rural hospitals.

A pproximately one in four Americans lives in a rural area. In the past, rural populations were defined by their dependence on farming and by their differences from urban populations in family size, lifestyle, and politics. Today, clear distinctions between urban and rural populations no longer exist. Sweeping improvements in transportation and communications, migration both to and from rural areas, and diversification of the rural economy have replaced simple definitions of rural with the concept that both rural and urban areas exist along a geographical continuum (Hewitt, 1992).

Rural areas are commonly associated with such geographical characteristics as small population, low population density, and isolation from urban centers. They also may be defined by economic and sociodemographic characteristics of the populations that inhabit rural areas. Meade (1992) combines geographical, economic, and sociodemographic characteristics to reach this broad definition of rural: "It encompasses farm and nonfarm, lands contiguous to great metropolises and lands remote from any town, places of economic growth and those of decline, places of retirement and those of abandonment. Such differences are associated with differences in demographic structure, that is, the proportion of different ages, races, and sexes. Because age, race, and sex are characterized by different levels of risk of various morbidity or mortality conditions, great variation in need for services in 'rural' America exists" (p. 69).

It is no longer possible to talk about rural America as a monolithic unit. Rural populations vary widely, leading to differing needs for health services. Education, income, occupation, political orientation, and physical isolation are among the many variables that might affect the need for health care services and the actions taken and causes supported to obtain services.

Rural populations are also volatile, shrinking and expanding in response to economic and social changes. Reversing the trend of the 1980s, when rural America suffered a net loss of 1.4 million residents, in the 1990s (through 1996) it witnessed a 2 million person net increase in population, with 75 percent of rural counties reporting population increases. The counties with the largest upswings are those with retirement or recreational facilities or those in proximity to a major population center (Cook, 1997). At the same time, some rural areas are virtually withering away. According to the 1990 Census, twenty-four rural counties, concentrated primarily in the Great Plains, lost sufficient population between 1980 and 1990 to gain *frontier* status (frontier counties are those with a population of six or fewer persons per square mile).

Out of this turbulent environment several population subgroups are emerging as particularly important as potential rural health care followers.

Uninsured Rural Residents

Some predominantly rural industries provide limited, if any, health insurance benefits to their employees. For example agriculture, forestry, and fishing provide health insurance coverage for approximately 40 percent of their workers and workers' families. Mining (also a rural industry but, unlike the others, one that is highly unionized) provides coverage to over 80 percent of its workers and their families. Approximately 96 percent of rural residents over age sixty-five are covered by Medicare and 5.8 percent of all rural residents are covered by public assistance programs, including Medicaid. Overall, 17.4 percent of rural residents have no health insurance (Office of Technology Assessment, 1990). The amount of out-of-pocket expense rural residents incur for health care is likely to influence their attitudes toward the health care system and the health care positions they support.

Rural Residents Enrolled in Managed Care

Medicare and Medicaid patients in rural areas likely will be channeled into managed care programs in increasing numbers in the future. Although Medicare managed care enrollment in rural areas is currently low (0.7 percent compared to the urban rate of 10.8 percent), recent changes in the method of payment for risk contractors serving rural areas almost ensure a significant increase in rural enrollment in the near future (Moscovice, Casey, and Krein, 1997). A majority of states are also preparing to embark on extending Medicaid managed care to rural areas.

Private managed care enrollment in rural areas also appears currently to lag substantially behind urban enrollment. Moreover, the high costs of marketing in rural areas, the small populations, and the lack of large employers suggest that private managed care enrollment may not develop as quickly in rural areas as publicly financed managed care enrollment. As a larger proportion of the elderly and poor are covered by managed care programs, conflicts may arise between these residents and rural providers over levels of payment and access to services.

Old and Young Rural Residents

For many years, better-educated young people have left rural areas. One explanation for their flight is that older residents control the wealth and land in rural areas, limiting young people's opportunities to participate in business or farming and causing them to seek opportunities elsewhere (Cook, 1997). This so-called brain drain is often lamented for its impact on the quality of rural leadership, but it also affects the ranks of followers. The young people who remain are less well off and less educated than other rural residents. They have substantial health care and social needs, but in comparison to their neighbors they may be less able or willing to mobilize behind community leaders to make their needs known. The elderly, in contrast, often have time to spend in community activities and the life experience to know how to accomplish their goals (Hobbs, 1997).

New Rural Residents

There are two general categories of new rural residents, the elderly seeking a safe, attractive, affordable retirement destination and young professionals seeking to improve the quality of their lives in, often idealistically envisioned, rural settings (Pooley, 1997). These newcomers frequently are more affluent than the established residents and have had their health care desires and expectations shaped by urban experiences. In some rural communities, clashes have resulted when *old-timers* perceived that newcomers were attempting to impose their cultural values upon them and the community at large. Many newcomers judge the quality and direction of rural social institutions such as schools, civic organizations, and hospitals as lacking and seek to reform them according to more urban standards, often meeting with resistance from long-time residents. Many key health care providers such as physicians and health services administrators have immigrated into rural communities from elsewhere.

These population subgroups implicitly and explicitly establish health care goals and select leaders. Conflicts among these goals are likely to become apparent as subgroups pursue them. How these conflicts are resolved is, in part, the job of leaders.

GOALS: LINKING FOLLOWERS AND LEADERS

Goals link followers and leaders. Burns (1978) observed that "persons are often perceived to be leaders simply because they reflect the needs and attitudes of their followers" (p. 265). Goals equalize leaders and followers: followers do not submit to a leader as a person but agree to join that leader in the common pursuit of a goal (Wills, 1994). Goals also serve as standards to evaluate policies, practices, other goals, and even leader performance. The performance of leaders is assessed by their contribution to change, as measured by goal attainment. Goals, then, are the principle organizing components of leadership: they bring followers and leaders together, direct their joint actions, and form the basis for evaluating leader performance (Burns, 1978).

Health care goals are formed by a variety of individual aspirations: economic (for example, a wish to lower expenditures or increase income), spiritual (for example, a desire for respect and dignity), and personal (for example, the hope of relieving one's own or a loved person's suffering). These individual desires find expression as the goals of a group, a community of interest. The goals of a particular group, however, are not static. They may change as intermediate steps are taken to attain them. As an interest group becomes larger, its goals may also become more diffuse or more grandiose. A larger group also faces the possibility of internal conflict that results in a modification of its original goals (Burns, 1978).

Rural areas' health care goals are numerous and vary widely from community to community. The population diversity described previously conveys to some degree the possible range of these health care goals. Examples of the likely goals of emerging subgroups are greater access to health care services (the uninsured and underinsured); lower out-of-pocket expenses and greater freedom of choice of providers (the insured); maintenance of local control of rural health care services (the *ruling elites*); and local access to a wider variety of health-related services and products (newcomers accustomed to the greater choices available in urban areas).

The various health-related interest groups in rural areas and the different goals they embrace provide many opportunities for the development of health care leaders.

LEADERS: WHO WILL LEAD?

Many different health care interest groups exist in rural areas, but each interest is not represented by a leader in every community. The lack of leadership to better define goals and to formulate and take actions to attain goals may result from a sense of powerlessness among followers in a community, a lack of information about possible courses of action, a lack of leadership ability, or the dominance of other issues.

Because many issues command rural residents' attention, health care goals are pursued by local leaders only to the extent that they are not eclipsed by other goals judged more immediate by leaders and followers. Health leadership, however, may be awakened by a catalytic event, or the perception of an impending catalytic event, such as the closure of a hospital service or an entire hospital, the loss of physicians to below the number acceptable to residents, the acquisition of local health care assets by interests outside of the community, or community awareness of a significant health care quality problem. For example, citing declining admissions and emergency room volume, the not-for-profit system that owned the hospital in Smithville, Missouri, converted the hospital to a skilled nursing facility. Community leaders emerged who attempted to gain ownership of the hospital through eminent domain. The not-for-profit system reopened the emergency room and is reevaluating its decision to close the acute care beds (Scott, 1997). Catalytic events are not only negative occurrences. A positive catalytic event, for example, would be the new availability of grant monies for community-based health planning.

When leaders emerge in rural areas, they typically adopt one of two leadership roles. They function either as specialized leaders, taking a narrow, subject-dominated view of community affairs, or as generalized leaders, expressing and coordinating a broad range of community interests. Specialized leaders, on the one hand, perform important community functions. They carry out task-oriented leadership activities that focus on the accomplishment of specific follower goals. Economic development, education, and recreation matters, for example, benefit from specialized leadership and so do local health issues. Specialized leadership, however, can lead to fragmentation when the special interests of the group are viewed as greater than the interests of the community as a whole. Generalized leaders, on the other hand, fill structure-oriented leadership roles aimed at coordinating and integrating the goals of various special interest groups for the benefit of the entire rural community (Israel and Beaulieu, 1990).

Health care leadership in rural areas often is dominated by specialized leaders. Health care providers, health care facility trustees, and large employers frequently form the cadre of rural health leaders. They lend their clinical, administrative, and political expertise to planning, organizing, and controlling the local health care system. This is an appropriate role. Their leadership becomes counterproductive, however, when these leaders' and groups' private interests are pursued over the public interests of the greater community or when their goals are not or cannot be integrated with community goals. In the former case they benefit one segment of the community at the expense of others. In the latter case their specialized goal may serve multiple segments of the community, but failure to integrate the goal into the political and economic fabric of the entire community may undermine the community's overall effectiveness.

Rural health care providers, large employers, and health facility trustees may pursue goals particular to their occupational or fiduciary role, unaware of the possible negative consequences for other segments of the community or for the community at large. For example, a local manufacturing plant manager's primary health care goal may be to control premium prices, and that manager may be unaware or unconcerned about the consequences of her actions on the local availability of services or local health care provider income; local physicians motivated by the goal of maintaining their income may argue against the recruitment of needed additional health care providers; or a hospital trustee may lead a fund drive to keep the local hospital open even though it is underused, another hospital is located less than twenty miles away, and it requires a continuing subsidy from county tax revenues.

Individuals outside the community also provide rural health care leadership. In an effort to maintain or increase their market share, urban providers and health plans recently have accelerated a trend, begun in the mid-1980s, to expand their influence in rural areas. Their strategies include forming strategic alliances with existing rural providers, offering previously unavailable health services locally, and competing with local providers within the rural community. One example of this trend is a clinical oncology outreach program at rural Kershaw County Memorial Hospital, offered in partnership with Richland Memorial Hospital in Columbia, South Carolina. Administrative staff, nursing administrators, medical staff, and pharmacists from both hospitals developed this chemotherapy clinic at Kershaw. The planning committee that directed the joint effort decided that the clinic would initially treat relatively stable patients using routine protocols but that patients requiring radiation therapy would still travel to Columbia. Richland Memorial made available its clinical and planning expertise to provide a previously unavailable service to Kershaw County, and it benefits from this arrangement by receiving referrals from Kershaw County (Moscovice and others, 1995).

Outside influence on local health care systems is a highly contentious issue. There are segments of rural communities that welcome the expansion of urban health care providers and plans into rural areas, in the belief that access to services will improve, facilities will be upgraded, and quality of care will be enhanced. Others view the increased presence of urban health care providers and plans as a challenge to local control of health care services and doubt the long-term strength of the urban commitment to rural health. For example, in the Smithville example cited earlier, the not-for-profit system owner closed the hospital when it was no longer profitable to operate. Whether or not they currently hold title to the hospital, many rural residents believe that they still *own* it. "We started the community hospital," a local leader in Smithville is reported to have said, and indeed, many rural hospitals would not exist but for the efforts of the parents and grandparents of current rural residents (Scott, 1997). Whether or not urban health care providers and plans maintain their interest in rural health care in the future, for the time being they are likely to have an impact on health care leadership in many rural communities.

These "outsiders" may serve as catalysts, encouraging the development of local leaders to support or oppose their presence in the community. Nevertheless, some local health care decisions will now be made by individuals residing outside the rural community. Effective community leadership may ameliorate the potential negative consequences of this external decision making by developing agreements with urban health care providers and plans that outline a role for the community in decisions that affect its well-being. In the anecdotal evidence that exists to date, there is little to suggest that urban health care providers and plans adopt a public-be-damned attitude when they enter rural areas. On the contrary, to the extent that they are made aware of rural residents' needs, desires, and values, they attempt to incorporate these issues into their business plans. They are, after all, in the business of selling products and services in a competitive market, and aggressive disregard for consumers is not a useful marketing strategy.

The health care system in many rural communities for the foreseeable future will feature a mixture of local and extralocal ownership of health care resources. Effective rural health care leaders will attempt to find ways that these interests can coexist and will avoid exploiting their differences for the particular benefit of a narrow segment of the rural community.

THE FUTURE OF RURAL HEALTH LEADERSHIP

It is common for rural health advocates to lament the lack of health care leadership in rural communities (Amundson, 1993; Amundson and Rosenblatt, 1991). In the past decade, private philanthropic organizations such as the Kellogg Foundation, the Northwest Area Foundation, the Colorado Trust, and the Kansas Health Foundation have sought to correct this situation by investing considerable effort and money in programs to develop rural community health care leadership. These programs have encouraged grant communities to organize themselves into broadly representative community bodies, select leaders, assess community health care needs, develop plans to address identified needs, and implement projects designed by community leaders. The communities that participated in these programs benefited not only from the grant dollars that flowed into the community but also from the outside technical expertise provided directly by the foundations or by consultants funded through the grants. In some cases the technical assistance took the form of leadership development. In other cases consultants played the role of knowledgeable but disinterested parties who were able to bridge gaps among special interests and focus attention on the entire community. Despite the programs' usefulness and the sums of money spent on them, the number of communities that received grant support was relatively small.

The vast majority of rural communities have received neither grant money nor technical assistance from outside the community to address local health care issues.

A growing body of research examines the characteristics of *effective* rural communities. Findings from this research indicate that the communities best able to act on local concerns have leaders skilled in involving a diverse set of actors in local decision-making activities, operate on democratic principles, and place the welfare of the whole community above the needs of any special interest (Israel and Beaulieu, 1990). The research goes on to show that these communities not only make better use of their own resources but are also better able to identify and use specialized outside resources. According to these studies, the most effective rural leaders are those who participate in networks beyond their communities (Hobbs, 1997).

These findings seem to suggest that the most successful rural health care leaders view health care in a broad social context. This is not to say there is no role for specialized leaders, but to be truly effective, they must pursue the interests of the public at large and be able to coordinate and integrate community health care decisions with the interests of other specialized leaders in the community.

The interest urban providers and plans have in rural areas may have a beneficial effect on rural health care leadership. On the one hand the entry or anticipated entry of an urban provider or plan may catalyze the development of local leaders. On the other hand, if local leaders reach out to the urban interests, they may find technical and financial resources equivalent to those provided by philanthropic foundations. What is viewed by many as the loss of local control of rural health may result in a revitalization of local health care leadership.

References

Amundson, B. "Myth and Reality in the Rural Health Services Crisis: Facing Up to Community Responsibilities." *Journal of Rural Health,* 1993, 9(3), 179–187.

Amundson, B., and Rosenblatt, R. "The WAMI Rural Hospital Project: Overview and Conclusions." *Journal of Rural Health,* 1991, 7(5), 560–574.

Burns, J. M. *Leadership.* New York: HarperCollins, 1978.

Cook, R. "America's Heartland: Neither One Mind Nor One Heart." *Congressional Quarterly,* Sept. 20, 1997, pp. 2243–2249.

Hewitt, M. "Defining 'Rural' Areas: Impact on Health Care Policy and Research." In W. M. Gesler and T. C. Rickets (eds.), *Health in North America: The Geography of Health Care Services and Delivery.* New Brunswick, N.J.: Rutgers University Press, 1992.

Hobbs, D. "The Context of Rising Rates of Rural Violence and Substance Abuse: The Problems and Potential of Rural Communities." [http://www.ncrel.org/sdrs/areas/issues/envrmnt/drugfree/v1hobbs2.htm]. Feb. 28, 1997.

Israel, G., and Beaulieu, L. "Community Leadership." In A. Luloff and L. Swanson (eds.), *American Rural Communities.* Boulder, Colo.: Westview Press, 1990.

Meade, M. S. "Implications of Changing Demographic Structures for Rural Health Services." In W. M. Gesler and T. C. Rickets (eds.), *Health in North America: The Geography of Health Care Services and Delivery.* New Brunswick, N.J.: Rutgers University Press, 1992.

Moscovice, I., Casey, M., and Krein, S. *Rural Managed Care: Patterns & Prospects.* Minneapolis, Minn.: Rural Health Research Center, Division of Health Services Research and Policy, School of Public Health, University of Minnesota, Apr. 1997.

Moscovice, I. J., and others. *Building Rural Hospital Networks.* Ann Arbor, Mich.: Health Administration Press, 1995.

Office of Technology Assessment. *Health Care in Rural America.* OTA-H-434. Washington, D.C.: U.S. Government Printing Office, 1990.

Pooley, E. "The Great Escape." *Time,* Dec. 8, 1997, pp. 52–65.

Scott, L. "Communities Strike Back: Residents Oppose Ceding Control to Outside Not-for-Profit Chains." *Modern Healthcare,* 1997, *27*(17), 26–32.

Wills, G. *Certain Trumpets: The Call of Leaders.* New York: Simon & Schuster, 1994.

PART FOUR

Technology Leaders

CHAPTER TWENTY-ONE

The Evolving Role of Health Information

Charles W. McCall

Ellen S. Dodson

Charles W. McCall is chairman of the board, president, and chief executive officer of HBO & Company (HBOC). Since he joined HBOC in 1991, its revenues have grown approximately 550 percent, with 1997 revenues totaling $1.2 billion. He previously served as president and CEO of CompuServe and is currently a director of EIS International, and WestPoint Stevens, AMERIGROUP, and National Service Industries.

Ellen S. Dodson is vice president of strategic planning for HBO & Company (HBOC). She has spoken at numerous conferences on topics related to the development of clinical informatics strategies, Year 2000 issues, strategic uses of data, community health information networks, and health care financial management.

H ealth care today is an information-driven indus-
try. Witness the role that information technology is playing in reshaping the access to care providers, the activities contained within a
routine visit, and the electronic flow of funds among parties. The
vision of health care as a totally paperless arena seems imminent. It
seems a reasonable expectation that information on individual health
histories will be streamlined, standardized, and available globally in
the twenty-first century.

THE VISION OF HEALTH CARE INFORMATION

The mission-critical role that information plays in the health care
industry was foreshadowed early in the twentieth century. Back then,
a Massachusetts physician named Ernest Amory Codman observed
that there are many "products" of the hospital and the patient care
process: public health service to the community, medical education,
social service, and contribution to science and the body of medical
knowledge. Management responsibility for these disciplines, Codman
proposed, was to be fed by an "end-result system," a manual approach
to abstracting, classifying, comparing, and measuring the quality and
outcome of patient care (Codman, 1990 [1914], 1996 [1917]).

Of great concern to Codman was accountability for outcomes,
which he called end results. Codman wrote that "trustees of hospitals
should see to it that an effort is made to follow up each patient they
treat, long enough to determine whether the treatment given has per-
manently relieved the condition of symptoms complained of." Furthermore, "they should see that all cases in which the treatment is
found to have been unsuccessful or unsatisfactory are carefully analyzed, in order to fix the responsibility for failure on . . . the physician
or surgeon . . . the organization . . . the disease or condition . . . [or]
the personal or social conditions" (Codman, 1996 [1917]).

Codman's thoughts and observations were radical in his time, causing him to lose his positions at the Massachusetts General Hospital
and the local medical society. But his pioneering work ultimately
resulted in the formation of the American College of Surgeons. The
college's Hospital Standardization Program, in which Codman par-

ticipated until 1917, is considered an early forerunner of the Joint Commission on Accreditation of Healthcare Organizations (DePalma, 1961; Neuhauser, 1990).

Although Codman's work stood relatively unheralded for generations, no study of the role of information in health care would be complete without acknowledging his contributions. It is in his writings—completely devoid as they are of any knowledge of computer technology—that Codman unwittingly discovers the greatest challenges of clinical automation. How detailed and granular must a medical record abstract be to provide quick and meaningful information to a wide array of end-users, whether they are giving care or financing it? How can various caregivers describe and compare their experiences with similar cases without consistent and standard classifications of disease and observations? How can an organization distinguish the different causes of adverse outcomes—whether based on diagnostic skills, surgical skills, equipment failure, or the natural course of disease? How can a provider organization reasonably follow through on the course of a patient's condition when the encounter overlaps only briefly with the complete episode of illness?

Fast forward to the end of the twentieth century. Computer technology has infiltrated every aspect of clinical practice and health care management. Most hospitals in developed countries are becoming automated, from admission to discharge, and a growing number of physicians' practices, clinics, and home care agencies are moving to computerized medical record and billing systems. At the same time, the health care industry (for it is no longer simply the medical profession) has developed several administrative layers responsible for reconciling issues of funding, rationing, cost, and quality. This is as true in nations with socialized medicine, where there are strict governmental controls on access, as in the United States, where health care is nurtured by an interesting hybrid of federal regulation, standards compliance, and competition.

USING INFORMATION TO SUPPORT RESTRUCTURING

By its very complexity health care invites debate. It is this debate—among those who have scientific knowledge, those who provide care, those who finance care, those who require care, and those who would regulate the others—that frames the requirements for health care information.

There are many uses and users for each type of clinical information. What was once as simple as a doctor-patient relationship now looms as an intricate mega-structure of professionals involved in community public health management, scientific discovery, commercial buying and selling of goods and services, and government-sponsored oversight of cost and quality. The data used to support each of these activities derive from clinical and financial information systems. As questions of medical necessity, clinical appropriateness, and cost to society become broader and more global, these same systems are driven to be more granular, more detailed, and closer to the patient.

No one can predict what shape the health care industry will take in the coming decades, although the structuring and restructuring of health care will continue to follow the world's political and economic waves closely. Fortunately, technology has lived up to its promise to outperform itself with each succeeding generation, providing a capacity for handling and processing volumes of data that were unthinkable even five years ago. Until recently it was remarkable to have the on-line capability to evaluate data summarizing how many tests of each type were ordered, what types of patients were treated, and which ones had good outcomes. Today, organizations are building high-capacity repositories that store clinical data in enough detail to evaluate each step in the care process, regardless of where it is performed. The various accountable parties working along the health care continuum might raise questions like these:

Who ordered the test?

What clinical information was known at the time the test was ordered?

Who performed the test?

When were the results available?

When did the physician read or acknowledge the results?

What actions were taken as a result of the test?

Was the patient's condition improved as a result of those actions?

Was there a less expensive test that could have produced the same outcome?

The administrative layers of the health care system—those organizations that mediate cost, quality, and access—rely more and more on individual caregivers for the information they use to perform their primary functions. How do such organizations calculate their risk for caring for certain populations of patients? How do they understand the cost effectiveness of a medical regimen as compared to a more aggressive surgical treatment? Each of these organizations, whether a hospital or clinic, a delivery network, a purchasing health maintenance organization (HMO), or the Health Care Financing Administration, studies information that first accrues as a by-product of direct patient care.

SPREADING INFORMATION
TECHNOLOGY ACROSS THE INDUSTRY

Today the most highly evolved information systems in health care are found in hospitals. For over a generation, hospitals have invested in automated charge capture and billing systems to ensure they get paid for the work they do. In addition, automation produces great economies for these organizations in which negotiated or prospective payments limit the amount of cost that can be passed on to third-party underwriters. These economies have spread into clinical areas, where information technology, on a single platform, delivers improved workflow, virtual access to a wide range of capabilities, and rules-based functionality. This means clinicians are finding it easier and more productive to use a computer as a clinical tool at the time when the industry most needs them to keep a complete audit trail of their activities.

The opportunities arising from information technology are spreading across the continuum of care. Low-cost alternatives to hospitalization are increasingly used, but having recently caught the attention of the government, these services are now facing the same pressures of prospective and negotiated rate-setting as inpatient services. Consequently, outpatient centers, clinics, physicians' offices, and home care agencies are following closely behind hospitals in the automation of their clinical and financial activities.

INTEGRATING THE
HEALTH CARE INDUSTRY

Automation among the principal settings of care is fortuitous for those parties who value information about the effectiveness of health care services. They include many types of organizations that today play a role in shaping how health care services are and will be delivered. These organizations follow a variety of models—community-based integrated delivery networks, national chains and consortia, contracting health plans, provider-based HMOs, and federal and state assistance programs, such as Medicare and Medicaid. Despite their differences in mission or structure, they share a need for the same types of health care information. Each of these organizations depends on the industry's developing a new infrastructure, moving from a visit- or encounter-oriented framework to one that promotes *wellness*.

Gone are the days when hospitals, physicians, clinics, and home care agencies operated in separate market segments, optimizing the dollars available to each care setting. Within the space of a single presidential administration, the health care industry and society as a whole have shifted to embrace the notion that the way to reduce the overall cost burden of health care is to focus on *health* rather than *care*. This has sent the entire industry to the drawing board, devising ways to integrate the independent information systems of each health care setting into a virtual system that offers a logically integrated view of clinical activities across the continuum of care. Furthermore, as the unit of revenue in health care spirals upward from rate-based care to per-member per-month payments, there is a newfound requirement to reconcile people's lifetime risk of health care cost to their cost of coverage.

This raises two important questions. What information technologies are essential for accomplishing this latest set of challenges? And how will an industry so pressured to reduce its overhead absorb the necessary cost of this new information infrastructure?

Essential Information Technologies

In planning information systems for today's health care organization, the to-do list is a mixed bag of mature mainstream technologies and emerging concepts and initiatives. Broadly speaking, these fall into four main categories: connectivity, person identification, optical imaging and storage, and point of care applications.

CONNECTIVITY.   Physical connectivity is a mission-critical consideration when planning and budgeting for information technologies. The extent to which an organization can share data among its interested parties is determined by its ability to connect its entities and users on a single network. As information becomes more plentiful, more available, and more complex, an organization requires significant increases in bandwidth (data transfer capacity) across its network to ensure timely delivery of mission-critical knowledge.

Good network planning ensures three important benefits. It helps facilitate the type of collaboration among caregivers and other parties that results in cost-effective utilization of services. It also connects those in need of information to external networks and databases, such as those for electronic claims adjudication, medical reference, and patient registry, or to the Internet. Finally, a well-connected organization has fewer growing pains when merging or affiliating with other networked organizations.

PERSON IDENTIFICATION.   Health care is adopting successful network technology from other industries, but logical connectivity among information systems is something the health care industry must master on its own. The stand-alone information systems of major health care providers are adequate for handling encounter-oriented clinical and financial transactions. Consider, however, what happens when one provider affiliates with several others and needs to track the activities of a patient across multiple settings of care. Each provider's system creates a unique tracking number for each visit, making it almost impossible to use those tracking numbers to connect a person's activities at one facility with those at another.

This challenge has given rise to a new application, the *person index.* The primary function of this software is to assign a unique and permanent identification number to an individual and to manage each individual's relationship to encounter-based transactions across the health enterprise. If the information systems in different facilities assign different visit codes or patient IDs for each transaction pertaining to the same individual, it is the job of the person index to reconcile these codes back to the person's permanent identification number.

In a managed care environment, a person is enrolled as a member in a plan. The system's member record often contains clinical profile and demographic information similar to that which a hospital system would require upon admission. The person may never have been a patient at any of the plan's facilities, but the plan's financial risk for that person's care creates the need for a record with a person identification number.

Whether an organization maintains a strict provider focus as an integrated delivery network, operates as an insurance entity with a network of providers on contract, or integrates the insurance and provider functions fully into a single enterprise, it needs to align clinical encounters across a variety of health care settings with the identity of an individual. The creation and validation of this unique computer identity will become increasingly important. Moreover, technology will improve the ability of the person index to guarantee identity, from complex algorithms that use demographic data (alternate spellings, word transposition, maiden names and aliases, and social security and driver's license numbers) to smart cards, fingerprint matches, and voice recognition devices.

OPTICAL IMAGING AND STORAGE. The challenges inherent in the rapid proliferation of complex data types are of growing interest. A great deal of health care information cannot be entered into electronic screens that mimic paper forms. This information includes the text documents, electronic tracings by medical monitoring devices, photographs, x rays, diagnostic images, clinical specimens, and audio- and videotapes that also must be considered part of the integrated record of care. Each of these types of data has special creation and storage needs. Each has implications for both physical and logical connectivity as well.

High-density, high-capacity optical storage makes it possible to store complex multimedia data on-line, but because of the vast size of these information objects when converted to digital format, the information system must have extremely broad bandwidth across the organization to give a large population of users routine access to them with reasonable response time. In addition, because different data types normally require unique access and storage platforms, the organization's ability to provide the user an integrated view of a record containing multiple data types (image, voice, and video) depends on its ability to link these elements logically to a single person.

POINT OF CARE APPLICATIONS. Even in handling the more routine types of information (those easily captured by typing them into a computer or by pointing and clicking at items on the screen), there is also a revolution of sorts taking place. Data entry was once a task performed by administrative users, but now more and more clinicians are using computers directly as part of the patient care process. Use of these *point of care* systems, so called because they make data collection a by-product of caring for a patient, is replacing the process of filling out paper charts or dictating notes.

Point of care systems are the product of hardware that remains unobtrusively in an exam room or at the bedside and software that simulates the clinician's normal workflow and does not require complete clinician reeducation. Point of care access contributes to overall system integrity because information is captured and displayed as close to real time as possible.

Simply collecting information at the point of care does not ensure that information's value to the organization, however. For this reason, organizations are asking that their clinical systems promote *structured data* capture and storage. Structured data extend "the benefits of collected data to the community of clinical information users by ensuring that . . . [these data are] organized in an orderly fashion for persistent storage across multiple users. The scheme for storage of clinical data ultimately will determine whether a clinician's documentation can be the basis for queries and cross-sectional studies, as well as contribute to information on population health and wellness, outcomes, and treatment efficacy" (Dodson, 1997, p. 25).

It is through this multipurpose use that organizations seek to realize a return on their investments in information technology. Furthermore, because structures for health care delivery continue to change and evolve, collecting data at their most granular ensures an organization's flexibility when it is faced with unexpected mergers, affiliations, or alliances.

Barriers to Information System Deployment

There are some barriers that challenge the deployment of information systems, and many of them are not technological. As in Codman's time, there remain clinical areas where the industry has yet to reach consensus on a common vocabulary. This makes aggregating and summarizing many types of data difficult at the regional and national levels. In addition, security remains a political tug-of-war between the traditional value system that protects the sensitivity of patient medical information and the new globalism that views health care information as a commodity in a consumer-driven world.

Putting data to use in a managed care environment often means adopting clinical guidelines and imposing clinical standards for care.

To support this, systems will allow clinical rule sets to be applied to the workflow of caregivers, evaluating their scientific process against preestablished norms and offering only those clinical options that are plan approved. Developing rule sets that can span demographic, problem, functional, and disease categories requires the knowledge that will result only from studying the continuous, detailed, structured data of systems not yet in widespread use.

FUNDING NEW INFORMATION TECHNOLOGY WITH CHANGE

It is easy to get caught up exploring the possibilities that technology affords an industry as complex as health care. More important, however, is to consider how the health care industry can acquire the information it needs to support its own restructuring without having the cost of the technology outstrip the potential economies. It is critical to understand what information is used at each level of health care delivery, where that information gets harvested, and who bears the cost of producing the information.

Health plans and insurance companies use information for authorization and claims processing that is similar to the information used by providers for delivering care and submitting bills. The fact that the information needs of payer and provider are closely related is diagnostic as well as prescriptive. Here is an area where collaboration among payers and providers can remove administrative redundancy and bring corresponding benefit.

Those who underwrite health care require clinical information in order to determine what they will and will not pay for. Consequently, health plans need to drive their own internal systems to the same level of clinical granularity that providers now seek. The cost of these technological enhancements will be passed on to providers, consumers, or both.

Populating such systems on the health plan side will still require the cooperation of the providers for crucial information captured at the point of care. These providers deserve consideration from health plans for bearing the administrative costs of producing information of value to both parties. Perhaps it is time for providers and payers to eliminate what distance still separates them, enhancing the information on hand in the provider community rather than establishing an overlying, competing health plan infrastructure with related or redundant systems.

Another way to relieve some of the cost burden to the industry is to mobilize information, to push it out to the health care consumer. Current experiments in *community access management* seek to demonstrate that health screening and proactive management of individuals with chronic conditions can result in more appropriate use and timing of health care encounters. Information technology brings health care organizations a cost-effective way to influence the health of individuals for whom they are at risk. Protocols for care, normal ranges for test results, information on self-monitoring and screening, guidelines for use of over-the-counter medications or emergency facilities, and educational materials can all be distributed to individuals and households via desktop software or Internet technology. In addition, the organization can provide a managed care feedback loop that includes telephone or E-mail triage and referral links back to its own facilities.

The key to consumer-based models is to recognize the long-term importance of capturing self-managed care information as ordinary encounters. Just as care was driven from hospitals to alternative settings of care, cost pressures will continue to drive patients to assume more responsibility for their wellness. Although accessing information may someday replace the need to visit with a clinician, the industry must first harvest the information that helps assess how and when it is safe to let individuals do so.

CONCLUSION

In 1900, a humble physician named Codman, joined by his chief of service, began documenting his clinical experiences with an insightful look at the value this information would provide, even beyond his own relationships with patients. He would later write, "This routine tracing of every case, interesting or uninteresting, had brought to our notice many things in which our knowledge, our technique, our organization, our own skill or wisdom, and perhaps even our care and our consciences needed attention" (Codman, 1934, p. xii).

Nearly a century later, computerized information technology makes it possible to record and link the activities associated with health and care across a wide variety of settings. The building blocks laid by Codman will continue to determine whether the health care industry meets its ongoing social and political challenges. Perhaps even Codman himself would be surprised by the extent to which information plays a pivotal role in shaping the delivery systems of a complex industry and in managing cost, quality, and access at every level.

References

Codman, E. A. *The Shoulder.* Boston: Thomas Todd, 1934.

Codman, E. A. "The Product of a Hospital." *Archives of Pathological Laboratory Medicine,* 1990, *114,* 491–496. (Originally published in *Surgery Gynecology and Obstetrics,* 1914.)

Codman, E. A. *A Study in Hospital Efficiency as Demonstrated by the Case Report of the First Five Years of a Private Hospital.* Joint Commission on Accreditation of Healthcare Organizations, 1996. (Originally printed privately, Boston, 1917.)

DePalma, A. F. "Ernest Amory Codman (1869–1940): A Biography." *Clinical Orthopaedics,* 1961, *20,* 1–7.

Dodson, E. "Structured Data: Smart Medicine for Today's Clinical Systems." *Group Practices Journal,* Oct. 1997, 24–27.

Neuhauser, D. "Ernest Amory Codman, M.D., and End Results of Medical Care." *International Journal of Technology Assessment in Health Care,* 1990, *6,* 307–325.

CHAPTER TWENTY-TWO

Wiring the Health Revolution

Morton H. Meyerson

Morton H. Meyerson has more than thirty years experience in the information technology services industry. He served as chairman of the board for Perot Systems Corporation from 1992 to 1998. A believer in strategic partnering with clients, Meyerson increased revenue at Perot Systems an average of 40 percent a year. He began his career in 1963 at Bell Helicopter and in 1966 joined Electronic Data Systems, where he served as president from 1979 to 1986.

$\sim\!\!\!\sim\!\!\!\sim$

Business activity in every industry can be made more efficient or effective through the application of information technology and new business processes. The typical pattern of technology-enabled innovation follows a cycle of

1. Reducing costs by replacing labor and scarce resources with capital

2. Leveraging investments and the efficient use of assets

3. Enhancing products and services for new or restructured markets

4. Enabling decision making

5. Reaching the consumer

Many people have written about and forecast an additional cycle in which new products or services created through "informationalizing an existing business" can "break away and become free standing businesses that can ultimately grow to rival or surpass the original business in revenue, profits, and market value" (Davis and Davidson, 1991, pp. 52–53). American Airlines' reservation system, Sabre, is a frequently used example.

In health care several companies are just beginning to use information content generated by hospitals and insurance and managed care companies to develop new Internet-based information businesses whose success may eventually rival health care enterprises as we know them today. However, health care has traditionally lagged behind other industries in efforts to improve business activities. Much work is still required to reduce health care industry costs by making basic business processes more efficient. This is especially true for emerging integrated health networks, in which processes for enrolling members in health plans, scheduling resources and patients, and managing care across a continuum of settings all have significant potential for technology-enabled process improvement.

FIRST SIGNS OF
TECHNOLOGY IMPROVEMENTS

Use of information and information technology is just beginning to enhance services for a restructured health care market. For example:

• Many managed care companies now offer health care information delivered through a system of triage call centers staffed by nurses as an enhancement to their traditional health care administration services.

• Some health care providers use various forms of interactive media to deliver information to support informed decisions and choices about alternative courses of action for chronic and acute diseases and medical conditions.

• Other innovative health plans are offering interactive applications to help their members master stress, in an attempt to reduce the estimated 40 to 60 percent of physician visits that are stress related (Davidson, 1998).

However, we are just scratching the surface of the fourth and fifth phases of the technology innovation cycle in health care: enabling clinical decision making and reaching the consumer. *Information appliances* are not yet a common fixture on the desktops of clinicians, and even in the early 1990s only 3 percent of the total national health expenditure went to prevention (Centers for Disease Control, 1992).

The health care information technology lag exists in part because health care has traditionally spent less than other industries on information technology. Hospitals and integrated delivery networks dedicated an average of 5.4 percent of their overall budgets to information technology in 1996, up from 4.8 percent the previous year, according to a survey conducted by the College of Healthcare Information Management Executives (1997). These figures are well below the estimated 15 percent of revenue spent on information technology by securities, brokerage, and asset management companies ("Spending Levels . . .," 1998).

The root cause of this low rate of expenditure lies primarily in the history of an industry that has been characterized by employer-sponsored benefits and governmental subsidies on the one hand and a fee-for-service payment scheme on the other. In this environment, little economic incentive existed to improve business activity. However, the environment has now changed. The U.S. health care market is now highly competitive, with significant economic incentive to improve business activity. Clinicians are assuming financial risk through risk-based pricing models, and consumers are becoming increasingly responsible for their health care costs.

In this restructuring process, health care enterprises must move quickly through the technology innovation cycle to the point of enabling clinical decision making and reaching the consumer through technology. Indeed, this is the holy grail quest of health care and the future of technology.

ENABLING CLINICAL DECISIONS

To get a sense of the potential impact of using technology to enable clinical decision making and reach the consumer in health care, it is helpful to consider both the pricing model and the cost structure of the health care enterprise.

Health care enterprises, today's managed care organizations and delivery networks, are either currently receiving fixed fees for the delivery of health services to a defined population or for the treatment of a specific disease or condition, or they will be moving to a fixed-fee structure in the future. From this fixed fee, health care enterprises spend relatively small amounts, 10 to 15 percent, on administration and overhead. In addition, both for-profit and not-for-profit entities have operating margins in the range of 2 to 15 percent. The vast majority of enterprise costs, 75 to 90 percent, are for medical delivery ("Market, Financial, and Operating Statistics," 1997a, 1997b). For health care enterprises, medical delivery is the equivalent of cost of goods sold and because these enterprises no longer operate in a cost-plus pricing mode, they must give significant attention to the medical delivery portion of their cost structure.

There are two primary drivers of medical delivery costs—consumer decisions to enter the health care delivery system and clinical decisions about the ways individuals should proceed through this system. Moreover, these consumer and clinical decisions have some interesting characteristics.

Fully informed consumers usually choose less risky and less expensive options than do those with little information. The effect of the availability of information in modifying consumer behavior was illustrated in a 1994 study by the Harvard University School of Public Health (Leavenworth, 1995). The study found that when nurses provided twenty-four-hour health information by telephone, 82 percent of privately insured callers and 92 percent of Medicaid callers who were about to use a hospital emergency room selected a lower level of care. More than 20 percent decided to treat their problems at home, without further assistance. According to another study, 89 percent of insured callers and 75 percent of Medicaid callers who planned to see a physician chose less costly alternatives (Leavenworth, 1995).

Clinical decisions show wide geographical variations in practice style, with corresponding differences in cost and quality outcomes

(Wennberg, 1996). Research from the Rand Corporation has demonstrated that a number of common and costly procedures are often unnecessary and inappropriate (Rand Corporation, 1991a, 1991b, 1992a, 1992b, 1992c, 1993a, 1993b). The reality is that clinicians can make errors of omission and commission that reduce clinical effectiveness and increase costs. However, many, if not most, errors are related to a lack of information rather than a lack of education or training.

This presents an interesting situation and challenge. Consumer and clinical decisions drive approximately 80 percent of cost and quality results in health care. Spending on health care in the United States during 1995 reached approximately $988.5 billion (Levit and others, 1996), and is expected to reach $1,472 billion by the year 2000 (Congressional Budget Office, 1995). The evidence suggests that significant cost reductions and improvements in quality can result if we can enable clinical decisions, and reach the consumer through information and information technology. Yet we have not even begun to penetrate the potential that exists. This is the link between health care and the future of technology.

Consider the nature of clinical decision making as we know it today. Most clinical decision making is still completely dependent on the judgment of the individual medical practitioner. Basing decisions on their training and experience, physicians select the course of treatment to follow and how to apply this treatment. The use of information technology in this process is still fairly limited, although the use of clinical decision rules in patient care is starting to expand. For example, many health care enterprises have developed clinical pathways that attempt to standardize certain aspects of care. Actual outcomes of patient care are compared against these standards, and changes may be suggested or discussed. The pathways are the result of analyzing large numbers of patient records and determining what may work best for a patient or for a specific disease. The fundamental purpose of the pathway development process is to look for evidence that supports specific clinical interventions as the best ways of treating an illness. In this search, which typically uses computer-based data, it is common that existing practices are found to be neither optimal nor representative of the best patient care. Because more data are available for larger groups of patients, information technology can be employed to develop the evidence that supports best clinical practices.

This information revolution is beginning to change the everyday practice of medicine. By tracking what treatments work best, we are beginning to get answers to long-standing questions. What are the chances that a patient will regain normal functioning? What are the results (morbidity, mortality, costs) of various treatment options in treating a specific condition? The amount of data needed to answer these and other fundamental questions illustrates why more than half of all medical treatments have never been validated by clinical trials.

A number of companies have taken clinical knowledge and embedded it in information systems. The hypothesis behind such systems is that many medical errors are due to a physician's intrinsic limits rather than to remedial flaws in knowledge. Information theory states that to eliminate such errors, one must commit more time to the processing of the relevant data (McDonald, 1976). The following example illustrates how a computer, given the necessary decision logic (protocols), can provide the processing time necessary to reduce clinical errors.

Clement McDonald, M.D., codirector of the Regenstrief Institute for Health Care and one of the pioneers in the development of computer-assisted medical decision making, performed an experiment in which he measured the response rate of residents in an outpatient clinic to indications for more than 150 different clinical indications. Believing that patient outcomes could be improved, McDonald created a computer-based clinical reminder program, based on physician-authored rules, that recommended particular steps to the residents when a clinically significant indication occurred. The responses of control and study groups of residents to the 15 most common indications were examined in detail.

For example, a control group of residents had a response rate of only 22 percent for the indication of occult blood in a stool sample. The response rate to the same indicator of a group of residents using the reminder program was 55 percent (McDonald and others, 1984). A previous study by McDonald (1976) also showed that a control group of physicians reacted to only 22 percent of certain events but that the group using protocol-based computer reminders reacted to 51 percent. These studies concluded that the amount of data presented to the physician per unit of time is more than one person can process without error. They demonstrate how the computer augments a physician's capabilities and thereby reduces error rates.

INFORMATION TECHNOLOGY'S FUTURE IMPACT

Now consider clinical decision making in a future in which there is significant and widespread use of information and information technology. As a result of systematic collection of clinical data, it will become possible to start the process of determining what actually constitutes good patient care. With the explosion of new technology and the expanded collection and linking of data representing the patient's entire experience (inpatient, outpatient, physician's office, and so forth) and the outcomes of different treatments, we can derive new knowledge of the optimal treatment for a patient or a disease.

The challenge is to apply this knowledge at the point of clinical decision making in a manner that truly influences the decision. Once the clinician has a more complete set of data points about a patient's specific condition, an evidence-based body of knowledge about treatment options and results will facilitate a customized approach to patient treatment. Nuances in a specific patient's disease symptoms, genetic makeup, and treatment options will be more easily synthesized and then assessed against the clinical knowledge base to determine which options are most likely to result in the desired patient outcome.

The patient will have access to the complete set of options tailored to the specifics of his disease and condition. The physician will have access to a much greater evidence-based body of knowledge that simply is not available today in an organized format. This is likely to lead to more focused and better-quality care simply because additional knowledge and insight are available to both patient and physician. Information technology will be able to distribute this knowledge to the point of care for use by the physician and patient and to the patient at home as he considers what treatment options might make the most sense given his preferences.

REACHING THE CONSUMER

The state of consumer decisions regarding personal health matters, both prevention issues and specific diseases or conditions, is also undergoing a dramatic and very rapid change, currently marked by a significant rise in active health consumerism.

For example, it is estimated that 50 to 60 percent of the general Internet user population has accessed health care information via the Internet (personal communication with Steve Shaha). The 1997 American Internet Users Survey (Miller, 1998) found that of the Internet users, 43 percent of men and 50 percent of women say they routinely access health care information on the Internet. According to Thomas Ferguson, M.D. (1996), one of the architects of the self-care movement in the United States and author of the book *Health Online,* the World Wide Web has more than twenty-five thousand health-related sites. However, today's consumers are still largely on their own; collection and delivery of health care information from and to consumers via technology is still fragmented and ad hoc. Also, the information that is available is often disease specific and presented in formats not generally easy for consumers to interpret.

Equipping the consumer with information via technology facilitates her participation in managing her demand for health care services, which in turn reduces health care expenditures and increases consumer satisfaction. This is a managed care model based on reaching and engaging the consumer rather than a model based on access control.

CONSUMER-ORIENTED HEALTH CARE

Consider a future in which health care enterprises consistently and systematically reach the consumer with information via technology. The *customer health care center* of the future will provide demand management products, services, and technology solutions for its entire member base, with an objective of serving and empowering the consumer rather than denying access to the delivery system. For example, an advanced customer health care center will offer these services.

- *Health history, health risk, and functional status reports:* self-administered and nurse-assisted health evaluations to assist in identifying consumers at risk of certain health disorders and also to set a baseline for the surveyed consumer population. Automated evaluation tools will enable direct consumer input via the Internet or private intranet and can be used by the customer health care center during one-on-one conversations with consumers.

- *Health reporting and management plans:* consumer population reports and individual management plans created subsequent to the health evaluations. Specific population-based and individual health solutions, target marketing, and physician referrals will be developed from evaluation information, with the consumer's consent. Computerized tracking will allow the center to automatically generate the appropriate follow-up activities and correspondence.

- *Interactive self-triage and health education:* consumer self-care systems, which include self-triage and on-line health education information and allow consumers to access the same consistent set of tools used by health care professionals. This knowledge will have widespread implications for the patient. Rather than being largely dependent on the practitioner's opinion, the patient will have access to the same information that was once the exclusive domain of the practitioner. This information about the outcomes of care will allow patients to assume a greater level of responsibility for their healing processes and have potentially better outcomes.

- *Health forums and support groups:* on-line health forums, support groups, and bulletin board services to enhance consumer-provider relations and consumer-physician loyalty. This strategy will be consistent with the way existing Internet forums operate but will be greatly enhanced by structured applications that will match consumer needs with the most appropriate discussion area.

- *Health transactions and communications:* enhanced communication among consumers, physicians, hospitals, and the customer health care center. This communication will increase efficiency as well as loyalty across the customer and referral base. Information about locations, services offered, and availability will be transmitted electronically, as will such specific transactions as determining eligibility, scheduling, and sending electronic mail.

Timely access to information and services is a win-win state of affairs for both the consumer and the health care enterprise. For the consumer empowered with health information the result is improved self-care skills, a sense of belonging to a health community, and assurance of access to the most cost-effective disease management and treatment protocols. For the health enterprise, there is not only a reduced demand for health care services, and therefore a reduced cost

of goods sold, but a corresponding increase in consumer brand awareness and loyalty.

References

Centers for Disease Control. "Estimated National Spending on Preven-
     tion—United States, 1988. *Morbidity and Mortality Weekly Report,*
     1992, *41*(29), 531.
College of Healthcare Information Management Executives.
     "Financial/Budget Profile." In *H.I.S. Desk Reference: A CIO Survey*
     (1996 ed.). [Joint study by College of Healthcare Information
     Management Executives and HCIA, Inc.] 1997.
Congressional Budget Office. "CBO Projections of National Health
     Expenditures Through 2005." In *The Economic and Budget Outlook:
     An Update.* (Appendix D). Washington, D.C.: Congressional Budget
     Office, 1995.
Davidson, J. "Slowing the Hectic Pace of Stress." *Public Management,* 1998,
     80(4), 14ff.
Davis, S. M., and Davidson, W. H. *20/20 Vision: Transforming Your
     Business Today to Survive in Tomorrow's Economy.* New York:
     Simon & Schuster, 1991.
Ferguson, T. *Health Online: How to Find Health Information, Support
     Groups, and Self-Help Communities in Cyberspace.* Reading, Mass.:
     Addison-Wesley, 1996.
Leavenworth, G. "Informed Employees Make Better Consumers: Improved
     Medical Information Services Needed; Preventive Medicine:
     Strategies for Quality Care and Lower Cost" (Illustration).
     Business and Health, 1995, *13*(3), 7.
Levit, K. R., and others. "National Health Expenditures, 1995." *Health Care
     Financing Review,* 1996, *18*(1), 175.
McDonald, C. J. "Protocol-Based Computer Reminders, the Quality of
     Care, and the Non-Perfectibility of Man." *New England Journal of
     Medicine,* 1976, *295*(24), 1351–1355.
McDonald, C. J., and others. "Reminders to Physicians from an Introspec-
     tive Computer Medical Record: A Two-Year Randomized Trial."
     Annals of Internal Medicine, 1984, *100,* 130–138.
"Market, Financial, and Operating Statistics" [Tables A and B]. *Pulse,*
     Nov. 1997a.
"Market, Financial, and Operating Statistics" [Tables B and C]. *Pulse,* Dec.
     1997b.

Miller, T. (study director). *American Internet User's Survey.* New York: Cyber Dialogue and Find/SVP, 1998.

Rand Corporation. *Coronary Artery Bypass Graft: A Literature Review and Ratings of Appropriateness and Necessity.* Santa Monica, Calif.: Rand Corporation, 1991a.

Rand Corporation. *Percutaneous Transluminal Coronary Angioplasty: A Literature Review and Ratings of Appropriateness and Necessity.* Santa Monica, Calif.: Rand Corporation, 1991b.

Rand Corporation. *Abdominal Aortic Aneurysm Surgery: A Literature Review and Ratings of Appropriateness and Necessity.* Santa Monica, Calif.: Rand Corporation, 1992a.

Rand Corporation. *Carotid Endarterectomy: A Literature Review and Ratings of Appropriateness and Necessity.* Santa Monica, Calif.: Rand Corporation, 1992b.

Rand Corporation. *Coronary Angiography: A Literature Review and Ratings of Appropriateness and Necessity.* Santa Monica, Calif.: Rand Corporation, 1992c.

Rand Corporation. *The Appropriateness of Hysterectomy: A Comparison of Care in Seven Health Plans.* Santa Monica, Calif.: Rand Corporation, 1993a.

Rand Corporation. *Cataract Surgery: A Literature Review and Ratings of Appropriateness and Cruciality.* Santa Monica, Calif.: Rand Corporation, 1993b.

"Spending Levels Do Not Indicate Business Value." [Research notes COM-05–0316]. GartnerGroup RAS Services, Aug. 1998.

Wennberg, J. M.D. "The Diagnosis and Surgical Treatment of Common Medical Conditions." In Dartmouth Medical School, Center for the Evaluative Clinical Sciences, *The Dartmouth Atlas of Healthcare.* Chicago: American Hospital Publishing, 1996.

CHAPTER TWENTY-THREE

Strategic Health Care Computing

Russell J. Ricci

Russell J. Ricci, M.D., is general manager of IBM Global Healthcare Industry, a multibillion-dollar global industry and one of eleven major industry organizations within IBM. He leads a diverse team of IBM executives and business partners engaged in the delivery of strategic consulting services and information technology solutions to payers, providers, pharmaceutical companies, and other health care organizations.

Today the financial risks associated with the delivery of health care are shifting from payers to providers. To survive and succeed—and ultimately to fulfill their mission of service—providers must embrace an information technology (IT) strategy that can drive improved outcomes at a lower cost, becoming the silver lining in what some perceive as the otherwise gloomy cloud of managed care.

To get a taste for the possibilities, consider an analogy with an entirely different profession—banking. Laden with complex, sensitive, labor-intensive, and time-consuming transactions, banking was once boxed in with tedious and expensive administrative burdens. Twenty years ago the obstacles to improved service and lower cost seemed daunting, and given the issues of security and confidentiality, a computer networking solution would have seemed unlikely. Yet such a solution has occurred through the automated teller machine (ATM). Today, a person can use a bank ATM card at numerous street-corner machines around the world—anytime, anywhere networked banking. More important, the ATM solution not only streamlined banking for greater efficiency, it opened the door to new strategic opportunities, such as the inexpensive expansion of convenient twenty-four-hour banking locations and the use of the ATM card as a point-of-purchase debit mechanism.

RIVERS MEET: THE CONFLUENCE
OF NEED AND CAPABILITY

Like banking, health care is poised to benefit tremendously from developments in network computing. But the advantages here go far beyond efficiencies in administration and into the very heart of care; IT places valuable information at the point of care and thereby improving the quality of care.

Consider the need. According to a Deloitte & Touche study in 1996, a small fraction of all patients, a mere 3 to 6 percent, often in the last months of life, accounted for 65 to 70 percent of the total cost of care. With the health care industry comprising 14 percent of the 1997 U.S. gross domestic product (becoming the second largest component of the GDP) at $1 trillion in expenditures, there is a crystal-clear economic imperative to improve the delivery and quality of care to the chronically ill and the very sick, the 3 to 6 percent of the whole.

At the University of Texas M. D. Anderson Cancer Center, a well-known comprehensive cancer center in Houston, the clinical staff participated in the development of a Lotus Notes application to help physicians identify best practices—those that led to the most favorable patient outcomes—for various difficult and costly disease states. Staff members using this application identified dozens of disease-specific best-practice treatment models, which reduced inpatient length of stays without any appreciable decrease in patient satisfaction.

For patients receiving cancer-related hysterectomies, for instance, M. D. Anderson reduced the costs of tests by 35 percent, costs of prescriptions by 72 percent, and length of stays by 30 percent. Patient care was enhanced, and the hospital and health care system saved millions, according to Anderson.

In St. Louis, Missouri, BJC Health System (born in a 1993 merger of Barnes Jewish and Christian Health Services) has launched Project Spectrum, a Web technology-based solution uniting existing, disparate legacy patient records systems into one easy-to-use system accessible to physicians and researchers. An ambitious plan to improve individual patient care and enhance physician access to medical information, Project Spectrum faced the daunting task of integrating information systems from fifteen BJC hospital sites and more than 3,500 affiliated physicians. In 1997, BJC commissioned Ernst & Young to define, quantify, and project the costs and benefits associated with Project Spectrum. In its second year of operation, Project Spectrum is expected to produce cost benefits in the millions of dollars.

There is no longer any doubt that IT can and will have a large role in making managed care manageable and in changing care delivery patterns in all environments. The remaining issues involve the scope and nature of the tasks and the commensurate means for handling them.

CHALLENGES

In many ways the contemporary state of health care IT resembles a vast sea studded with islands of information. Among the islands are important sets of data—but the natives speak different languages, no one has a good map, and the boats needed to get from one island to the next are missing their compasses. Successful health care IT must translate the languages into a common tongue, develop an easy way to navigate through the information, and create vehicles that make it easy for the user to get from one set of information to the next.

In sum, health care IT needs to integrate many fragmented systems into one connected network. The successful network must:

- *Address all the constituents:* they include physicians, patients, insurers, employers, vendors, managed care organizations, suppliers, governmental regulators, and others.

- *Be easy to connect and cost effective:* from legacy systems to desktop PCs, everything must interconnect without being prohibitively expensive.

- *Employ open standards:* they must allow different systems to interface without obstructions.

- *Combine technologies:* the Internet can be joined with intranets (internal organizational networks) and extranets (highly secure networks administered by a third party to admit only qualified users) to form one fluid network, accessible anywhere.

- *Create an adequate network infrastructure:* the average medical record consumes four megabytes; the average chest x ray, six megabytes. Medical information, especially imaging (x rays, MRIs, CT scans, sonograms) tends to be data intensive, and you cannot squeeze a flood of information through a garden-hose network.

- *Offer remote connections, to provide immediate information, regardless of location:* this is a critical issue for mobile health care providers, such as those in home care, and for the distribution of patient information and education.

BRIDGES

The common denominator is integration. The current state of data and information—stranded on various islands such as admittance reports, lab reports, patient histories, and discharge summaries—runs counter to the need to manage costs, manage outcomes, market products and services, expand customer outreach, and provide wider information access to providers and consumers. In order for any of these initiatives to succeed, health care stakeholders must be able to draw on information culled, analyzed, and distributed across all the previously isolated computer sources: the islands must be bridged, interconnected, and bound by a common power to communicate in a secure environment.

This vast transformation of content will involve a parallel, and welcome, transformation of access. With information rooted in a solid network of computing power, users will no longer need closed proprietary systems to access information; in computer parlance the trend is away from *fat* clients (hardware- and software-intensive PCs, for example) and toward *thin* clients (Web TVs or smart phones, for example) that are less expensive to run, easier to maintain, and best of all, easier to use.

The amounts of information contained in these systems will become an invaluable resource, a veritable treasure trove of business and health gems that can and should be used to improve care models and patient outcomes as we evolve toward evidence-based medicine. The technology to be used is called *data-mining*. In health care it is currently being used successfully to ferret out fraudulent claims at several major payer organizations, including the Health Care Financing Administration. Other industries, such as banking and utilities, mine customer information for gold, using it to identify trends and products to sell to the customer base. Why not mine the accumulated data on patient outcomes to assess the effectiveness of care your organization provides or to identify best practices that can enhance patient care and cut costs? The technology exists today to get started.

ON THE HORIZON

Recent market research reveals two dominant themes for the future: first, a movement toward greater clinical productivity and focused, consistent delivery of provider services and, second, the rising empowerment of consumers, who will demand clinical products and services designed to fit their specific needs and delivered at their convenience (according to a 1997 IBM/Wilkerson study). The resulting confluence of these trends generates market pressure: pressure to create flexible health care products and services to meet consumer demands and pressure to deliver the same at the consumer's convenience—any place, any time.

How can health care providers respond to these and other pressures? The most promising method is e-business.

Just as the standardization of the track gauge for railroads in the nineteenth century spurred the rise of nationwide enterprises, Web technology is making global enterprise an obtainable, present reality. But in a significant departure from any previous means of distribution, collaboration, and communication, the Web is personal, direct, and inexpensive and capable of delivering services tailored to the exact needs of an organization's consumers and constituents. That is the true power of the Web; that is the real promise of e-business.

With the expansion of the World Wide Web, the Internet is no longer the domain of a technological elite but a familiar and growing force in the U.S. home. Internet use among adults continues to climb; the demographic group showing the fastest growth in activity is also the group with the fastest growing need for health services and information: the over-fifty-five age group. In addition, a recent study by MediConsult.com revealed that up to 40 percent of all adults "surfing" the Web seek medical or health information (Sutcliffe, 1997).

Finding information at sites in a computer network is not only appealing, it is inexpensive. The banking industry, for instance, lowered its per-transaction costs dramatically. According to a study by Booz-Allen & Hamilton, the typical bank branch transaction costs $1.08. The same transaction costs $0.54 on the telephone and a mere $0.26 through PC software. But the Web topped them all, with an average transaction cost of only $0.13.

The advantages for health care are obvious. Given a cost of $8.00 to $9.00 to pull a medical record manually, health care has an immediate incentive to improve its records retrieval capabilities. And record retrieval is just the tip of the e-business iceberg. However, to leverage the full power of network computing to improve clinical quality and develop greater market flexibility, the health care industry must embrace a new role in technological leadership. Moreover, network computing must be conducted in a secure, confidential environment. Concern over personal privacy and the confidentiality of patient information is a hotly debated issue in health care these days. Although there are those who contend it cannot be done, technologies developed for the encapsulation encryption of highly confidential and valuable intellectual capital now provide the answer to this concern.

INTO THE FUTURE

With so many of the critical technologies already in place in other industries, now is not the time to wait and see; now is the time to see and act. Several provider organizations have already launched major Internet-based initiatives that are reshaping both the nature of their care and its delivery.

In 1997, Allina Health System, an integrated system of clinics, hospitals, and health plans in Minnesota, western Wisconsin, and North and South Dakota, developed Allina HealthVillage, an Internet site that provides twenty-four-hour-a-day, seven-day-a-week access to medical, drug reference, and health plan information. Allina had two major goals: to provide plan members with information that would empower them to make informed decisions about their own health care, and to cut administrative costs by providing members with direct access to benefit information. Through Allina HealthVillage, members can now access a directory of providers, find health and wellness information, and receive updates on classes and seminars sponsored by Allina. In the future, members will find expanded appointment scheduling, access to Allina's library services, a personal health diary, and other tools that will allow them to take greater control of their health.

A secure extranet can also be a crucial provider-to-provider pathway. VHA, Inc., a national alliance of more than 1,600 not-for-profit health care organizations, needed a practical way for members to carry out business transactions and share patient information and best practices. Although VHA members recognized the competitive advantage they would gain by sharing information and the clinical advances they could make by sharing best practices, they seemed trapped by incompatible legacy systems.

VHA collaborated with IBM Global Network to create VHAseCURE.net, an extranet that links members' current internal networks through Web sites. Without having to invest in whole new systems, members now enjoy real-time communication with one another, sharing information about practices, products, and services. Clinicians, researchers, and administrators can participate in health care forums, analyze supplier contracts, distribute community health information, and provide performance improvement programs. VHA estimates that the bigger health care systems might save millions of dollars every year from the greater efficiency allowed by the network.

The interest in innovative network computing is not limited to the United States. In Milan, Italy, for example, the Istituto Nazionale per lo Studio e la Cura dei Tumori, a major cancer center, sought a way to reduce high costs and lengthy patient stays as it maintained a culture of caring for long-term, terminally ill patients. A live video system provided the solution by allowing caregivers to monitor cancer patients at home. Linked to the institute by the Internet, the video system lets physicians monitor their patients on regular morning and evening rounds. The virtual rounds offer not only an inexpensive means of ensuring quality care but the patient intimacy and reassurance needed to sustain the institute's personal care mission.

OPPORTUNITIES AND LESSONS

The examples in this chapter have illustrated the power of network computing to improve both the practice of medicine and the business of health care. By sharing clinical information, providers can create data warehouses, mine that data, and then determine and distribute best clinical practices for improved quality and outcomes. As on-line participants in the distribution of knowledge, consumers can participate in therapeutic communities of interest, retrieve critical information, and take greater control of and responsibility for their health. Internet-based solutions give health care organizations extraordinary but relatively inexpensive opportunities to leverage administrative efficiencies, establish their brand, increase market share, and become more immediately responsive in an increasingly dynamic and flexible marketplace.

To realize these advantages, however, we need to learn from the technology leaders—and then become leaders ourselves. Stasis is not an option. In an environment of consolidation and growing demand for clinical and financial accountability, health care organizations must develop the IT resources that allow instant, organization-wide access to critical information, and they must do so fast. This information can then be used at the point of care to change physician behavior, to alter our present model of clinical care to a true evidence-based paradigm.

Reference

Sutcliffe, I. "A Glimpse of the Future: Consumer Marketing on the Web and Beyond." Speech at IBM seminar, Palisades, N.Y., Sept. 16, 1997.

CHAPTER TWENTY-FOUR

Technology-Induced Ethical Questions

Stephen R. Latham

Stephen R. Latham is director of ethics standards at the American Medical Association. A graduate of Harvard Law School, he practiced health law in Boston and San Francisco before receiving his Ph.D. degree from the University of California at Berkeley. Latham has taught ethics and political theory at Brown University, legal ethics at Harvard Law School and Berkeley, and health care business law at Berkeley and the University of Chicago.

At this writing my grandmother is in rehabilitation for knee surgery. When she was born, there was no penicillin or insulin or cortisone, no polio vaccine, no technique for separating and storing blood, no intravenous shunt—to say nothing of microsurgery or lithotripsy or coronary artery bypass graft or organ transplant. Peo-

The views expressed in this chapter are the author's own and not necessarily those of the AMA.

ple alive today have witnessed a stunning expansion of what medicine is capable of doing, an expansion largely though not entirely due to technological advance. Our shared experience of this explosion in medical progress necessarily frames our conceptions of medicine and of the ethics that must govern its practice.

In this chapter I offer what amounts to a rather breathless tour of some (certainly not all) of the issues that I predict will face biomedical ethics as a result of this continued explosion of technological progress. I have stayed entirely away from issues (such as abortion) that seem to me not profoundly affected by technological change. In the interest of brevity I have also sacrificed discussion of such hot topics as cloning in favor of touching on issues more likely to affect more readers. I offer the following predictions hesitantly, knowing that recent experience of rapid change is hardly the best basis for confident prognostication.

RESEARCH ETHICS

Our recent experience of explosive progress in medicine has given us a reasonably well-grounded faith that a large number of present medical problems—the absence of a vaccine for HIV disease, the need for more cancer cures, the technical problems of genetic manipulation—will, eventually, be solved. In light of this faith it is not difficult to reach the dangerous conclusion that medical research is just as-yet-unrecognized medical progress. Some patients are anxious to enroll in research protocols because they think that research is just another name for cutting-edge medicine. But research is research; it often involves unpredictable risks and uncertain benefits, and in many cases enrollment in a research protocol means enrollment as part of the control group or as a placebo recipient. Researchers and institutional review boards will have to exercise great care to ensure that subjects do not consent to enrollment in research protocols due to false hopes or to misconceptions about the risks of medical research.

GENETICS

Scientific knowledge about the links between genes and medical problems is growing at a tremendous rate. This poses quite a few problems. Most practicing physicians know very little about genetics and genetic diseases; many older physicians never even had to take basic human genetics in medical school. There is a chronic shortage of trained genetic counselors. These facts combined mean that it is difficult for patients to get the accurate information they need in order to give (or withhold) informed consent to genetic testing or to procedures (such as prophylactic mastectomy) based on genetic test outcomes. We need to conduct educational and outreach programs to ensure that patients and their physicians can understand both the utility and the limits of genetic tests and can interpret test results properly. We need also to inform patients and the public of the import that a genetic test result may have for family members who share genetic traits with the test taker. In some instances we may need to offer genetic counseling not just to individual patients but to whole families. Finally, physicians and patients will need to be aware that genetic test results may expose patients to discriminatory practices, and they will need to take care that test results are kept confidential.

No discussion of the ethics of genetic medicine is complete without some mention of the risk of eugenic practices. The use of genetic therapy to cure specific conditions in specific patients seems not unlike other medical therapy, but the use of germ-line genetic therapy to eliminate specific conditions from a family's genetic inheritance is more problematic. It is a small step from there to germ-line genetic enhancement and from there to discrimination against the nonenhanced. Moreover, it is not clear that we know enough about genetic interactions, or about the interactions between genetics and environment, to justify widespread use of germ-line interventions. Experimental design in this area will require close monitoring.

PRIVACY, SECURITY, AND CONFIDENTIALITY

More and more medical records are being kept in computers. People sitting at other computers very far away can copy and open those records. This has tremendous medical advantages—records can be forwarded from a physician's office to an emergency room at the press of a button—but it also poses grave threats. This increased technological opportunity for obtaining confidential medical information is matched with an increasing motive for obtaining it. Recent advances in our understanding of genetic illness mean, among other things, that a well-taken medical history or the results of an appropriately given genetic test can have strong predictive power. In other words, medical records will increasingly contain information not only about how healthy a person has been and is but about how healthy the person will be years in the future. The financial incentive for insurers and employers to identify and select away from potentially costly insureds and employees is strong. We need to develop techniques to ensure that patient records are secure and that patient rights to privacy and confidentiality are not violated.

An important ethics issue is raised when patients waive their rights to privacy and confidentiality. There are a number of legitimate purposes for examining patients' medical records. They include insurance utilization review to establish whether a health care provider is following proper medical and record-keeping procedures; peer review to establish the qualifications of a physician on the basis of her track record; and retrospective medical research to discover, for example, whether earlier cases of a given disease had gone unnoticed. Law enforcement officials sometimes need access to medical records for the purpose of documenting abuse or medical insurance fraud. It is all too common for patients to be asked to sign blanket waivers of confidentiality authorizing release of records for all of the above purposes and more. This effectively eliminates the confidentiality of medical records. Patient waivers should instead be as narrowly framed as possible. Redacted or disidentified versions of medical records should be substituted for full records whenever the purpose of the review allows such substitution.

COST CONTROL

The urgent need to control the costs of medical care is only a few decades old. Prior to World War II, for example, a physician could "do everything" for a patient, and the cost would not be staggeringly high. Our recent experience of explosive medical progress has changed all that. Doing everything today involves doing a great deal more than it used to. The last few decades' medical progress is in large part tied to the development of expensive technology. Hospitals' desire to provide the best medical care was translated into a desire to acquire the latest and best capital equipment; this in turn was largely responsible for double-digit medical inflation rates in the 1980s. That inflation led to various methods of cost control: utilization review, Medicare prospective payment, managed care, and practice group financial incentives to limit referrals for costly inpatient and specialty care. These techniques have sparked debate that will undoubtedly continue into the next decades. There are two important elements to the debate about health care cost control. The first is setting health care budget constraints, and the second is encouraging efficient use of budgeted resources.

Few of us, as individuals, are interested in purchasing every bit of medical care that could be of some benefit to us. We prioritize, purchasing only what seems to us to be the most important and necessary medical care, because we have other pressing uses for our limited financial resources. Most of us do not, however, simply set a budget constraint on our medical purchases and force ourselves to live within it. Rather we reevaluate our medical needs from time to time and compare them to our other pressing needs in light of our available resources. Importantly, we also evaluate our needs differently from one another, partly because we have differing levels of wealth, partly because we have differing levels of susceptibility to illness, and partly because we have differing tolerance for various symptoms. Markets are very good at delivering medical services to different consumers at levels responsive to such varying preferences. For this reason, many believe that the budget constraint element of health care cost control should be determined one person at a time, in a free market. Each of us can decide what he wants to spend and can join with others with similar preferences to ensure that the group's dollars are spent efficiently.

The difficulty with this analysis is that markets are not very good at delivering medical services to the poor. There are well-known ethical arguments to the effect that a wealthy society such as ours should supply at least some basic medical services to those who cannot afford them on their own. Such a policy affords the poor a measure of dignity and security and increases their ability to raise their socioeconomic status through study and work. The obvious ethics problems here are how are we to pay for the supply of basic medical services and which medical services are to count as basic? These are the fundamental questions of health system reform, and although I have preferences among policy options, I cannot begin to argue for them here. I feel safe in predicting, however, that for at least the next decade we will be working with a complex combination of private and public payment systems. Private systems will allow the market to set their budget constraints, and public systems will set their constraints politically.

Suppose, for a moment, that the public and private systems have solved their budget constraint problems. They have determined what resources their enrollees will spend on health care. They have achieved this by setting (politically or through the market) a dollar figure representing the total revenue for the enterprise and perhaps also by ruling out certain procedures considered high cost and low return (for example, experimental therapies, cosmetic orthodontia, and transplants for the elderly). Public and private systems will still be faced with the need for cost control to ensure that the funds they are willing to spend are spent efficiently and that the more expensive medical techniques on their approved lists are not overused. The difficulty here is to establish methods that eliminate unnecessary high-cost care but do not prevent any patients from receiving high-cost care that they really need.

Both the budget constraint problem and the problem of efficient use of allocated resources demand good social science thinking. We need to know more about the application of cost-benefit analyses to health care, about the effects on practice of various financial incentive schemes, and about the effectiveness of various techniques of retrospective utilization review. But these problems also require sophisticated clinical ethics thinking. Whatever limits we set upon access to costly medicine will affect the way medicine is practiced within those limits. The act of placing certain therapies off limits for cost-control reasons may affect physicians' ability to speak with full candor about them; it may even affect their ability to consider them real options. The incorporation of cost and financial incentive considerations into physicians' evaluations of their patients may affect patients' trust in their physicians. That may in turn affect patient compliance, satisfaction, and even health outcomes.

Medical progress comes literally at a price. The needs to set budget constraints and to encourage efficient use of resources will become ever more pressing in the next years. In meeting those needs we must continue to bear in mind the classic arguments for social justice in the allocation of scarce resources. We will also need to bear in mind that medicine is as much art as science and that in setting limits to it we do not leave it unchanged.

IATROGENESIS

Iatrogenesis refers to illness that results from medical care. The classic example is that because hospitals are full of sick people, a certain number of hospital patients catch new diseases as a result of their inpatient stays for other diseases. The problem of iatrogenesis is getting more and more serious, however. Treatment of tuberculosis patients with antibiotics and of AIDS patients with antiviral cocktails can result in the creation of treatment-resistant strains of disease. We may yet see a resurgence of infectious disease as such resistant strains increase. This is a technical problem, but it gives rise to a number of serious ethics problems. Should physicians offer antibiotic or antiviral treatments to patients whose ability to comply with treatment regimens is open to serious question? How invasive may physicians be in attempting to ensure patients' compliance?

Xenographic transplantation (transplantation of organs from nonhuman animals, including genetically altered animals) raises other important concerns about iatrogenesis. We are on the brink of being able to use genetically altered pigs, for example, as organ donors. But our understanding of the risks of introducing animal organs into human bodies is incomplete. Might we transfer previously unknown diseases from animal populations into human populations that are unequipped to resist them? The risks are grave and require careful study.

REPRODUCTIVE TECHNOLOGIES

Medicine's technical progress is perhaps most obvious in the area of reproduction. The legal and ethical issues raised by new reproductive technologies are legion: Who owns the deceased's unused frozen sperm? How may we dispose of nonimplanted frozen embryos? Is it permissible to engage in selective reduction of multiple pregnancies in order to avoid the gestational dangers of carrying multiple fetuses? Is it permissible to have artificially implanted multiple embryos in the first place?

There are deeper questions here as well. Bioethicists have often inquired whether it is legitimate to spend resources on complex reproductive technologies simply to indulge potential parents' desires to have children to whom they are genetically linked. There are further inquiries worth making: Has our society created some fertility problems by pushing back the age of reproduction? Does the high cost of fertility treatment raise questions of class preference in reproduction?

END-OF-LIFE CARE

Medical progress now allows people to live through events that would have killed them only a generation ago. In part as a result of this change, we can reasonably expect that more of us will live to be old and that in our elder years we will be more productive than ever before. However, we are also more apt than members of previous generations to live for large numbers of years with significantly diminished physical function and to die of multiple causes than of simple one-shot causes such as heart attack or stroke. Finally, we are far more apt than past generations to die under medical care.

The biomedical ethics problems presented by these developments are well known. Decades of work in bioethics have also armed us with an impressive number of solutions. The principle problems in end-of-life care are now practical: we need to get the solutions implemented. Patients have the right to decline unwanted end-of-life care, but we need to develop better ways to inform patients of that right and to encourage them to document their preferences. Physicians are required by law to honor their patients' preferences, but we need better ways to ensure that physicians understand the law and that they learn patients' preferences in time to act upon them. We have excellent techniques for management of pain and other symptoms at the end of life, but we still need to provide better education about those techniques to physicians out in the field.

Finally, the issue of assisted suicide is not apt to go away. People fear loss of control and loss of dignity; they fear pain; they fear being a burden to their friends and relatives. For all these reasons they will continue to consider ending their lives. In the next few years we will need to work hard to ensure that assisted suicide is not embraced as a simple and cost-effective alternative to listening to patients' fears, tending to their needs and desires, managing their symptoms, and assuring them of our love. Physicians, friends, and relatives must all beware of offering their patients and loved ones control over their deaths as a substitute for the more difficult task of granting them control over what is left of their lives.

PART FIVE

Clinical Leaders

CHAPTER TWENTY-FIVE

Challenges to Physician Leaders

Thomas R. Reardon

Thomas R. Reardon, a general practitioner from Portland, Oregon, is chair of the American Medical Association (AMA) Board of Trustees. A member of the board since 1990, he has served on its executive committee, as AMA secretary-treasurer, and as vice chair of the board. He has also served on the Congressional Physician Payment Review Commission, the National Committee for Quality Assurance Board of Directors, and the President's Commission on Patient Rights and Quality of Care.

I n a profession such as medicine, where progress is made minute by minute and is measured in millimeters and micro-surgeries, a century is a long time to contemplate. For the physician, each day's successes advance the frontier; each new challenge builds on the achievements of the past. From mapping the human genome to developing the marvels of telemedicine, one medical advance leads to the next in rapid and logarithmic succession. Today, astounding developments in medical care are occurring alongside remarkable changes in how that care is delivered.

As we come to the close of the twentieth century, we face a complexity of health care plan options unprecedented in human healing history. From traditional fee-for-service medicine to managed care, from employer-provided plans to state and federal entitlements, and from hospital practice plans to the most recent innovation, physician-run health plans, the options are almost as many and varied as patients and physicians themselves. What is more, these options continue to change and expand with every passing day. Years of focus on cost cutting are now giving way to a renewed concern with quality; in the meantime the consolidation and integration of physician practices continues unabated as single and multispecialty group practices become the rule of the day.

Such sweeping professional change, however, does not take place in a vacuum. Medicine's challenges for the twenty-first century echo enormous changes in the larger society and in patients themselves. Ethical challenges, demands for greater choice, and the necessity of responsibly financing care for the future must all be counted as part of the equation. Given such rapid movements in the modern medical marketplace, the single greatest challenge for those of us who are physicians today lies in finding ways to lead the pace of change, ensuring that evolving delivery systems and shifting priorities do not undermine the essential values of our ancient healing relationships.

Fortunately, patient and physician alike have a champion in this task. More than 150 years ago, the American Medical Association (AMA) was founded to "advance the art and science of medicine and to promote the public health." Ever since that time, AMA physicians have taken the leadership role in making U.S. medicine the very best in the world. It is a mission that is as strong on the eve of the twenty-first century as it was in those long-ago days before antibiotics, CT scans, and other tools of modern healing. Here now is a look at that continuing mission as it evolves for the future.

THE CHALLENGE OF PATIENT CARE

For physicians, for 2,500 years and more, all of medicine has ultimately begun and ended with the relationships we share with our patients. Since antiquity, each member of the medical profession has sworn a solemn oath to keep her patients' priorities foremost in the daily exercise of her profession. This ancient mission has been increasingly complicated, however, by recent changes in the U.S. health care system.

For the past twenty years, this nation has witnessed phenomenal growth in the managed care arena in the form of health maintenance organizations (HMOs), preferred provider organizations (PPOs), and an entire alphabet of additional plan and program types. In that time, managed care has proven itself economically efficient insofar as it reduces care of marginal value in the system and eliminates redundant practices. As physicians have increasingly become employees of these large, integrated delivery systems, however, their autonomy, unsurprisingly given system goals, has decreased. Health care bureaucracies have succeeded in reducing costs by driving down demand through administrative rule making and by simultaneously shifting risk from insurers to providers. At the same time, efficiencies have often been driven by financial incentives, such as targets for resource utilization.

Today the combined strengths of patient preferences and medical professionalism and ethics are causing physicians to fight back against purely dollar-driven restrictions on care. In addition, the courts have been holding plans legally responsible in cases where necessary care is denied. Patients themselves are also creating a strong impetus for change. Disillusioned by restrictions on coverage and care, they are increasingly demanding choice of physician, hospital, and even type of health plan. More than ever, patients see physicians as the essential point of trust in a changing system, and demand choice and stability in their vital relationships with their doctors. As a point of stability in a sea of change, the patient-physician relationship is seen by patients to be truly significant.

At the same time, patients themselves are becoming better educated, not only about their insurance options but also about medical treatments. Today, thanks to the Internet, trends in product advertising, and the massive proliferation of medical information, patients are better equipped to take part in their care than ever before. Rather than simplifying the physician's job, however, this increased patient knowledge base is creating new challenges.

First, there is the challenge of accurate information. With so much health data available, it is especially important that resources be reliable; physicians can be an ideal checkpoint and important help in prioritizing and interpreting key concepts and research for their patients. More than ever, physicians will need to keep abreast of new developments and help educate patients about various treatment options. Second, if the current trend toward insurance coverage of alternative care increases, physicians will need to become familiar with a larger, and often foreign, perspective on wellness, guiding patients to sound, scientific solutions that will maintain and ensure their health.

A QUESTION OF COST

Expanding health care options have traditionally meant expanding health care costs. Clearly, discretionary dollars are few and far between in a day when health care costs have already surpassed the $1 trillion mark. Solutions still must be found, however, to the plight of the forty-two million Americans who lack health insurance coverage today. Certainly this is an AMA priority for the future and a social priority as well. Learning how to accomplish this objective will be one of the signal challenges of the twenty-first century, not only for physicians but for all Americans.

The push is on for new solutions, and the AMA, for one, believes choice is the key. Patients must be allowed to choose how to pay for care and how much coverage they desire. Options like medical savings accounts and defined contributions are part of the profile. New models of care also demand consideration.

For instance, on the one hand, patients are increasingly opting for point of service packages, which allow them to go outside plan networks for care, and for insurance that allows them direct access to specialty care. On the other hand, physicians are increasingly joining group practices and, on the more sociopolitical end of the spectrum, recognizing the need to organize to create bargaining power and greater physician unity. Physician-sponsored health plans, a longtime AMA priority, are also on the rise, strengthened by a renewed emphasis on patient needs and protections and the primacy of the patient-physician relationship. Clearly, cost has ceased to be the sole consideration, but it is and will remain a key factor in all models of care.

THE AGE OF ACCOUNTABILITY

The emphasis on cost that has characterized health care for two decades and more is now giving way to an increased focus on quality. In fact, quality of care is now being addressed across the United States by initiatives like the new Presidential Commission on Quality in Health Care, a body charged from the highest level with protecting patients and ensuring that quality is not lost in the continuing drive to cut costs.

The president's commission is not only examining questions of quality in care, it is establishing clear measures and standards for the future. That is the focus behind the so-called Patient Bill of Rights the commission has delivered to the White House. It is also the focus of a number of new AMA programs, including AMAP, the American Medical Accreditation Program.

AMAP is a voluntary, comprehensive physician accreditation program aimed at measuring and evaluating individual physicians against national standards and peer performance in five key areas: credentials, personal qualifications, environment of care, clinical performance, and patient care results. AMAP's goal is to develop a new national benchmark of physician quality. For physicians it means they can look to one single, reliable standard-bearer of quality in the care they provide, rather than deal with an endless parade of investigators, each with a different measuring stick in hand. For patients it means that by choosing an AMAP-accredited physician, they can be sure they are getting the highest-quality care, regardless of practice setting or delivery system.

Patients are also getting a new voice for quality in the form of the new National Patient Safety Foundation at the AMA. Based on the simple premise that any preventable error in the medical workplace is one error too many, the program emphasizes physician accountability and implements changes in practices and procedures in order to avoid doctor and hospital errors. Meanwhile the AMA also continues to work with various other organizations—the National Committee for Quality Assurance, the Joint Commission on Accreditation of Healthcare Organizations, the Health Care Financing Administration, and the Agency for Health Care Policy and Research—to develop coordinated approaches to the evolving science of measuring health care quality and outcomes.

The AMA is making these and other efforts to improve and protect quality because it is an important issue for patients and absolutely essential for our profession. Physicians are taking a leadership role quite simply because they must. Only the medical profession has the medical expertise to develop the tools of tomorrow—tools of quality management for the twenty-first century.

Defining quality has never been easy, but today more than ever, physicians must make defining quality in health care their priority. The effort will go a long way toward reassuring patients that their good health is a top priority and in making sure medicine remains committed to the core values on which it is founded.

ETHICS AND PROFESSIONALISM

Chief among the medical profession's core values, of course, is the ethical code that guides physicians. This code sets medicine apart from all other enterprises; it states simply and clearly that here is a profession bound to serve a higher good: the health and welfare of patients. However, medical ethics today faces challenges that our professional forebears could never have imagined. From physician-assisted suicide and end-of-life care to patient confidentiality and brave new proposals for cloning, the changing landscape of care is driving medicine to establish new ethical guidelines to accommodate the new day of medicine.

Patient records, like all information, are entering the electronic age. As this patient information is increasingly used to measure performance, we must develop methods that allow us to extract the generalized data that will be of help to the entire health care system without jeopardizing patients' confidentiality and the sacred trust of the patient-physician relationship. In the same way, as our knowledge of the human genome continues to grow, we will need to discover means of managing new potentials that emerge, such as genetic testing. Physicians of the twenty-first century will need to be prepared not only to offer genetic counseling but to ensure that patients are protected against loss of insurance coverage following genetically related diagnoses.

Physicians must also prepare to expand their historical role as guardians of life, giving equal attention to fulfilling the needs of patients at the end of life. Continuity and compassion will be the watchwords as patients live longer and more medical technology exists to support life. It will be up to physicians to guide their patients through these emerging ethical labyrinths.

That is why the AMA has recently launched its new Institute for Ethics, which is helping to sort through the array of ethical challenges facing modern medicine. Under the leadership of medical ethicist Linda Emanuel, the institute is conducting research on ethics policies and establishing practical outreach for physicians. More important, it is advancing the place of ethics in medicine's professional activities and safeguarding the professional standards that are at the very heart of the patient-physician relationship.

A VISION FOR THE FUTURE

All these AMA actions come down to a single key concept: a vision for the future of health care in the United States. We all want a health care system in which patients have a voice and a choice in their care, one in which the patient-physician relationship is protected and preserved as the cornerstone of the medical profession.

We seek a system that gives physicians the autonomy and freedom to make the best decisions for their patients without intrusions or interference from outsiders; a system that promotes professionalism, integrity, and the highest ethical and educational standards—in short, a system that remains the envy of all other countries and continues to distinguish itself as the very best in the world.

Physicians too want these things, and in the summer of 1997, the American Medical Association board developed the *AMA Vision,* a document that the AMA is working to make a reality. This vision reaffirms the AMA's 150-year commitment to patients, physicians, and the medical profession and provides the AMA with a moral compass to guide its actions in 1998 and beyond. Grounded in the AMA's core purpose—to promote the art and science of medicine and the betterment of the public health—the AMA vision is aimed at creating a future in which the AMA is a leading force in pioneering solutions, knowledge, and tools that promote health, from information on health and medical practice to standard setting to advocacy for physicians and their patients.

Such a vision is important for all physicians as they enter the twenty-first century. More than ever, organized medicine will take the leadership role in creating the future of health care. Tools like the AMA vision will guide physicians as they recognize, cope with, and shape change for tomorrow.

Yet no matter what challenges we may face on the road to the twenty-first century, one essential endures: the value and the primacy of our patient-physician relationships. Change is not the only constant, after all. Young people entering medicine today, just like generations of physicians before them, will know and be enriched by the sanctity and the trust which characterize these healing relationships. From the days of Hippocrates to the present, patients remain our priority. For physicians, meeting their needs will remain the challenge of our future—for this and every century.

CHAPTER TWENTY-SIX

Core Competencies for Physicians

Edward O'Neil

Edward O'Neil is associate professor of family and community medicine at the University of California, San Francisco, where he is codirector of the Center for the Health Professions. He is also executive director of the Pew Health Professions Commission and founding partner of O'Neil & Associates, a consulting firm that assists its clients with policy, management, and training solutions to the challenges they face in today's health care market.

There is little that has been written about leadership in medicine or the health professions in general that will be of much practical use as a guide for action over the next decade. The next ten to fifteen years will witness a fundamental realignment of health care in the United States. In this process the sources, functions, competencies, and measures of success for leadership in health care will change just as dramatically as the context in which that leadership operates. The reasons for such a transformation in the health system have been discussed in other settings and are beyond the scope of this chapter on physician leadership. But three dimensions are so essential to our understanding of the changing nature of physician leadership as to merit examination at the outset.

THE NEW EPOCH

The *power base* that undergirds all of health care has already experienced a shift and will remain unstable into the future. The professions have been the dominant source of power in health, with medicine playing the predominant power role among the professions. On one level this dominance by the professions seems obvious and natural, but on another level it has excluded other voices from helping to form critical decisions about health care. Such voices include communities, individual consumers, corporate purchasers, and public policymakers. For myriad reasons these other health care players are now vying for more power and voice in the decision-making processes surrounding health care. Those that are growing in power are the corporate purchasers (both public and private), individual consumers, and health plans. Communities, public policy bodies, and public health delivery structures seem to be holding their own with little gain or loss in power. The professional groups (doctors, nurses, and allied health workers) and the delivery organizations (hospitals, home health agencies, and clinics) seem to be on a path to giving up some of their power in the change (O'Neil and Coffman, 1998).

A second shift in the health care environment that is impinging on physician leadership is a change in the *rules of how the system works.* Up until the late 1980s, health care was a highly structured system of formal and informal rules and regulations that informed the behavior of the people and institutions that made up the system. Increasingly, this traditional pattern of relationships and behavior simply does not correspond to reality. Who delivers care? Who assumes risk and responsibility for the patient? Who decides what is quality care? Who is in charge? Who finances care? These and other basic questions are up for review and redefinition. Perhaps more alarming to old system incumbents is the dawning reality that as the power shifts in health care, others may have legitimate answers to these questions. Or even more revolutionary, they may have a new set of questions that they want answered.

As power changes hands and rules are altered, the system is slowly but inexorably beginning to exhibit *a new set of goals,* or outcomes, that it desires. They are largely inchoate at this point, but the broad outlines are knowable. For medicine, the most dramatic of these shifts will be the move to balance its traditional focus on treating individuals who present with acute care needs with an equal or even predominant focus on understanding population health needs. As part of this new focus, medicine will have to deploy educational and management strategies against the growing chronic disability burden in the nation. This shift will represent a dramatic new challenge to the next generation of physician leaders.

CORE LEADERSHIP COMPETENCIES FOR THE NEW EPOCH

A redistribution of power, new rules for playing the game, and new outcomes will be essential realities for the physician leader in the emerging epoch. In this period of transformation, when what was certain and established will become vague and unpredictable, the essential leadership task will be to bring coherence, structure, and meaning to a world of changing norms and expectations. What leadership skills and competencies will be needed to understand, survive, and thrive in such an environment? Will they be tied to those that have existed before, or will this new epoch be a period of discontinuity with the recent past (Taylor and Wacker, 1997)? Myriad skills, values, and competencies exist with which to equip a future leader. However, if we focus on what is critical for the physician in this new age, both what must be learned and what must be unlearned, we come to a manageable array of four basic and interrelated competencies that should be present to ensure leadership success in the future: the abilities to develop a vision, practice alignment, partner with other organizations, and manage change.

Develop a Vision

Given the demands of the rapidly evolving health care system, knowing how to develop a vision is the core ability because all other leadership attributes must be understood and used in relation to the vision. What is emerging as the U.S. health care system will be dramatically different from what is being left behind. For fifty years health care in the United States has been a series of breathtaking expansions and enlargements, all on the same theme: the application of biomedical knowledge to the treatment needs of individuals. Physicians, nurses, and other professionals and hospitals and other institutions provided this application through a rather fixed set of behaviors and practice patterns. It was highly innovative but in a very narrow band. The system that is emerging does not look to the old patterns for direction and inspiration. It increasingly asks of itself, What are the outcomes to be achieved, and what is the least costly, most effective means to these ends? The less one depends on the established ways of doing things, the more one needs a vision to drive and create the reality of the future world. The fact that these changes are being driven, not by a uniform public policy, but by the workings of a dynamic market means that there are literally thousands of health care entrepreneurs creating their visions in every area in which health care services are provided (Grudin, 1990).

Successful leadership visions in health care require four dimensions:

1. Focusing on the future

2. Founding the vision on core values

3. Making the vision genuinely creative

4. Aligning efforts in implementing the vision

First, the vision must focus on the future not the past. This seems an obvious point; a vision seems to be by definition a direction into the future. But because many incumbents in health care are satisfied with the status quo, oftentimes their visions are merely ways to return to the past. How do we keep our economic position? How do we sustain our power prerogatives in relation to other professions? How do we continue to control these institutions? True vision liberates itself from these impediments, embraces the reality of a changing environment, and pushes through to create a different world. As much as is humanly and institutionally possible, leadership vision creates this world by suspending self-interest and reforming around genuine public interest.

This public interest points to the second dimension of vision: it works best when it is moored to core individual, professional, or institutional values (O'Neil, 1997). These values may be inwardly oriented toward fulfilling one's own needs and desires or externally focused on responding to the needs of others, whether patients, customers, or the broad public. Health care is moving away from a period in which it produced what it wanted to supply to a period in which it must respond to the demands of a varied public. Leaders will do well to ensure that their values and the corresponding vision are responsive to such demands.

Third, the emerging system of health will place a premium on visions that are creative. Those leaders who are able to step outside the confines of existing relationships and patterns and reveal new ways to configure health care will be in demand. Successful leaders will have the intuition to see the emergent patterns. Most leaders live at the operating core of the institutions and organizations that they shape. This is where they both draw and use their power. In stable times the core and the vision are aligned; in times of transition the core becomes discontinuous with the organization's future. Leaders will do well to leave the core behind and look toward the periphery of their organizations for the new and creative.

Practice Alignment

Finally, leaders will find that vision alone is not sufficient to transform their institutions. Leaders must also implement the vision and align the efforts of those within the health care organization so they move in a consistent new direction. This is a complicated undertaking and will require the concerted effort of the leader on three key tasks: communication, involvement, and focus.

Communication during times of transition is absolutely critical, and failing to communicate adequately is a shortcoming of most leaders. Being open and responsive is relatively easy when things are under control and leaders know the answers to the questions and are clear about the directions of the organization. When matters become shadowy, most leaders respond by shutting down communication and covering up their insecurity about not knowing. Many leaders think, "Better to have them guess whether or not I have the answers, rather than opening my mouth and confirming that I am lost." But in times of transition, silence just breeds speculation, a form of communication that is almost always worse than truth because it is by definition beyond the control of the leader.

Communication begins by conveying the vision of the organization and changes as that vision unfolds and develops. At first, communication from the leader should be general, educative, positive, and reassuring. Leaders often forget that the experiences they have gone through to develop a vision of the organization's future have been involved and complex. They reduce the vision to an elegant few words, which may mean volumes to the speaker but little to the message recipients. Effective leaders, in contrast, translate the vision into stories that explain the changing environment, tie the organization's traditional values to these changes, and point to the ways in which the work of those inside the organization can and should change. These changes should be consistent with both the new external demands and the new internal directions that come from the vision.

Internal communication must be two-way and actively involve the entire organization. First shared in a general manner, the vision becomes more specific through the development of a strategy and operating plan. Strategies and operating plans are excellent devices for educating people about the vision, reshaping parts of the vision, and achieving buy-in as people relate their work to the vision. Leadership during this phase is a balance between supplying overt directions and encouraging participation. Leaders should be very conscious of their role and their own attitudes as they move communication from the visionary to the operational.

Finally, the leader must provide reinforcement to those involved so they remain constant to the organizational vision and purpose. As dynamic as the health care environment is, there is a natural tendency for organizations to jump from one good idea to another, seeking the same kind of stability they had in the past. Such stability is a false goal. What organizations need and what leadership must provide is a guiding vision, one that evolves over time and that informs the creative responses of those who work inside the organization. Achieving internal alignment of this sort is the second task of physician leaders.

Form Partnerships and Alliances and Make Acquisitions

The third task is the external corollary of achieving internal alignment: developing partnerships, alliances, and acquisitions. The old approach to structuring health care permitted a considerable amount of independence for professionals and organizations. One of the principle forces transforming health care today is the movement to engage all the elements of health care in an integrated program. The exact form of this integration will vary from program to program, but all health care leaders will need new skills in assessing, developing, and sustaining partnerships, alliances, and acquisitions with other organizations.

The benefits of a prospective partnership, alliance, or acquisition must be assessed in relation to the needs of both parties. These needs can be known only when the respective leaders have achieved clarity of mission and strategy. With this knowledge the core assets of potential partners can be assessed. The questions are all pretty straightforward: What will be needed to achieve the vision? What do we have? What do we need? What does the partner bring to the work? Without the discipline of a vision and strategy that inform the decision, the leader will find it difficult to be successful.

Another key to developing successful relationships is to understand the differences between alliances and acquisitions. Acquisitions are the easiest in some ways. Buying the core assets of an organization and applying them where they are needed is quick and efficient but requires capital investment up front and may produce a downstream integration cost, particularly if physicians are involved. Physician leaders have been particularly challenged by the task of aligning purchased practices to meet larger organizational goals.

Alliances are less costly initially but may ultimately be very expensive, as they demand continual maintenance to sustain the involvement of the partners. This may be particularly draining on leaders, as these relationships often require direct involvement by the executives on both sides. Alliances are particularly useful when both parties have similar or complementary interests. Partnerships are alliances of a more involved kind. They often result in the creation of a third mutually owned organization. They work when the partnership produces a win for both partners.

Regardless of the pathway—acquisition, alliance, or partnership—chosen by the leader, the work begins with that pathway's creation. Leaders invest a considerable amount of time in identifying and bringing these relationships to life. It is natural for them to pull back a bit when they are created. But when these arrangements fail, it is often because the leader has not allocated enough time to actively direct and manage them after their creation. During the first eighteen months, leaders must provide oversight and direction to nurture these efforts into the proper alignment with the direction of the larger organization.

Manage Change

The final task facing physician leaders in the next century will be how to manage change itself. That change is the only constant has become axiomatic in health care and other parts of our society and economy. The phenomenal crush of continual and fundamental change is perhaps the greatest leadership challenge. All that has been discussed here relates to the core competencies needed to bring direction to the bubbling chaos that health care has become. A creative vision, a disciplined strategy, effective communications that align and motivate internally, and the selection of allies that can assist in achievement of the vision—all these contribute to calming the turbulence of the white water facing health care leaders. But a few other skills are needed as well for leaders to effectively harness the power of this turbulence in order to meet the challenges of health care.

Self-knowledge is critical in managing change. No two leaders are alike, and each has a different composite of strengths and weaknesses. It is not the leader's responsibility to be strong or accomplished in every skill required to move a health care organization forward. However, it is the leader's job to know what skills are needed and the relative abilities possessed by the leader and the executive team. It is also the leader's responsibility to create a culture that recognizes diversity of ability, provides training and development throughout the organization, and ensures that individuals grow and develop in their professional work. Without linking the leadership agenda to the diverse and developing abilities of its members, an organization cannot manage change effectively.

The transitions in health care will not be easy or comfortable, particularly for system incumbents. They will experience loss of power, salary, prestige, and position. When the stakes are this high, conflict is inevitable. Physician leaders must develop an ability to manage this conflict. Many people believe that the relevant task is to *resolve* conflict. In many instances this will simply not be possible, but the effective management of expectations, processes for decision making and participation, and commitment to broader organizational goals and vision will help get the organization through the inevitable tensions of serious change.

Finally, the development of a diverse executive team that is aligned with the vision and strategy of the organization is critical to the success of any leader. As health care opens up to novel ways of doing business, develops new partnerships and alliances, and enters new fields of activities, the leadership team will require new skills and perspectives in order to be successful. Building and sustaining such a team will be one of the essential tasks in mastering the change management process. For the physician leader this will mean developing an ability to see the world from the perspective of other professions and to understand what the emerging system needs from the executive team. Active and sustained involvement with partners and customers will be the key to developing such perspectives.

—⁓—

Attention to the development of the four core competencies will be key to the success of the physician leader of the next century. With these skills the next generation of leaders will have a chance not only to survive but to master the health care white water of the next decade.

References

Grudin, R. *The Grace of Great Things.* New York: Ticknor & Fields, 1990.

O'Neil, E., and Coffman, J. (eds). *Strategies for the Future of Nursing.* San Francisco: Jossey-Bass, 1998.

O'Neil, J. *Leadership Aikido: Filling a Global Gap.* New York: Harmony Press, 1997.

Taylor, J., and Wacker, W. *The Five Hundred Year Delta.* New York: HarperCollins, 1997.

CHAPTER TWENTY SEVEN

The Future of Nursing

Marjorie Beyers

Marjorie Beyers is executive director of the American Organization of Nurse Executives (AONE), an organization committed to developing community-based, integrated health care delivery systems. A Fellow of the American Academy of Nursing, she has published extensively and consulted in the areas of nursing administration and health care quality and has presented over two hundred lectures to hospitals, schools of nursing, and professional organizations across the country.

T his discussion of the future of the nursing profession and the continued development of nursing as a profession is based on some assumptions:

- Nursing's rich legacy will propel it into the future. Its history is rich with examples of its mission to improve the health of individuals and communities, take care of the sick and ill, and attend to people in times of disaster, war, and crises.

- Future patterns of nursing care will blend past practice into future practice. Nursing's existing mission and values will continue to drive practice, and the way nursing care is delivered will reflect changes in the way the public uses nursing and health care services.

- The nursing profession will undergo significant development in the ways it meets its accountabilities to the public, both in practice and in methods for voluntary credentialing and taking professional accountability for practice outcomes.

- Nursing practice will be aligned with patient requirements for care in health care service sectors that incorporate the continuum of care. Practice will be enhanced and expanded as a result of technological developments in both health care and communication that will increase the use of nursing's capacity to provide patient care.

- The educational preparation of nurses will continue to provide opportunities for career mobility and expanded roles. Nursing will continue to be a unique profession with a growing science but will interface with other health professions in its educational processes. Continuing education will be as important as the basic educational program.

- The nursing workforce will continue to be pluralistic. Shifts in generalization and specialization will occur as patient demand and health care technology develop. Increased patient involvement in care and interdisciplinary care teams will influence staffing and thus workforce requirements, driven by patient demand for care.

- Public policy toward the nursing workforce will be based in newly devised supply-and-demand projection models that incorporate not only patient demand for care but also use of interdisciplinary team collaboration.

FUTURE PRACTICE

The mission of nursing and its values will remain constant, but its delivery modes and location of care will continue to change significantly. In the future, nursing services will be organized around the patient population groups found in three main settings—primary care centers, specialty care centers, and community service centers—connected through governance and administrative structures.

Primary care center nurses, working with health care teams, will provide patient assessment, education, and support with the goal of wellness. Primary care centers will be the basic level of health care for individuals and communities. This cadre of nurses will be responsible for clinical integration of care across the continuum of care and will coordinate each patient's care in collaboration with physicians and other health professionals. These nurses will work with comprehensive data banks containing information on patients' genetic assessment, health history, significant lifestyle factors, and estimation of health risk. The data will also include each patient's chronological record of health care with outcomes. One accountability of this group of nurses will require working collaboratively with physicians and other health professionals to systematically analyze patient data in order to discover ways to improve all aspects of patient care and to learn about causes and effects.

The nursing care role will involve care management over time for individual patients to ensure that assessments are timely and that follow-up is implemented. Primary care nurses will work with health care teams, connecting patients with the other types of care resources as needed. For example, individuals requiring diagnosis and complex treatment will be connected with physicians. Individuals with housing and daily living problems will be connected with community services. The health care team will comprise nurses, physicians, pharmacists, nutritionists, physical and occupational therapists, and rehabilitation specialists, available as needed by the patients. In addition, patients with similar problems and concerns will receive certain types of care in groups. Nurses responsible for a given patient population group will assess the care needed by that group. Members of the interdisciplinary care team will participate in group care as indicated by the group problems. The team, including nurses, will be responsible for the efficiency and effectiveness of care, using electronic communication and quality improvement methods (Parsons, Murdaugh, and O'Rourke, 1998). The nurses will also interface with other components of the health care system, including specialized care centers and community care services.

Specialized care center nurses will be associated with health care centers such as acute care and long-term care facilities, home care programs, and hospice and healing centers. In locations with high-density populations, each care center may be a separate entity, but in areas with fewer people, specialized care centers may be grouped in one facility. Care center nurses' roles will be similar to today's nursing practice. Leaders and clinical specialists will manage the organizational aspects of care and provide direct patient care. Specialized care center nurses will be responsible for the care environment and care management. Interdisciplinary teams will provide comprehensive care, with the nursing role focused on twenty-four-hour care and ongoing care management. The nursing staff will include chief nurses, advanced practice nurses, generalist nurses, and assisting staff. Although these care centers will look much like hospitals of today, they will be designed to meet patients' specialized needs and will be equipped accordingly. Some will be more like hotels, and others will resemble today's high technology hospitals. As in all types of care centers, patients will be actively involved in their care programs. The specialized care center nurses will interface with both primary care and community care nurses.

Community care nurses will be a blend of today's public health nurse, community health care center nurse, and health planner-educator. Community health assessments, plans for improving health, and special projects to deal with selected issues of the environment and ecology will be their main accountabilities. Clients will include community leaders (in schools, churches, businesses, and the other types of groups in which people cluster) who are undertaking special projects to improve the environment for health, to deal with particular health issues, to garner resources in times of crises, and to promote and support neighborhood health groups. Thus community care nurses will often accomplish their work as part of project teams. Community members will participate in designing and implementing projects. One of the important interface groups for community care teams will be the public officials, police and firefighters, and persons whose work brings them into close contact with the grassroots community members (Parsons, Murdaugh, and O'Rourke, 1998). The community care teams will also work closely with the primary care teams, to provide services and support for the chronically ill, elderly, and disabled persons who need assistance. They will work hand in glove with the primary care teams in community-based care centers.

FUTURE ARCHITECTURE

In the future the architecture of the nursing profession will be designed to incorporate the components of education, practice, administration, policy, and research. Because care will be delivered in clinical organizations with less infrastructure than today's organizations have, key relationships within nursing will evolve around education, research and development, and new ways of practice. The profession will have a common core of activities for continued development of its science, evaluation, and improvement. Education, research, and regulation will be specialized functions associated with universities, institutes, and virtual groups sharing the same specialties. Each nurse will develop a professional career profile in each of the five basic dimensions of nurses' professional role: education, practice, administration, policy, and research. Professional leadership will be provided by nurses with doctoral degrees in one aspect of the full professional role. These nurses will be closely associated with professionals in other disciplines who share their areas of focus.

Educators will specialize in delivery of basic and continuing education and will provide expertise in educational interventions for individuals and community health initiatives. They will be conversant with cognitive patterns and theories of learning. They will use new technology to deliver education, designing curricula that can be used in local areas. They will coach and guide others in the use of learning materials and in educational processes.

Administrators and executives will focus on resources and organization. They will participate in the organizational design and operation of patient care delivery, ensuring that structures for patient care are relevant to patient requirements. They will focus on design, decision making for effective use of resources, competency, and outcomes. They will also engage in continual study of care delivery and outcomes, technology assessment, and development of ways to detect when changes should be planned and introduced. They will manage change and work with broad-based teams in all sectors of health care.

Policy experts will continue to be a major force in analyzing public need for quality patient care and in ensuring that policy fosters health for all citizens. Nursing's policy experts will contribute to international, national, and state policy initiatives in unique ways evidenced in patient care. To fulfill a strong patient advocacy role, nursing will establish a learning loop from the care experience to the policy table.

Researchers will continue to develop the science. They may be aligned with specific types of practices, and their research priorities will be to advance nurses' capability to provide quality patient care. Part of their role will be to make research findings accessible to practicing nurses, facilitating application of research to practice.

FUTURE WORKFORCE

Nursing's future architecture includes a design of relationships among the members of the nursing profession workforce and among nurses and the members of other health care workforces. In the future there will be a shift toward higher qualifications, new staffing configurations, and more explicit clarification of the roles and functions of nurses in relation to their educational preparation. In the future the nursing workforce projections will concentrate on qualifications to meet patient requirements for care rather than on numbers in a staffing matrix. Nurses will have more uniform preparation in the respective undergraduate and graduate programs. Graduate preparation will be required for practice in complex situations requiring extensive planning, negotiation, discovery, and analysis in decision making (American Organization of Nurse Executives, 1997, 1998). Higher degrees will be necessary for effective collaboration with other nurses and other health professionals for health care service design, delivery, and evaluation.

Undergraduate preparation will be essential for nurses who wish to specialize in care processes in highly defined situations. These nurses will participate in interdisciplinary care teams and participate in management of care resources to ensure efficient and effective care. The majority of them will practice in specialized care centers, working with patients experiencing acute illnesses or requiring support in managing chronic illnesses. Nursing assistants will provide support for nurses in these sectors. In the future, patients and their families or other personal caregivers will also be active participants in patient care.

FORCES SHAPING NURSING'S FUTURE

Of the many strong forces now shaping health care, four have special implications for nursing's future: the unbundling of health care organizations, the capabilities of health care and communication technology, the development of integrated care delivery systems, and the growth of consumer involvement.

The unbundling of health care delivery into many more organizations and settings than before is setting the stage for future health care. The current redesign, reorganization, and restructuring in health care organizations is being driven by multiple events, including health care financing changes, quality improvement initiatives, and shifting resources. However these events are overshadowing events of greater continuing importance such as the development of health care technology and communication. New technologies and means of communication will eventually be viewed as a pathway to new definitions of care (Hiebeler, Kelly, and Ketteman, 1998). And technological and communication changes will be seen as necessary to keep the growing bureaucracy in health care from restricting development of clinical services useful to patients.

The emerging models of health care delivery have great potential for using nursing's capacity for care. Technology is often overlooked as a major force in health care change, yet it remains the one constant that allows and supports new care delivery methods. Technology can be viewed as supporting or enabling change or as a source of change. Both views have merit. Technology has enabled much of the health care reorganization to date. The increased volume of outpatient surgery, for example reflects advanced health care technology that permits less invasive procedures and shorter patient recovery times. Ongoing introduction of new technology has also changed people's perspective on continuing education. Learning new competencies is now an accepted norm, to keep up with the change.

Technology will continue to mature in ways that will make today's health care system seem primitive. Work now under way in genetics promises to yield genetic diagnostics for detection of specific diseases, treatments using gene-based pharmaceuticals, and genetic therapies. Health care will continue to be challenged by ethical and moral dilemmas created by genetic interventions. At the same time, high-technology lifestyles will create needs for caring services. Healing centers and many of the healing methods used in the past will continue to gain prominence in society as health care is expanded to holistic care.

Introduction of new communication technology is also affecting nursing practice. Nurses along with other health care professionals now provide care through telemedicine, which connects specialists, nurses, and patients in their different settings. Interactive television can also be used to support patients in their home settings. Another example of technology use is *ask-a-nurse* service. These telephone arrangements began as triaging services, were used for marketing, and now are again being used for patient teaching and counseling and also early initial assessment and referral. Many people now use the Internet to obtain information about their illness or disease, information formerly available only to health professionals. As a result, health care professionals must adapt patient information and counseling to the patient's knowledge base. Nurses are using computers to obtain resource information, transmit patient reports, and make arrangements for patient care. Communication technology also enables seamless care; patient records can be transmitted to multiple settings, thus saving time and travel, and more important, enabling decision making. All these innovations influence the way nurses establish patient relationships, design patient education, and participate with others to manage care.

The development of integrated care delivery systems is tapped into nursing's strengths in patient care. The nursing perspective on integrated care delivery is the continuum of care, that is clinical integration of care processes. Nurses understand the continuum of care, and they have processes in place to coordinate care over time and among health care settings. The nursing process, nursing care plans, and clinical pathways contribute to managing care and are used in most care settings. As organizational structures are consolidated and redundancy is reduced, clinical processes become more visible (Institute of Medicine, 1998).

Consumer involvement has been instrumental in making the health care environment more user friendly. In nursing practice, consumer awareness is resulting in an emphasis on service and increased patient participation in care (Morath, 1997). Practices that increase patient satisfaction with service have to some extent replaced previous restrictions on what patients could or could not do, should or should not know. The environment for care is now more conducive to patient involvement in decision making and also facilitates the helping relationship. In this new environment there will be a new focus on the patient and on meeting patient needs across the continuum of care. One of the outcomes is that patients will have more choices about their care. In many instances these choices will be beneficial, but patient choice will also raise new ethical and moral issues, particularly when a patient refuses care known to be helpful. A strong benefit of increased consumer participation in care is that health care team members will become increasingly interdependent.

Another effect of increased consumer choice is the ongoing resurgence of healing remedies from the past, the establishment of healing centers, and the use of non-Western interventions like acupuncture. Nursing science has incorporated many of the *alternative* therapies and documented that such interventions enhance patient outcomes.

FOUR INITIATIVES

Four major initiatives will be prominent in nursing's journey toward the future. They include nursing professionals' relationships with physicians and other health professionals, the way the profession meets its accountabilities to the public, the composition and development of the nursing workforce, and the adaptation of nursing science to changing practice.

Nursing will not be alone in making changes in these areas, and turf battles about overlapping areas of practice and primary accountabilities will increase during the transition. Prescription privileges will be debated, for example. These battles will lead to the charting of new territory as practices and the complementary roles of the various health profession change, and who does what in the new practices is sorted out. In the future, patients and communities will initiate much of their care and will have access to many interventions now managed by health professionals (Center for Health Leadership, 1997). Health care professionals will increasingly be called upon for counseling, guidance, support, and assistance with decisions about health care. Not all professionals will be comfortable with patients' increased control.

The way nursing now meets its accountabilities to the public is largely centered on licensure, certification, and accreditation of services, agencies, and facilities—activities grounded in peer review and expert judgment. Nursing has already begun to consider standards of care across hemispheres, develop multistate compacts for licensure, and organize certification programs through the American Board of Nursing Specialties. These initiatives will converge into a unified approach to monitoring and evaluating the competence of nurses in areas of practice and quality of care. A new structure for professional regulation will emerge. One feature will be a unified focus on entry to practice based on educational preparation, and another will be increasing use of specific competency certification for selected areas of practice. Nursing will also be engaged in the effort to define specialization and generalization in practice. Centralized data banks will contain nurse profiles with data on individuals' basic education, certification, and practice outcomes. Issues of confidentiality, practice opportunities, and useful evaluation will be paramount in determining how the data banks will be used.

The composition of the nursing workforce is varied and complex. Struggles to define the education required for entry to practice and the appropriate education for advanced practice have dominated the field in the past decades (National Advisory Council on Nurse Education and Practice, 1997). In the future, nursing will become comfortable with its pluralism. The profession will continue to include nurses with different types of education, from the basic short-term course to the doctoral program (American Association of Colleges of Nursing, 1998). The trend will be toward eventual consolidation of the baccalaureate and master's programs, however, with associate degree programs preparing nursing assistants, baccalaureate and master's degree programs preparing clinical nurses, and doctoral degree programs preparing nurses with advanced, specialized knowledge. But diversity will continue because nursing will be in the mainstream of education and will be shaped in part by educational opportunities. Adding to the current pluralism in nursing will be the access to self-study and advanced preparation through virtual education on-line. Problems with program availability will be resolved by these virtual programs.

The nursing workforce will be profoundly affected by the trend toward interdisciplinary care. Basic curricula will become more broad based. Schools may develop a core health professional education that is followed with specialized education for a specific discipline such as nursing. This could make more nursing education a master's degree endeavor. In addition, the health professions can be expected to regroup according to patient requirements for care and technology. In the future there will be basic health professions such as physician and nurse and a number of technical programs that prepare these professionals for specific care functions. All the professions will grapple with their identity, their science, and their continued research and educational functions.

The adoption of new science into practice will be equally challenging because in a virtual society many of the quality controls and methods once used to test new practices will not be relevant. Nurses will have access to new information more quickly and will adopt new technology more routinely. The former dependence on rules, regulations, and policies will be replaced with a strong orientation to the ethics of practice, to working in communities of health professionals, and to discerning the effectiveness of care practices through outcomes measurement and analysis. The greatest challenge will be deciding how to deal with process and structure in this outcomes evaluation, because diversity in the ways care is delivered will only increase in the future (National Institute of Nursing Research, 1998). A new way of defining accepted behaviors will include process and structure, with focus on appropriate practices. Increasingly, standards of practice will be developed and adopted worldwide (Commission on Graduates of Foreign Nursing Schools, 1996).

References

American Association of Colleges of Nursing. *Enrollment and Graduations in Baccalaureate and Graduate Programs in Nursing.* Washington D.C.: American Association of Colleges of Nursing, 1998.

American Organization of Nurse Executives. *The Evolving Roles of Nurses in Executive Practice.* Issue brief. American Organization of Nurse Executives, 1997.

American Organization of Nurse Executives. *Refining the Art of Nurse Executive Practice.* American Organization of Nurse Executives, 1998.

Center for Health Leadership. *Exploring Alternative Futures.* Berkeley, Calif.: Center for Health Leadership, Western Consortium for Public Health, 1997.

Commission on Graduates of Foreign Nursing Schools. *The Trilateral Initiative for North American Nursing: An Assessment of North American Nursing.* Philadelphia: Commission on Graduates of Foreign Nursing Schools, 1996.

Hiebeler, R., Kelly, T. B., and Ketteman, C. *Best Practices: Building Your Business with Consumer Focused Solutions.* Simon & Schuster, 1998.

Institute of Medicine. *Primary Care: America's Health in a New Era.* Washington D.C.: National Academy Press, 1998.

Morath, J. (ed.). *Patients as Partners.* Chicago: American Hospital Association, 1997.

National Advisory Council on Nurse Education and Practice. *Report to the Secretary of the Department of Health and Human Services on the*

Basic Registered Nurse Workforce. Rockville, Md.: U.S. Department of Health and Human Services, Health Resources and Services Administration, Bureau of Health Professions, Division of Nursing, 1997.

National Institute of Nursing Research. *Community Based Health Care: Nursing Strategies.* Washington D.C.: National Institutes of Health, 1998.

Parsons, M. L., Murdaugh, C. L., and O'Rourke, R. A. *Interdisciplinary Case Studies in Health Care Redesign.* Gaithersburg, Md.: Aspen, 1998.

CHAPTER TWENTY-EIGHT

Transforming Nursing Leadership

Marilyn P. Chow
Janet M. Coffman
Robin L. Morjikian

*Marilyn P. Chow is vice president, patient care services, at
the Summit Medical Center, and dean for clinical affairs,
at the Samuel Merritt College in Oakland, California.
She is program director for the Robert Wood Johnson
Executive Nurse Fellows Program, a leadership development program, and she serves on several advisory boards,
including the Division of Nursing's National Advisory
Council on Nurse Education and Practice.*

*Janet M. Coffman is associate director for workforce
policy and analysis at the University of California at
San Francisco Center for the Health Professions. She serves
on the advisory committee for the California Strategic
Planning Committee for Nursing, and her publications
include* Strategies for the Future of Nursing *(coedited
with Edward O'Neil, 1998).*

*Robin L. Morjikian is deputy director of the Robert Wood
Johnson Executive Nurse Fellows Program at the University*

*of California at San Francisco Center for the Health
Professions. She also oversees other leadership development
activities of the center's Training and Consulting Division,
including a program for physicians.*

C hange has been the one constant in health care in
the United States in the 1990s. Although the pace and characteristics of
this change vary significantly, certain general patterns have emerged
in virtually every region across the nation. Since the early 1990s,
private and public purchasers have looked to managed care organizations to enhance the value of their health care dollars. The growth of
managed care has in turn prompted increased competition and consolidation among health care providers.

These new dynamics have fostered the growth of for-profit organizations, which have set new standards of efficiency by lowering costs
while achieving patient outcomes as good or better than those attained
by their not-for-profit competitors. Success in this environment
requires health care organizations to improve work efficiency, with
focused attention to the concerns of increasingly assertive and sophisticated consumers. These developments are facilitated in large part by
information technology advances that are expanding access to information for both providers and consumers (O'Neil, 1998).

As a consequence the field of health care has become increasingly
complex and chaotic. Health care organizations are constantly revis-
iting the range of services they offer and the means by which they furnish these services. In effect, the system is requiring leaders and
professionals to master the new roles and responsibilities needed to
fly an airplane that is being designed and constructed while it is in
flight.

The authors gratefully acknowledge the contributions of Janis P. Bellack,
Senior Fellow, University of California at San Francisco Center for the Health
Professions, and senior consultant to the Robert Wood Johnson Executive
Nurse Fellows Program, for her contributions to this chapter. We also thank
Edward O'Neil, Catherine Dower, Beth Mertz, and Jean Ann Seago for their
helpful comments during the chapter's preparation.

The ramifications of these and other developments are especially pronounced for registered nurses because theirs is the largest health care occupation in the United States, with 2.1 million active practitioners in 1996 (Moses, 1997, p. 33). Consequently, many efforts to improve efficiency involve changes in the configuring of the nursing workforce. The most dramatic reconfigurations are occurring in hospitals, the institutions that employ the largest numbers (60 percent) of the nursing workforce (Moses, 1997, p. 45). Decreasing health care dollars and challenging clinical imperatives to reduce patient length of stay in spite of increasing patient acuity require hospital executives to reevaluate the work of registered nursing personnel. Hospital executives are increasingly challenged to ensure that the right person delivers care at the right time for the right cost. One result is that the role of the registered nurse must focus on tasks that can be performed safely and effectively only by licensed professionals.

Several additional factors compound the challenges facing nursing leaders. First, nursing is probably the most diverse health profession. Multiple points of entry into practice and multiple pathways for career development make it difficult for nurses to reach consensus on appropriate roles for members of the profession. Second, nurses tend to view health care exclusively from the clinical perspective. They are excellent at identifying and responding to the multiple factors that affect the health and healing of individuals and their families, but are not accustomed to considering the economic, political, and social factors that affect health care organizations. Third, the nursing workforce is aging, prompting concerns, particularly among hospital nurse executives, about the system's ability to retain sufficient numbers of experienced registered nurses in increasingly demanding inpatient settings (Fralic, 1998). Finally, in many organizations, turnover among nurse executives is quite rapid, which compromises continuity and generates tension in the relatively stable workforces they are called upon to lead.

PERSPECTIVES FOR SUCCESSFUL NURSING LEADERSHIP

These rapid and dramatic changes in nurses' roles and responsibilities are generating much disruption and anxiety among nurses. Yet they are simultaneously providing nurses with greater opportunities to develop new and cost-effective models of improving the health and well-being of individuals and their communities. One of the most important contributions nursing leaders could make today would be to articulate a coherent vision of the future of both the profession and the health care delivery system. To do so, leaders will have to adopt three complementary perspectives:

Focus on core values

Welcome change as opportunity

Adopt a cosmopolitan outlook

Focus on Core Values

The nursing profession has a strong set of core values that emphasize concern for consumers' needs. Collins and Porras's observations (1997) about successful organizations suggest that nursing would do well to focus on preserving those core values: "Those who build visionary companies wisely understand that it is better to know WHO YOU ARE than where you are going—for where you are going will almost certainly change" (p. 222). This perspective is especially critical in health care today, where the pace of change is rapid. The nursing profession will serve the public best if it concentrates on maintaining and articulating its core values in the wake of these changes.

Welcome Change as Opportunity

However, nursing leaders must not confuse preserving core values with preserving specific roles and staffing patterns. Nursing has an exquisite challenge to educate, mobilize, and motivate a huge, diverse workforce to be flexible and to be welcoming of the ever changing demands of a system in the midst of chaos. Striving to preserve a status quo that will inevitably disappear diverts nursing leaders' valuable energies from creating the profession's future. Rather the nursing leader must become a *transformational* leader, one who "willingly lets go of old patterns and assumptions, and invites new thinking and behaving" (Kohles, Baker, and Donaho, 1995, p. 275). Transformational leadership requires a vision of the future and the capacity to articulate and implement innovative, coordinated strategies to achieve it.

Adopt a Cosmopolitan Outlook

Maintaining core values while looking toward the future will require nursing leaders to broaden their focus. Rosabeth Moss Kanter has observed that traditionally leaders succeeded by concentrating on the interests of their own profession or organization. The new environment in health care requires *cosmopolitan* leaders, ones "who are comfortable operating across boundaries and who can forge links between organizations" (Kanter, 1996, p. 91). This competency is consistent with Murphy's finding (1996) that exceptional leaders "provide a larger structure within which individuals and teams come together to achieve a whole greater than the sum of its parts" (p. 223).

Cosmopolitan leadership in nursing calls for greater engagement at three levels:

Among professional nursing organizations

With other health professionals

With leaders outside health care

PROFESSIONAL NURSING ORGANIZATIONS.   Nurses have organized themselves into myriad professional organizations, each with a different mission and agenda. The American Nurses Association seeks to represent all registered nurses, but the growth of specialty and role-based organizations (for example, the American Association of Nurse Anesthetists and the American Organization of Nurse Executives) suggests that many nurses display greater allegiance to such organizations than to the profession as a whole. At this critical juncture the nursing profession cannot afford such fragmentation because it impedes nurses' ability to reach consensus about the profession's future. Initiatives such as the National Federation of Specialty Nursing Organizations and the Nursing Organization Liaison Forum, which aim to unite nurses around overarching professional issues, must be expanded.

OTHER HEALTH PROFESSIONALS.   Nursing leaders must also work more closely with leaders in other health professions. Enhancing the cost effectiveness of clinical care will require all health professionals to work collaboratively to improve efficiency and patient outcomes. Collaborative leaders also serve as important role models for health professionals in the growing number of organizations that employ interdisciplinary teams to deliver services. In addition, forming common cause with leaders in other health professions to address policy issues of mutual concern will increase nursing leaders' ability to promote legislative and regulatory reforms.

LEADERS OUTSIDE HEALTH CARE. Finally, nursing leaders must also engage more frequently and systematically with leaders outside health care. Building and sustaining healthy communities requires health professionals to look beyond the walls of their institutions to the communities in which they operate. Dialogue with leaders outside health care is critical to identifying community needs and the roles that health care organizations can play in meeting them. In addition, many ideas for innovation are likely to come from those not bound by traditional assumptions about health care delivery.

STRENGTHENING LEADERSHIP DEVELOPMENT

The new dynamics of nursing leadership necessitate a recommitment to educating nurses for leadership roles and a rethinking of traditional patterns for teaching leadership skills. New and complementary strategies, particularly executive-level initiatives, are needed to ensure that nursing leaders acquire needed competencies.

The Need to Develop Executive Leaders

Given the nursing profession's unique position in the health care system, development of strong executive leadership is a paramount concern. Most nurses in leadership positions have been taught leadership only as part of their basic nursing education. At that time, however, they have no professional experience upon which to reflect. They can only absorb general principles and observe the actions of other nurses in leadership roles. As a consequence, many are unprepared for their later leadership roles and responsibilities.

Nurses' frontline roles in care delivery provide them with intimate knowledge of clinical operations. From this experience, they also gain a number of competencies critical to leadership, including cultural awareness, community focus, and conflict management and teamwork skills. However, experience alone is not sufficient to augment the nursing leadership courses taught at the basic level. Nurses require additional leadership competencies if they are to meet the challenges of institutional transformation and system change. In particular, they need a systems perspective and competencies in developing strategic visions, risk taking, innovating, and managing change.

Ultimately, leadership development must be conceived as a lifelong process that encompasses multiple episodes of formal training that build upon prior professional experience. Individuals do learn from their experiences, but formal leadership development programs facilitate focused self-assessment and mastery of new leadership competencies.

The Benefits of Leadership Development Programs

A number of formal professional development programs have been established for nurses. Some programs seek to enhance nurse executives' management and business skills. An example of this approach is the Johnson & Johnson–Wharton Fellows Program in Management for Nurse Executives. Launched in 1983, this intensive three-week summer program is geared toward giving nurses an understanding of the personal and organizational dynamics of decision making. It covers such topics as marketing, organizational behavior, the economics of health care decision making, financial management, and mergers and acquisitions.

Such business and management-oriented programs are quite valuable but must be complemented by initiatives that focus on leadership competencies. Executives need more than strong business skills to lead health care organizations in these turbulent times. They must also be able to manage change and communicate their vision of the future to employees, members, consumers, and community leaders.

Recognizing this need, nursing organizations have established programs and initiatives that emphasize leadership competencies, including the Center for Nursing Leadership, which is a partnership of the American Organization of Nurse Executives and the Network for Healthcare Management. The Center for Nursing Leadership enhances executive nurses' leadership effectiveness through a series of experiences such as the Journey Toward Mastery, a yearlong leadership program. Two other initiatives are Sigma Theta Tau's Leadership Institute and the American Association of Colleges of Nursing's Executive Development Series, which includes the Academic Leadership Workshop.

One of the newest leadership development programs for nurse executives is the Robert Wood Johnson (RWJ) Executive Nurse Fellows Program. Sponsored by the Robert Wood Johnson Foundation and directed by the Center for the Health Professions at the University of California at San Francisco, this three-year fellowship program is open to outstanding nurses in executive roles in health services (including patient care services, integrated delivery systems, health plans, and other health care organizations), public health, and nursing education. The program aims to prepare participants for leadership roles at the highest echelons in health care.

Building on the leadership profile advocated by the leadership experts who call for greater collaboration and innovative partnerships, the RWJ Executive Nurse Fellows Program focuses on five key leadership competencies for the next century:

- *Self-knowledge:* the ability to understand self in the context of organizational challenges, interpersonal demands, and individual motivation
- *Strategic vision:* the ability to connect broad social, economic, and political changes to the strategic direction of institutions and organizations
- *Risk taking and creativity:* the ability to transform self and organization by moving outside traditional and patterned ways of success
- *Interpersonal skills and communication effectiveness:* the ability to translate strategic vision into compelling and motivating messages
- *Managing change:* the ability to continually create, structure, and effectively implement organizational change

These five competencies are the program pillars and will infuse the learning experiences of each Fellow. Once appointed, each Fellow will follow a three-year course of study, completing a core leadership curriculum and an individual learning plan and being mentored by a senior executive. Each program component will promote acquisition of the five key competencies. The core curriculum will provide a solid grounding in leadership theory and techniques. The structured mentoring experience will nurture competencies in alliance building, partnership development, communication, and change management through one-on-one interaction with senior executives in various industries. Self-directed activities like peer coaching and journal writing, critical components of the individual learning plans, will foster each Fellow's increased self-knowledge and greater awareness of personal leadership style.

One of the unique features of the program is that it will engage the participating Fellow's employing organization as the Fellow completes a leadership project in that institution. Finally, the program is committed to creating and sustaining an ongoing leadership network composed of current and former Fellows, past and present mentors, faculty, scholars, and other leaders.

References

Collins, J. C., and Porras, J. I. *Built to Last: Successful Habits of Visionary Companies.* New York: Harper Business, 1997.

Fralic, M. F. "How Is Demand for Registered Nurses in Hospital Settings Changing?" In E. O'Neil and J. Coffman (eds.), *Strategies for the Future of Nursing.* San Francisco: Jossey-Bass, 1998.

Kanter, R. M. "World-Class Leaders: The Power of Partnering." In F. Hesselbein, M. Goldsmith, and R. Beckhard (eds.), *The Leader of the Future: New Visions, Strategies, and Practices for the Next Era.* San Francisco: Jossey-Bass, 1996.

Kohles, M. K., Baker, W. G., and Donaho, B. A. *Transformational Leadership: Renewing Fundamental Values and Achieving New Relationships in Health Care.* Chicago: American Hospital Association, 1995.

Moses, E. B. *The Registered Nurse Population, March 1996: Findings from the National Sample Survey of Registered Nurses.* Rockville, Md.: U.S. Department of Health and Human Services, Health Resources and Services Administration, Bureau of Health Professions, Division of Nursing, 1997.

Murphy, E. C. *Leadership IQ.* New York: Wiley, 1996.

O'Neil, E. "Nursing in the Next Century." In E. O'Neil and J. Coffman (eds.), *Strategies for the Future of Nursing.* San Francisco: Jossey-Bass, 1998.

PART SIX

Gaining New Skills

CHAPTER TWENTY-NINE

Leading Across
the Network

Marshall Goldsmith

*Marshall Goldsmith is a founding director of
Keilty, Goldsmith & Company (KGC) and a
cofounder of the Learning Network, an association
of the world's top leadership development consultants.
His clients have included many of the world's leading
corporations, and the leadership feedback processes
that KGC has helped develop have been used by over
one million people in seventy different organizations.
The coeditor (with Frances Hesselbein and Richard
Beckhard) of* The Community of the Future *(1998),*
The Organization of the Future *(1997), and* The
Leader of the Future *(1996), he serves on advisory
boards for Andersen Consulting's Strategic Change
Institute and the Josephson Institute of Ethics and on
the board of directors of the Drucker Foundation.*

A major trend already shaping health care leadership and likely to accelerate is the trend toward leading *across* a network of partners, as opposed to leading *down* a hierarchical organization of subordinates. Health care leaders of the future need to know why this trend is becoming so pronounced, and (even more important) they need to understand how their capabilities need to change if their organizations are to succeed in tomorrow's networked world.

CHALLENGES OF LEADING ACROSS THE NETWORK

Here are a few key reasons (of the many that could be listed) why networked health care organizations will become more important in the future:

The dramatically increased cost and complexity that suppliers will face in getting products and services to market. Almost all the major organizations involved in the discovery and development of drugs are scrambling to build networks. These networks are being built through mergers, joint ventures, alliances, and even deals with competitors. Major pharmaceutical firms are investing in university relationships and start-up companies at a record pace. All innovation requires a willingness to take risks and to face the possibility of failure. The cost of failure in tomorrow's world may be so great that spreading the risk is becoming an increasingly prudent business strategy.

The issue of cost and complexity does not exist on just the developmental side of business but on the distribution side as well. Global distribution will become increasingly important in tomorrow's health care market. Several leading companies are building partnerships with their former competitors to ensure that their products receive high-quality global distribution without incurring prohibitive costs. As the cost and complexity of getting new products to market increases, the networked organization will begin to become the norm. Companies will be increasingly unwilling to go it alone, and leaders will need the skills to build and manage alliances.

The increased formation of customer alliances at every level of the health care value chain. The ultimate consumers of health care products, the patients, are increasingly organized in large groups. The individual consumer as the sole maker of the health care decision is becoming the rarity as opposed to the rule. Small businesses, historically independent, are now forming cooperatives that can give them the same purchasing power as major organizations (the state of California even organizes small businesses for this purpose). Medical doctors are forming alliances to reduce the cost of doing business and to negotiate (or even compete) with health maintenance organizations (HMOs). Independent pharmacies, which were getting badly beaten on price by major chains, have joined together in purchasing cooperatives. Individual hospitals, which can not afford all the specialized equipment they would like, are forming partnerships with other hospitals to spread the cost of new medical technology. The increased importance of customer alliances will require tomorrow's health care leaders to have very different skills from the leaders of the past. These new leaders will need to form many more partnering relationships with customer groups and to structure much more complex, multiparty customer agreements.

The impact of new information technology.   New information technology can connect formerly disparate entities into one network without incurring prohibitive cost. A recent extreme example of the importance of information technology involves a huge health care provider who had a severe information system problem. When the magnitude of the problem came to light, the company's stock dropped by more than 50 percent, the CEO was asked to leave, and the organization was purchased in a turnaround sale by another organization (which believes that it can fix the system). The degree of importance that information technology is coming to have in the health care field could not have even been imagined twenty years ago. In the future the ability to improve networking by using information technology will be a major competitive issue for many health care organizations. Leaders will have to have not only a knowledge of their health care field but the technological savvy to successfully implement new information systems.

The demand for integrated solutions, not stand-alone products. Tomorrow's consumers in a variety of fields will be demanding integrated solutions, not stand-alone products. This trend can be observed in fields as diverse as telecommunications, banking, and travel and leisure. The health care world is definitely no exception. Sophisticated customers are increasingly asking for comprehensive agreements that meet complex needs, not just simple products that fix simple prob-lems. The old days in which the detail man sold a product to an in-dividual physician or pharmacist are quickly being replaced by a future in which a highly trained consultant calls on a team of cus-tomer representatives who consider many complex factors in making a purchasing agreement. Integrated solutions frequently involve mul-tiple organizations and may call for a completely different set of net-working skills compared to the comparatively simple need to sell a product. The knowledge required for understanding complex cus-tomer needs (including financial needs) will be quite different from the knowledge required for understanding how to sell stand-alone products.

The increased pressure on cost and time.   The health care industry was able to pass increased costs and inefficiency on to the consumer for years after this was no longer possible in most other industries. Those days are gone and will not return. Tomorrow's health care orga-nizations will either be intensely competitive or will disappear. The stocks of many health care companies in the United States and Europe are selling at record levels. Shareholders have grown accustomed to high returns in general and are now expecting returns commensurate with the very high premiums they have paid for these stocks. Under-performing companies will be bought (with or without the consent of their boards). Reengineering, restructuring, and continuous improvement have become ongoing processes as opposed to one-time events. The flexible networked organization will become a require-ment as the time and cost of yesterday's bureaucracy becomes impos-sible to support. Leaders will need to be able to use flexible networks to get the job done quickly and efficiently. Leaders who can not adapt to these changing requirements will be replaced quickly and efficiently.

The new high-potential employees have very different expectations. The *knowledge workers* in the health care field of tomorrow will have very different expectations of their leaders than the knowledge work-ers of the past had. In the past even the high-potential employees were willing to pay their corporate dues and play the organizational game. Very few of today's high-potential employees expect (or even want) to work in one large corporation for their entire careers. According to Prof. Reggi Herzlinger in a 1998 conversation at the Harvard Business School, almost half of the students at Harvard Business School today want to be entrepreneurs. The new high-potential employee wants to be given challenge, involvement, and opportunity—not certainty, direction, and security. High-potential employees of the future will have to be treated more like partners than subordinates. The ability to attract and retain these key knowledge workers will become a critical factor in the long-term success of the organization.

KEY CAPABILITIES FOR HEALTH CARE LEADERS

The successful health care leader of the future may well need to possess a much broader range of capabilities than the leader of the past. These new capabilities will include a greater breadth of knowledge, a greater depth of knowledge, and a significant increase in required interpersonal skills. As has been discussed, leading in a complex networked organization will be significantly more challenging than leading in a simpler, more hierarchical organization.

The health care leader of the future may need these key capabilities:

The skills to form partnerships inside the organization.   In a networked global organization, leaders will need the skills to effectively influence people without having direct line authority. Product managers may need to convince country (or regional) managers to commit to a strategic global plan that may benefit the entire corporation but not be in the short-term best interests of the individual country. Decisions about the use of new technology will have to balance the organization's need for consistency with the unit's need for customization. People at all levels of the company may become involved in decisions formerly reserved for executives. Skills at developing win-win relationships across the organization will become more important than ever. Dictating to people what to do and how to do it may not get them committed, but it is simple. Involving people across the organization as partners is a much more complex process and may well require increased cultural sensitivity and a significant upgrade in leadership skills.

The ability to form alliances outside the organization.   Even the largest organizations in the health care field realize that they will need to form strategic alliances in order to maintain a competitive advantage in tomorrow's marketplace. Forming a large-scale business alliance requires the ability to conduct an in-depth analysis of both companies' strengths and weaknesses, a relatively deep understanding of finance, and (perhaps most important) the interpersonal skills to negotiate a deal between executives who may have reasonably large egos. Many leaders in the health care field today may not have the business or negotiation skills necessary to build large-scale alliances.

The subtlety and sensitivity to take a new approach to competitors. Aside from a change in skills, future leaders may also need a change in orientation. Historically, the health care executive has focused largely on *winning* for his or her organization. The leader of the future may have to exhibit a great deal more subtlety and long-term sensitivity toward competitors. When today's competitors are tomorrow's business partners or customers, the entire rules of business change. The concept of *destroying* the competition may become dysfunctional. Leaders will need to ensure that their organizations have reputations for fairness and integrity and that competitors will regard them as good potential partners.

The ability to understand customers at every level of the value chain. The health care organization of the future will often have to learn to deal with a number of different customers who may well have competing agendas. Governmental agencies and HMOs may be pushing for decreased costs, physicians may be asking for more autonomy, patients may be pressing for more flexibility, and investors may be demanding a greater return on investment. The effective leader will balance the costs and benefits so that they will be shared by all groups in the network. This will be far from easy. The leader will be required to understand not only the health care issues at every customer level in the value chain but also the business issues. Understanding each network member's financial needs and resources was much less critical in the past than it will be in the future. Many leaders in the past were not trained to deal with the complexity or the pressure that they may face in the future.

The technological savvy needed to produce a competitive advantage. It is unrealistic to expect the leader of the future to be an expert in all the health care and information technology that will affect the organization. The rapid pace of technological change will make that level of technical knowledge almost impossible to achieve. Nevertheless, the leader who does not know how to use e-mail and says, "I don't understand that stuff," when answering technology questions is a thing of the past. Leaders will have to *understand the impact* of technology and *speak the language* of technology. They will have to have the savvy to see how new developments in technology will affect their organizations. This technological savvy will require not only learning new skills but continually upgrading existing skills.

The ability to hire and retain knowledge workers. As Peter Drucker noted in a Drucker Foundation meeting in 1997, the ability to successfully manage knowledge workers will be a key variable that differentiates the most successful organizations of the future from their competitors. This ability will be especially important in the health care field. As knowledge workers have become more *important* to keep, they have also become much more *difficult* to keep. Health care leaders of the future will have to make hiring, developing, and keeping great people one of their top priorities. Ralph Larsen, the CEO of Johnson & Johnson, for example, told the author in a 1997 meeting that the development of capable leaders (at all levels of the organization) is one of his greatest challenges in achieving the long-term growth that he knows J&J can produce. The skills needed to retain tomorrow's highly mobile knowledge workers will be very different from the skills required to retain yesterday's more stable knowledge worker. Leaders who make this skills transition may produce a huge long-term advantage for their corporations.

Leading the health care organization of the future will be a much more complex and difficult task than leading the health care organization of the past. Tomorrow's leaders will need to learn to thrive in a new networked world. Compared to the more traditional, hierarchical organization of the past, the networked organization will follow different rules and require different capabilities. Leaders of the future will have to develop new capabilities and skills not just once but continually throughout their careers. The pace of change is not going to slow down. Leaders who can not adapt to the new world of health care management will be quickly replaced. Leaders who can adapt to the new networked structure and develop new capabilities will thrive.

CHAPTER THIRTY

Four Dimensions of Lasting Change

Karen Golden-Biddle

R. Mark Biddle

Karen Golden-Biddle is associate professor of organizational analysis at the University of Alberta in Edmonton, Canada. A founding member of the Center for Healthcare Leadership at Emory University School of Medicine, she conducts executive education and development seminars for North American and international managers in for-profit and nonprofit organizations. Her primary area of research and consulting is culture and change management, particularly in health care organizations.

R. Mark Biddle is a consultant with a concentration on private career counseling. He was the founding director of Emory Clergy Care, a program providing health care, career counseling, and crisis intervention. A United Methodist minister and a licensed professional counselor, he has written articles and designed workshops in the areas of leadership development, wellness, and health care.

The recent changes in health care have garnered a great deal of interest and discussion and also consternation. The ways leaders address these changes will shape the concepts and practices health care organizations will ultimately stand for and the organizational structures the health care industry will use to deliver care in the future.

To ensure short-term survival in today's turbulent health care environment, much leadership attention has been directed toward identifying external changes (for example, reimbursement and fee schedules) and then responding by initiating adaptive internal changes (for example, streamlining costs). Thus environmental change has been followed by organizational change. However, leaders will find that initiating change is the easy part of the health care transformation. The hard part is sustaining change.

How can leaders effectively sustain desired change once it is initiated? How can leaders sustain change when the former world of health care, characterized by fee-for-service, no longer exists and the future world is yet to be defined? How can leaders become more active in shaping their organizations' future missions and identities?

In our work with organizations over the past twenty years, we have observed that the more fundamental and far-reaching the implications of change, the harder it is to accomplish and sustain that change. Once the highly touted and visible phase of initiating organizational change is accomplished, it is followed by an often overlooked transitional phase. It is in this latter phase that the work of sustaining change occurs. The key to sustaining change is to navigate effectively through this period. It is in this phase of *liminality* (Turner, 1974), or organizational limbo, that organizational members confront not only confusion and anxiety but also the potential for tremendous creativity and scenario building. And it is this phase that requires energy and devoted effort from all affected by the changes, both inside and outside any single organization.

We have identified four dimensions of sustained change: reformulating organizational identity, establishing partnerships, institutionalizing trust, and developing structural participation. Underlying these dimensions is the recognition that no single organization can sustain desired change in isolation from the larger community.

REFORMULATING
ORGANIZATIONAL IDENTITY

Fundamental change of the type being experienced in the health care industry does not affect only practices, operating procedures, and other routines. It also affects organizational identity and structure. No change efforts can be sustained unless organizational leaders within and across specific health care organizations understand how an organization's identity is affected by change and are active in reshaping and reformulating that identity.

Organizational identity can be defined as that which is central, enduring, and distinctive about an organization (Albert and Whetten, 1985). An integral part of an organization's culture, or governing belief systems (Golden-Biddle and Rao, 1997), identity is a key source of organizational stability. It provides a sense of continuity in the midst of change. However, in the midst of fundamental change, even identity is affected. Leaders then must ask what aspects of the organization's identity need to change and what ones should remain the same. Here are two examples.

In the past a health care organization's identity and care delivery structure assumed that patients entered the organization when they were ill and sought medical expertise to be cured. However, this prevailing identity has been called into question by such changes as the advent of managed care, a better understanding of systemic causes of illness, and increased patient knowledge about personal illness. Whereas the old identity was based on a hierarchical model of the physician-patient relationship, the emerging identity needs to incorporate a more consensual model for the physician-patient partnership, seeing patients as responsible for their health and actively involved in their treatment. At risk is the belief in the authority of the physician and other health care professionals upon which the old identity of health care organizations has been based. Will health care organizations expand their identities to incorporate a belief in the value of an informed patient? If they do not, their identities will rest on conflicting models and become ambiguous, and the transformation of the health care organization will remain incomplete and ineffective.

The second example concerns the identity of academic medical centers. They were founded to provide specialty medical care based on the most recent research. In practice, this identity translated into the valuation of research over clinical practice. However, with the advent of managed care, the supremacy of research over clinical practice is being seriously challenged. What happens to the belief in the value of research? Can it coexist with an identity built on clinical practice? If these questions are not resolved, the centers' identity will become ambiguous, and lack of a strong identity will lead to the failure of changes in practices and the failure to work effectively with managed care programs.

Sustaining change necessitates, then, that leaders keep a watchful eye on an organization's identity. Deciding which aspects of an organization's identity should endure is often overlooked in the rush to initiate change, yet these aspects will give stability to the organization in an otherwise turbulent context. Likewise, discerning which aspects of the organization's identity should change is equally important; these changes help impel the organization into the future.

ESTABLISHING PARTNERSHIPS

More broadly, reshaping the identity of health care organizations is the responsibility of leaders in the field, both leaders of single organizations and leaders of larger groupings. Health care leaders must engage the broader community in dialogue that goes beyond public relations. They must support partnerships based on listening, understanding, and sharing with organizations, community members, and other stakeholders in the health care system. These partnerships are best characterized as interactive; all stakeholders are represented at the table of decision making. In this grand design of governmental, health, and community voices, often the least prepared for the dialogue and yet the most in need of health care are the members of the community, particularly those on the margins of power and influence.

Dialogue between a health care organization and community members starts with numerous difficulties. These include the bridging the disparity between medical language and public understanding, finding an adequate place to hold the dialogue, and overcoming the community's perception that the health care provider is insensitive to public needs, wants, and even values. However, these problems are not insurmountable. Dialogue (Senge, 1990) offers opportunities to fix broken places, one at a time. Leadership that can enhance such communication, not only in the organization but also in the community, will help legitimize that organization in the community. This task will not be simple but will build a foundation of trust.

The health care organization that does not attend to the vision of public health in the community will be viewed as uninterested. Partnerships based on the longings, hopes, and dreams of those served will give organizations more knowledge of community needs and help them adapt to those needs. The ability to adapt based on an awareness of the community needs, and not only on the changing demands of the health care institution, is instrumental in sustaining change. Those organizations capable of such adaptation are those likely to transform themselves successfully for the future.

INSTITUTIONALIZING TRUST

Institutionalizing trust is an integral dimension of sustaining change. Without trust an organization's efforts will be viewed with skepticism at best and as damaging at worst.

Trust at a basic level occurs in health care when individuals in the community believe that the medical profession will not do them harm. For example, such trust should exist between patient and health care provider from the moment the patient calls the physician's office or enters a hospital or clinic in the search for care.

When organizations incorporate such basic trust into health care delivery, they begin to institutionalize that trust. In essence, they build on basic trust by putting it into practice. One might call this *legitimized trust* (Greenleaf, 1977). Organizations that achieve legitimized trust will be perceived in the community as reliable, responsive, and ready to serve. In contrast, organizations that fail to develop it are likely to fail.

Institutionalized trust is particularly important when health care organizations are in the midst of fundamental changes because patients want assurance that the quality and reliability of care will be the same each time a patient seeks care. Indeed one of the major concerns expressed as health care organizations change is whether their increasingly financial focus has damaged the delivery of health care. When they address only the concerns of efficiency and fiscal survival, for example, they are likely to fail in their attempts to sustain change and to survive the fundamental transformation under way in health care. They will neither improve health care nor develop the requisite institutionalized trust.

Establishing and institutionalizing trust is not as elusive as organizational leaders might first imagine. Indeed an argument can be made that a deep and abiding sense of basic trust already exists between the community and the health care organization. In fact, in only a few institutions in our society is basic trust so strong. Nevertheless, in the midst of today's fundamental health care change, breaches in that trust can and do occur. Trust is perhaps the most precious of commodities for health care organizations. Leaders who are intentional about maintaining and increasing trust, especially during fundamental change, will go a long way toward ensuring their organizations' survival and readiness for the future.

DEVELOPING STRUCTURAL PARTICIPATION

Structural participation is perhaps the most elusive of the necessary dimensions for sustaining change. Structural participation is both a pattern of interaction and an ethical posture. It is the health care provider's disposition toward the health care recipient. Figure 30.1 illustrates structural participation, showing the possible combinations of the roles of the health care provider as colleague or expert and the roles of health care consumer as active or passive participant.

Traditionally, in the predominant form of structural participation, the physician is seen as the expert and the patient is expected to be passive. However, recent changes are challenging that pattern, and there

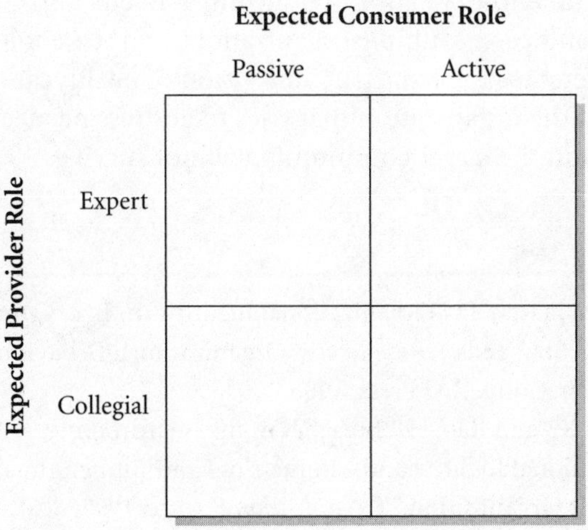

Figure 30.1. Forms of Structural Participation.

is a shift toward seeing the physician or other provider as a colleague and expecting the patient to be active. For this shift to become fully functional, the health care provider and health care consumer must develop an awareness of their *partnership* for better health. The organization takes on a greater responsibility for communication and education; the consumer takes on greater responsibility for prevention. Patients must be educated about their personal responsibility in reducing health care costs. Preventable accidents, physical fitness, and public health standards are vital concerns. Similarly, health care providers need to acclimate themselves to a more active consumer.

In response to the profound changes occurring in health care, organizational leaders have focused on surviving in these turbulent times. This has meant, for example, that they have necessarily focused on adapting to declining health care dollars by streamlining costs and establishing contracts for fixed dollars for services. Surviving by initiating such changes, we have argued, is the easy part; sustaining such changes is the more difficult challenge. Sustaining change requires health care organizations to reformulate their identity, establish partnerships with stakeholders in the broader community, institutionalize trust even as changes occur, and integrate a new form of structural participation for health care providers and recipients. More fundamentally, providers must engage in dialogue with recipients and other community stakeholders about community needs and the future delivery of health care. Multiple organizations and stakeholders need to form partnerships to reconstruct the vision of health care delivery. It is likely that the organization that tries to address needed changes in isolation from the larger community will not survive.

References

Albert, S., and Whetten, D. "Organizational Identity." In L. L. Cummings and B. M. Staw (eds.), Research in Organizational Behavior. Vol. 7. Greenwich, Conn.: JAI Press, 1985.

Golden-Biddle, K., and Rao, H. "Breaches in the Boardroom: Organizational Identity and Conflicts of Commitment in a Nonprofit Organization." *Organization Science*, 1997, 8(6), 593–611.

Greenleaf, R. *Servant Leadership*. New York: Paulist Press, 1977.

Senge, P. *The Fifth Discipline: The Art and Practice of the Learning Organization.* New York: Doubleday Currency, 1990.

Turner, V. *Dramas, Fields, and Metaphors.* Ithaca, N.Y.: Cornell University Press, 1974.

CHAPTER THIRTY-ONE

Developing Organizations by Developing Individuals

Elaine Franklin

Robbin M. Moore

Elaine Franklin is a managing director and director of assessment for career development programs at the Center for Healthcare Leadership at the Emory University School of Medicine. She is also director of assessment at Global Access Learning, an international executive education and management development consulting firm. She specializes in training and coaching managers of all levels in health care and other leading nonprofit and for-profit organizations.

Robbin M. Moore is associate administrator at Emory Hospitals in Atlanta, Georgia, administrator of Emory's Center for Rehabilitation Medicine, and also the coordinator for Emory Hospitals' participation in the Leadership Forum. She is a nominee for the 1998 International Emerging Leaders in Healthcare Award, a facilitator for the Covey Leadership Center, and a founding member of the Atlanta Quality Resource Center.

ompetent organizations view challenges as unique opportunities for learning and growth. But organizations do not really make learning and growth happen—*people* do! An imperative for survival is the continual encouragement of both individuals and organizations to identify, enhance, and lead from core learning strengths and core competencies.

One of the most formidable challenges facing health care organizations is defining and developing the new skill sets required to lead increasingly complex integrated systems of delivery. This chapter outlines the process used by a complex integrated system in an academic medical center to address this challenge.

DEFINING THE NEED

Emory Healthcare has formed the Learning Council, a group representing the major components of its integrated system: the hospitals, geriatric center, rehabilitation medicine center, and faculty practice plan consisting of over eight hundred physicians. The purpose of the Learning Council is to provide a forum through which council members anticipate and coordinate the learning needs of the system. In pursuing these goals the Learning Council engaged in a forecasting exercise aimed at anticipating the skill sets required to manage future challenges. For example, health care organizations in the twenty-first century will need to be considerably more agile and responsive to the changing needs of multiple customer groups. They will need to develop new services with speed and flexibility. This will require leaders to be learners who have developed the capacity to amass critical resources quickly in response to rapidly arising opportunities and demands.

The Learning Council identified multiple skill sets (management and leadership competencies) that are required of leaders in the organization. For example, from a project management perspective, particular skills will be needed to oversee new services initiatives begun by rapid response health care systems in the future. Initiative success will in large part rest on leaders' capacity to coordinate across traditional boundaries, bringing the necessary human and capital resources to bear on rapidly emerging demands and opportunities. From a leadership perspective, one of the skills required is cognitive flexibility, so that leaders can, for example, amass resources creatively in support of innovative, responsive solutions to changing constituent requirements. Another leadership skill needed is the competence to form effective interpersonal alliances across professional and functional boundaries.

Strategies can best be formulated and driven when baseline competencies clearly identify both successful behaviors from the past and prospective requirements for the future. Competency identification can also help create an organizational language useful in articulating strategies and identifying and developing high-potential performers. Because people create and drive strategies, competency criteria–based assessment of people's level of performance is a vital step in the individual's developmental process and the organization's developmental growth. Assessment, or diagnosis, of an individual's competency-based behaviors is the next step in the process of practicing preventive medicine within an organization. Following diagnosis, a prescription is offered for improvement and growth, accompanied by periodic checkups to monitor whether real, measurable change is occurring. Businesses have been relying on competency-driven development processes for several years, and a recent successful example in health care is the Emory Healthcare Learning Council's Leadership Development Process.

USING THE LEADERSHIP DEVELOPMENT PROCESS

It was specifically to ensure application of a formal, consistent approach to leadership development that John D. Henry, Sr., CEO of Emory University Hospitals, created the Learning Council. With top management's support the Learning Council embraced a truly strategic role that focused on several ways to facilitate learning. As one key project, the council members began a competency assessment feedback program. After extensive research for a methodology for assessing which competencies an individual does or does not demonstrate, they chose 360-degree feedback, a popular and widely used form of multirater appraisal. Most often used for developmental purposes, it gives individuals a perspective on how others with whom they work (boss, peers, reports, customers, and so forth) perceive their behavior in competency areas critical to success with specific jobs and strategies.

The Learning Council participants (educators, administrators, department heads, and key staff employees) began by identifying the core competencies of the health care leader, based on future organizational requirements; developing the 360-degree-feedback assessment tool; creating a survey feedback report; developing a developmental planning guidebook linking participants to a broad array of resources including the Internet; and designing a five-month coaching process to assist participants in formulating and completing a personal strategic plan based upon their feedback.

During the first phase of the 360-degree-feedback project, the Learning Council reviewed the many complex and diverse competencies required of health care leaders. Eight core competency dimensions were identified as critical at Emory Healthcare: self-management, management, leadership, interpersonal, conceptual, communication, organizational strategy, and technical. When defining these competency dimensions, forty-three specific competencies, or skill sets, emerged that would challenge individuals in all levels of the organization to learn how to anticipate and adapt to change.

In the second phase the Center for Healthcare Leadership (CHL) of the Emory Medical School worked with the Learning Council to create a feedback survey instrument with behavioral statements that reliably measured an individual's rating on the forty-three skill sets. For example, under the self-management competency dimension, time management was one of the specific competencies, and a time management behavior, "Insists that things get completed when they are promised," was rated for every participant, on a scale of 1 (strongly disagree) to 5 (strongly agree). Once the competency assessment survey was constructed, thirty-five people were selected for a pilot program; they included some senior administrative team members, volunteers from the department directors group, and a random selection of department leaders from each administrative division. At a kickoff seminar, each participant received a feedback survey about individual competencies, which the participant and his or her boss(es) were to complete. This was the diagnosis phase of the project. To ensure confidentiality, surveys were mailed directly to the CHL by the raters. In the next phase of the process, after all participant surveys were received and scored, a coach from the CHL set up an appointment to meet with each participant and to present the person with a survey report and the planning guidebook, *Guide to Development*.

During the three face-to-face sessions and as-needed telephone coaching sessions, each participant and the coach discussed perceived strengths and developmental areas, completed a plan for development, discussed specific challenges to implementing the plan, and looked at new ways to drive the participant's goal to completion. The plan for development, the prescription, contained a written goal that was specific, time-phased, measurable, and a bit of a stretch. Participants also defined the action steps required to attain their goals. They focused upon such potential activities as designing a new job assignment, fixing a problem, starting something from scratch, getting involved in a new or different project or task force, broadening scope of responsibility, and occasionally doing someone else's job. The action steps also required participants to identify mentors and coaches, sources of ongoing feedback, potential obstacles, learning opportunities, and ways to evaluate and measure progress. Each step had to support the goal, address critical personal developmental issues, and align with organizational strategic priorities. At each session, participants were asked about their successes and challenges and were encouraged to implement their plans to stay on task. Their CHL coach asked guiding questions intended to sharpen their focus, gave suggestions when appropriate, and discussed or provided resources related to their competency development area. Improvements, recorded on the planning sheet, were identified through observation by each participant and by the participant's coach, mentors, colleagues, and others. This feedback created the basis for the next phase of the participant's learning curve—enriching the current plan to develop a critical competency and using the work successfully undertaken to start a new learning curve.

A follow-up retreat was designed to address common competency development needs of the pilot group, and a session on coaching was presented to encourage all senior administrative staff and department heads to move from the old paradigm of *control-order-prescribe* to a new paradigm of *acknowledge-create-empower*. In this new paradigm, knowledge becomes shared power; it no longer resides exclusively at the top of the organization. Making a personal commitment to oneself and to another person is an extremely powerful piece of the process. The perspective of this additional person—who knows what the organization values, knows what skills are needed for a specific job, and offers specific, relevant information about the participant's performance—is invaluable. At this point in the learning process the person doing the checkup, whether a coach, mentor, boss, colleague, or some other person, can give feedback that promotes adaptation that can drive real change and move the process forward. Thus the people in the developmental program have the eyes of another to monitor progress and assist them in seeing when it is time to expand upon or conclude work being done in the selected competency area.

RECOGNIZING THREE
MODES OF LEARNING

Three modes of learning were present in the Emory Learning Council project and were important factors when creating personal development plans that helped participants navigate through myriad currents, some of which appeared unexpectedly, a few of which were not easily recognizable, many of which were out of participant's control, and all of which were demanding. The first mode is *shock learning,* or crisis problem solving, and it is the first meta-skill of learning. Because each of us faces a crisis at times, we must all learn techniques and skills for solving critical problems. Organizations and individuals tend to put an inordinate amount of focus on matters that may be urgent but are not necessarily important. Crisis problem solving is learning for what *has happened.*

Maintenance learning, the second mode, is often viewed as learning for improvement of current activities. It involves education and training, formal and informal, for work currently in progress or for work and work problems sometime in the near future. This type of learning is not only for general preparation but can also involve planning that prevents or avoids problems. Maintenance learning focuses upon what *is happening.*

In contrast, the third mode of learning, *anticipatory learning,* is learning for what *will happen* in the future. It involves not only getting ready for or predicting the future but also to some degree creating the future. Collecting and analyzing data that reveal cause-and-effect relationships over time enables organizations and individuals to understand what is happening now and what could happen in the future. The goal is to produce outcomes or results that are desired rather than determined by external factors and forces. At least three meta-skills are linked to anticipatory learning and required if individuals and groups within organizations are to develop. They are reaching out to obtain data, using new methods of display and analysis to construct valuable information, and applying new approaches to integrate and interpret information (Sashkin and Franklin, 1993).

Future-focused intelligence and anticipatory learning can be used to develop long-term action strategies. Anticipatory learning can drive significant individual and organizational development and change culture from the inside out, so it accords with the organization's purpose, values, and required competencies. A dynamic culture then emerges when shared strategic intent becomes an active process of articulating creative strategies that are invented by individuals to accomplish ambitious ends. In this ideal scenario, strategic intent is not driven by plans formulated at the top and pushed down throughout the organization (Hamel and Prahalad, 1989); it is birthed within a culture where lasting and significant contributions are made by those who are guided by a core ideology and shared sense of mission in their efforts to build a visionary organization (Collins and Porras, 1996). Future-focused individual and organizational transformation allows for interpolation backward to the present, making it easier to know now what competencies will be required in the future to achieve strategic intent.

References

Collins, J. C., and Porras, J. I. "Building Your Company's Vision." *Harvard Business Review,* Sept.–Oct. 1996, pp. 65–77.

Hamel, G., and Prahalad, C. K. "Strategic Intent." *Harvard Business Review,* May–June 1989, pp. 63–76.

Sashkin, M., and Franklin, S. "Anticipatory Team Learning: What Is It and How Does It Happen?" *Journal of Management Development,* 1993, *12*(6), 34–43.

CHAPTER THIRTY-TWO

The Changing Dynamics of Customer Satisfaction and Its Measurement

Charles D. Frame

Charles D. Frame is managing director of the Center for Healthcare Leadership and assistant professor at Emory University School of Medicine. His research and consulting interests center on assessment of perceptions of quality and satisfaction. He has served as a consultant to senior management at several Fortune 100 firms and also serves on the board of the Academy for Healthcare Quality, a joint educational effort of the Joint Commission on Accreditation of Healthcare Organizations and several leading universities.

Significant changes have taken place in the world of satisfaction measurement in health care. What was once the province of the marketing department and a small band of enlightened managers has now become a resource that is required, and used, by a wide range of the modern health care organization's constituencies. Leaders of successful health care organizations must understand the role that satisfaction measurement plays in the management process. Market and social forces are driving the evolution of health care organizations' measurement of constituent satisfaction from measurement of isolated, episodic events toward comprehensive, continuous assessment systems. The results of this evolution are of vital importance to current and future health care leaders, as they portend a future class of constituents whose decisions are increasingly information driven, and whose information sources are becoming increasingly real time, comprehensive, and accurate. This chapter offers some simple frameworks for looking at the quality of service provided by a health care organization at the ways organizations currently measure constituent satisfaction.

FORCES FOR CHANGE

In the era of predominantly small or solo physician practices and the fee-for-service model, the patient's perception was the most important measure; individual patients voted with their fee-for-service dollars, choosing either to remain loyal or to switch providers if dissatisfied. Although patient perceptions were important in the aggregate, the individual patient's perceptions were often overlooked; an individual patient's dissatisfaction and defection had little effect on a given provider's bottom line, and the ripple effects of that patient's defection seldom went beyond the borders of the provider's small practice.

The phenomenon of increasing scale on both the patient and provider sides has forever changed the relative importance of customer satisfaction in health care organizations. From the patient perspective the era of the patient as an independent decision maker, having relative carte blanche in the choice of provider, with the payer remitting without question, is gone. In most managed care packages, the patient gives up an element of autonomy, moving from being an independent agent to being a member of a group whose ability to choose is constrained. At the same time, the individual patient, previously unheard, may gain a significant voice through the leveraging of the scale of the covered lives in the managed care group.

To illustrate the difference in impact that increased patient scale brings, consider a solo practice physician whose lack of patient relationship skills drives off one hundred patients annually. In the fee-for-service indemnity scenario, the physician has lost the future fee stream from these patients, in all probability a small percentage of income.

In the managed care scenario, the potential negative effect of dissatisfying one hundred patients becomes significantly greater. If those patients' complaints trigger removal of the entire group of covered lives from the physician's care, the effect on the physician's bottom line could be significant.

In a similar vein, increasing provider scale has changed the importance of satisfaction measures. In the era of predominantly small or solo practices, the costs of failing to satisfy a customer were felt only by the individual physician or the small physician group; if the physician or group was willing to live with the reduced fee flow resulting from the dissatisfied patients' defection, no one else was affected economically. As physician groups get larger, the potential economic damage one dissatisfying physician can cause the other members increases significantly. In large physician groups, satisfaction measures serve a necessary function by allowing objective monitoring across a group of professional peers.

EMERGING CONCEPTS OF CUSTOMER SATISFACTION

As provider and payer systems have evolved, so too have the concepts and processes of customer satisfaction measurement. Early models of customer satisfaction tended to look at satisfaction as one-dimensional; patients had a certain level of satisfaction, and it was usually measured on a global scale, without considering its causal components. Using these models, research into customer satisfaction operated on what could be called the *direct approach,* assuming that customers would know a satisfying service when they saw it. Questionnaires based on these models were short and sweet, asking respondents point blank "how satisfied" they were with various attributes of a doctor or hospital.

This line of satisfaction measurement, though simple to administer, has several shortcomings. Principal concerns are the variety of definitions that respondents may have of the concept of satisfaction and the variety of drivers for that concept. Integral to any individual's concept of satisfaction is the set of expectations that he brings into the relationship. (Current models of satisfaction measurement, discussed later, take expectations into account, lessening the concern about differential definitions of satisfaction.) A second shortcoming of the direct approach is its lack of behavioral underpinnings. By asking the "how satisfied" question, the organization is not assessing the service provider behaviors that might be changed to increase satisfaction levels. If a respondent indicates a low level of satisfaction with Dr. X, it should be the responsibility of the satisfaction measurement system to indicate the areas in which the physician failed to meet the constituent's expectations. When a satisfaction measurement system evaluates employees of a health care organization and the results affect compensation, promotion, and continued employment, the system should be capable of pointing out the behavioral changes that need to be made to effect higher satisfaction ratings.

The work of Zeithaml, Parasuraman, and Berry (1990) has been instrumental in allowing organizations to develop more representative satisfaction measurement systems and obtain results on which they can act. Their model identifies perceived service quality as a function of the difference between a consumer's expectations for a service encounter and the customer's perceptions of the actual service she received. Their research has produced the SERVQUAL scale (Parasuraman, Zeithaml, and Berry, 1985, 1988, 1994), which measures customer perception of service quality on five dimensions:

- *Tangibles:* the appearance of the firm's physical facilities, personnel, and promotional material
- *Reliability:* the firm's ability to perform its promised services dependably and accurately
- *Responsiveness:* the firm's willingness to help customers and provide prompt service
- *Assurance:* the ability of the firm's employees to convey trust, confidence, knowledge, and courtesy
- *Empathy:* the extent to which the firm provides caring, individualized attention to its customers

EVOLUTION OF CONSTITUENT SATISFACTION

It is important to understand how the concept of satisfaction fits into the larger construct of quality, in both its objective and subjective senses. Leaders in health care organizations have traditionally been cognizant of, and comfortable with, the more objective clinical quality indicators available in the organizational reporting system. They have been less comfortable with the more subjective issues of patient and more broadly constituent satisfaction. This lack of comfort may be attributed to a variety of factors. Traditionally, health care organizations have been judged on data that were objectively measurable, with little perceptual bias: length of stay, readmission, mortality and morbidity, and so forth. These data were readily available from the existing management information system, were not subject to filtering through human perceptual processes, and were required by the payers and the relevant accrediting organizations.

But recently various forces have converged to increase the presence and importance of measuring satisfaction with perceived quality of health care organizations' services. One major driver is the increasing competition in the health care marketplace. As managed care wrings excess costs out of a market, providers will be driven to reduce their prices to what is referred to in traditional economic terms as the *market clearing price*, below which the firm will lose money and, in the long run, go bankrupt. In a competitive marketplace, once the competing firms have priced their products at the market clearing price, they need to look to other attributes by which they can differentiate themselves from the competition.

Even though quality is an obvious candidate for differentiating goods and services, health care organizations historically have had a difficult time signaling quality, and consumers have had an equally hard time determining what matters in their evaluation of health care quality. As Bell, Krivich, and Boyd (1997) state: "As the health care industry continues to move from price competition to competition based on quality and performance, patient satisfaction is likely to increase in importance relative to an organization's financial success. This new focus will help shift the conception of value from the traditional equation, or value $= f(\text{cost, quality})$, to a new understanding that value $= f(\text{cost, quality, satisfaction})$" (p. 30).

The research of Zifko-Baliga and Krampf (1997) provides a simple yet powerful framework for understanding how constituents of the health care system perceive quality. Although their research used a hospital setting, the framework should prove equally useful to a variety of provider organizations. Their model, shown in Figure 32.1, takes the input—process—outcome model used widely in the CQI (continuous quality improvement) literature and tailors it to the health care provider, redefining the input portion of the model as *structure,* defined as "the consumer's perception of the physical environment and physical facilities in which the service occurs. It also includes corporate image, appearance/aesthetics, cleanliness/tidiness, security, and tangibles. In the case of patient care in a hospital, structure is defined to be the hospital itself including the physical facilities and environment" (p. 29).

In this model, *perceived quality of process* is the consumer's evaluation of the interaction with the service personnel (and other consumers) during the performance of the service. *Perceived quality of outcome* entails an assessment by the consumer of the results of the service interaction. Although measures of traditional objective clinical outcomes remain important, Zifko-Baliga and Krampf are clear that patients' perceptions are also vitally important: "We have traditionally defined measures of outcomes in hospitals in terms of 'hard' data such as mortality or length of stay. However, outcomes also involve perceptions; if patients do not feel cured in their minds, then indeed they have not been cured" (p. 29).

Although the intent of this chapter is to give the health care leader a framework for understanding constituent satisfaction, enlightened leaders will realize the importance of having employees understand the components of quality and satisfaction. Most employees truly

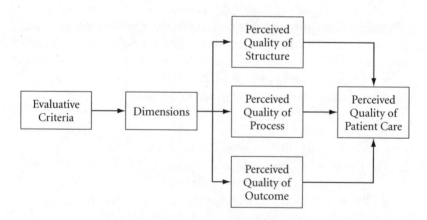

Figure 32.1.   Conceptual Model of Perceived Quality of Patient Care in a Hospital Setting.
Source: Zifko-Baliga and Krampf, 1997, p. 30. Reproduced with the permission of the American Marketing Association.

want to please the customer; the more specific an organization can be about the processes by which a customer is satisfied, the more easily an employee can be empowered to diagnose and correct service disconnects (the differences between expectations and perceptions noted by Zeithaml, Parasuraman, and Berry, 1990) before they work their way into a negative evaluation of quality.

The employee empowerment process should have two components: education and accountability. The educational element should be made part of the employee orientation and training process so that employees are made aware of the ways their actions shape customer perceptions and of their ability to effect changes in customer satisfaction by influencing elements of tangibility, reliability, responsiveness, assurance, and empathy.

After the organization has made employees aware of the importance of their actions in the creation of satisfaction, the employees need to be made accountable for those activities that create and maintain satisfaction. Reliable, understandable measures are vital for giving employees feedback on their satisfaction-inducing activities. It is extremely important that each of these measures be behaviorally based—it must draw the connection between an employee's action (or lack thereof) and a component of the customer's satisfaction. It is equally important that these measures not be used punitively. Penalties based upon satisfaction measures are nearly always counterproductive; employees become adept at managing their behaviors to meet the measures in use at any given time. Unfortunately, no set of satisfaction measures is as richly varied as the drivers of satisfaction in a service relationship, so leaders need to be aware that even with a lengthy survey, they are measuring the depth in only a relatively few spots in the satisfaction lake.

References

Bell, R., Krivich, M. J., and Boyd, M. S. "Charting Patient Satisfaction." *Marketing Health Services*, 1997, *17*(2), 22–29.

Parasuraman, A., Zeithaml, V. A., and Berry, L. L. "A Conceptual Model of Service Quality and Its Implications for Future Research." *Journal of Marketing*, 1985, *49*, 41–50.

Parasuraman, A., Zeithaml, V. A., and Berry, L. L. "SERVQUAL: A Multiple-Item Scale for Measuring Consumer Perceptions of Service Quality." *Journal of Retailing*, 1988, *64*(1), 12–40.

Parasuraman, A., Zeithaml, V. A., and Berry, L. L. "Reassessment of Expectations as a Comparison Standard in Measuring Service Quality: Implication for Future Research." *Journal of Marketing,* 1994, *58,* 111–124.

Zeithaml, V. A., Parasuraman, A., and Berry, L. L. *Delivering Quality Service: Balancing Customer Perceptions and Expectations.* New York: Free Press, 1990.

Zifko-Baliga, G. M., and Krampf, R. F. "Managing Perceptions of Hospital Quality." *Marketing Health Services,* 1997, *17*(1), 28–35.

CHAPTER THIRTY-THREE

Blending Health Care Organizations

Roderick W. Gilkey

Gary R. Lieberman

Roderick W. Gilkey is executive director of the Center for Healthcare Leadership at Emory University. He holds joint appointments in the School of Medicine, Department of Psychiatry, and the Goizueta School of Business and has received the university's highest teaching honor, the Emory Williams Award. The coauthor of Joining Forces *(with Joseph McCann, 1988) and a contributor to* Organizations on the Couch *(1991), he has also consulted to a number of global and Fortune 500 companies.*

Gary R. Lieberman is associate director of the Center for Healthcare Leadership at Emory University. He has worked with organizations such as Merck, IBM, Vitalink, Emory Health Care, and the Medical College of Georgia, providing consulting and education services on health care industry topics. He currently teaches at the Emory University School of Medicine and at the Goizueta School of Business.

W hen pharmaceutical companies are included, the health care industry has the highest level of merger and acquisition activity of any sector of the economy at this time. The resulting turmoil has placed the very substance and identity of health care organizations—their mission, purpose, vision, and values—at risk. Health care leaders must bring a superior level of psychological insight and managerial acumen to their work to ensure organizational viability into the twenty-first century.

This chapter addresses, first, the need to understand the particular challenges presented in a postmerger environment, which are similar to those found when two previously separate families must blend into one new family. Second, it provides a framework for managing or blending the new corporate family through transitional structures and processes.

BACKGROUND: THE CHANGING LANDSCAPE

Although provider corporations such as Columbia/HCA and Tenet continue to build large, national for-profit hospital systems, they represent only a small percentage of all hospitals in the country. The majority of health care delivery still is done by smaller, local or regional systems. On the not-for-profit side, VHA, the nation's largest alliance of hospitals, is starting Community Health Corp., whose aim will be to acquire hospitals in the Southwest that are considering converting to for-profit status. In order to compete, religious hospital systems also are concentrating on creating networks, both with other religious hospitals and with not-for-profit and for-profit community providers. Hospital networks are not the only areas of consolidation in the industry. Pharmaceutical companies are merging, and huge, publicly traded insurance companies are expanding their influence: for example, Aetna Insurance spent over $8 billion to purchase U.S. Healthcare in order to own a managed care organization and offer services directly as a health maintenance organization (HMO).

In addition, the time of the solo practitioner and small-group practice quickly is disappearing. Physicians are consolidating to maintain power: huge multipractice independent practice associations (IPAs)

and for-profit physician management companies (PMCs) are spring-
ing up across the country. Even two of the biggest PMCs, PhyCor and
Medpartners, the latter a combination of Medpartners and Mullikin,
at one point engaged in merger talks, although they called the talks
off after eight months for financial and cultural reasons. Even academic physicians, such as those at Stanford and the University of California at San Francisco, have been seeking mergers.

However, the real work comes after the marriage has taken place.
It takes two to three years for the trauma of an acquisition or merger
to subside. In many cases, the feeling of normalcy never returns. And
even though most new merger efforts make sense for strategic or
financial reasons, they fail to account for human factors. This was the
case with the failed merger between New York University and Sinai
Medical Centers in 1997, when cultural differences between NYU's
classic academic mentality clashed with Sinai's corporate style.

All organizations and leaders considering a new and closer relationship on any level face such human differences. A merger will not
produce that elusive *synergy* sought by organizations unless the crucial human factors are addressed.

THE PSYCHOLOGICAL CHALLENGE

A great deal of analysis, money, effort, and excitement are associated
with the structuring of any complex merger, acquisition, or alliance.
Unless comparable attention and assets are focused on making the
new relationship work, from the moment it is seriously considered by
the parties involved, the money and effort invested can be lost, and
any excitement generated can turn into disappointment, resentment,
confusion, and inefficiency. In the worst cases it can end in chaos, loss
of key leadership and management, and ultimately failure.

Significantly, business leaders use different language to describe the
merger and acquisition process at different stages. For example,
the language describing premerger activities is often highly roman-
tic and focused on conquest and winning. Terms such as courtship,
white knights, suitors, rivals, takeovers, rescues, plunderers, and poison pills seem better suited to an Arthurian romance than to a business transaction. The media often initiate much of this language and
imagery. But it gains popular acceptance presumably because it
speaks to people's fears or aspirations when they must give up the old
for something new and unknown. Once the actual transaction is

completed, the language moves quickly through references to a honeymoon period or a partnership, soon settling on the imagery of marriage and commitment.

Creating a sense of shared motivation within newly merged or acquired organizations requires a delicate balance between maintaining the autonomy and independence of the former entities and gaining a new sense of higher-level control. Leaders facing this challenge need to recognize and address the emotions that each organization is likely feeling.

- *Anxiety and uncertainty.* Perhaps the most pervasive emotion people feel in a newly blended organization is lack of understanding about the future. When their expectations of a stable environment in which they have operated traditionally are dashed, a sense of shock, bewilderment, and confusion follows. An ability to cope with continual transformation is becoming increasingly important for all managers, and it is especially critical during the aftermath of a merger, acquisition, or alliance of any kind.

- *Helplessness and rejection.* People will become stressed because they lack control over the circumstances that shape their lives in the new organization. And they often feel a sense of betrayal by their old group or business, stemming from this forced change of affiliation, a perceived lack of protection, and the loss of control. These feelings often are heightened in the health care environment, where the ultimate care relationships remain direct: physician-patient, nurse-patient, hospital–local community.

- *Divided loyalties.* Leaders are often viewed as parent figures. In mergers or other forms of blended organizations, new leaders emerge, often with different personalities and leadership styles. Old loyalties are challenged, and new authority relations are established. Individuals may more easily accept a strong leader, who clearly introduces the new set of expectations and sticks to the agenda, than one who is more patient and less definitive. But even under optimal circumstances—when the transition is sensitively and directly managed—conflicts over loyalty are inevitable.

- *Withdrawal and avoidance.* The unwritten psychological contract between employer and employee is often rewritten after the new relationship is finalized. Staff members can easily reduce their level of commitment and use their energy either to cope with their anxiety and confusion or to try to find new employment opportunities. Even when they remain in the organization they may withdraw or withhold their contribution, as part of a *psychological quit*. This can be a subtle process, but it is damaging. Consider the lack of motivation on the part of some primary care physicians whose successful practices were acquired. Incentives were structured in such a way that, once purchased, the physicians had already received their benefits and, as a result, lost the motivation and drive that once made the practices successful. Such attitudes can spread. They can impede the recovery period following an organizational shake-up. When an individual starts worrying about attracting attention and then pulls back, little risk taking or innovation is likely to take place, stifling long-term growth and success.

• *Conflicts over new values.* One of the challenges for members of blended health care organizations is, as one executive of an acquiring hospital described it, "getting along with a stranger from another planet." Each group entering the new organization has a different set of rules, values, and expectations. New leadership and new strategic direction creates loyalty and allegiance conflicts. Everyone is affected. At the extreme some employees are displaced and others are redeployed. On the community level, hospitals can shrink or disappear. Those less directly affected can be demoralized or angry when they see loyal coworkers suffer setbacks in their careers and lives. Besides wondering if they are next, they can easily feel *survivor's guilt,* questioning whether they really deserve to continue largely unharmed by the changes.

BLENDED AND NUCLEAR ORGANIZATIONS

Five dimensions distinguish the blended health care organization from one that has not experienced a major reorganization and still has a direct link to its original founders (Sager and others, 1983; Fulmer and Gilkey, 1988): the structure of the system, the purpose of the system, the tasks of the system, the influences on managers, and the forces that impinge on the system (Exhibit 33.1 summarizes the issues associated with each dimension).

Managing the blended health care organization can be as formidable as managing any part of the merger given the presence of legal constraints; financial concerns; structural differences; and divergent histories, rules, rituals, traditions, and ideals. The lack of a shared

Issues of System Structure
- Previous management systems and personnel exert continued influence on current employees.
- People have varied experiences of being managed (different leadership styles, systems, and personnel).
- Multiple systems are functioning.
- The system is more open to the outside, and new personnel come in; filling roles and relationships often initially unclear.
- Bonds uniting people are devised suddenly and often arbitrarily and are ill defined. There is no sense of historical continuity, no body of shared experience, no ritual to support the formation of a bonding unit or culture.
- Boundaries are fuzzy, and there are no precedents.

Issues of System Purpose
- People's sense of mission and understanding of strategy are often unclear and come in whole or in part from people considered outsiders.

Issues of System Tasks
- People must deal with inconsistency and incongruity as different groups in different phases of development address varying tasks in managing growth and maturity.
- Task definition comes from changed and multiple sources; roles are newly defined.

Issues of Influences on Managers
- Continuing contact with past systems, practices, and personnel can exert great influence and make the integration process more difficult.
- Ideals from the past, to the extent they have been internalized and lived, are often distracting.
- Career paths and plans are changed, raising concerns about fairness and future organizational memberships.
- The need to relocate is a major, often realistic, concern.
- Employee influence systems are disrupted, and significant forms or procedures for influencing the company are often lost, thus exacerbating all the previously cited issues (loyalty conflicts, loss of sense of purpose, and so forth).
- Because the limits for organizationally deviant behavior are not defined, risk averse behavior usually prevails, although the system may inadvertently encourage behind-the-scenes rebellions.

Issues of Forces That Impinge on the System
- Influence and control are suddenly exerted by new players outside the organization, whose language, methods, and purposes are often unclear and unpredictable.
- Locus of expertise is more external, creating confusion about the locus and the nature of power and influence in the system.
- New stakeholders are present, and their agendas are often unknown or unclear.

Exhibit 33.1.   Issues for the Blended Organization.

history with a common vision of both past and future is one of the most difficult challenges that a newly blended group must face. Here are some specific issues.

• *New structures and systems.* In merged organizations, authority structures and systems of control are in flux and unclear. Such basic issues as dress or grooming standards may need to be clarified or discussed. The question of who decides what must be addressed before equilibrium can be restored to the organization.

• *The power of outsiders.* A newly joined organization must conduct business in an arena where representatives of legal, financial, consulting, and community groups all exert power and influence, often to a greater extent than past opinion leaders. This problem is exacerbated by the fact that power is exercised by intermediaries and outsiders who ordinarily play a more minor role in the organization (if they have a role at all). This can undermine the effectiveness of the management systems. In addition, the appearance of outsiders from another organization disrupts mentoring relationships and career paths. New managers can feel resentment at having to take on additional management roles in the blended organization. The resentment between new managers and employees is often mutual. It is apt to arise particularly when the stronger party exercises power in a manner that is or is perceived to be insensitive.

• *Territorial battles.* Previous alliances and power structures persist, often overriding new authority structures or causing individuals to resist them. An informal organization can start operating alongside the formal one. In order to manage the transformation, leadership in the new organization will need additional formal structures.

• *Who will fit in?* Organizational membership is no longer clearly defined. The longer an employee has been part of the premerger organization, the greater the risk he or she will not fully integrate into the new organization. Adapting to new ways is most difficult for employees with the longest premerger tenure. Some of the most loyal employees in the old organization can easily become recalcitrant and unproductive in the new organization.

• *Start-up problems.* So that an operating system and infrastructure can be smoothly established, the new merged entity must work as a functional unit even though it has no historical precedent and even though it has no culturally transmitted rites of passage to assist it in bridging the transition from separate states to one blended state.

INTERVENTIONS

The key to managing postmerger dynamics is to procure the required resources to create the appropriate transitional structures and processes. Ideally, the blended corporate family is based on the strengths of each individual acting in an environment of mutual respect, shared values, and common mission.

For example, during the merger of a well-respected community hospital with a nationally known university-based teaching hospital, town and gown tensions were overcome through a transition management process that identified each partner's respective strengths, traditions, and values and then used them to create shared systems and mutual commitments on which to build the new organization and an effective blended corporate family. Less than three years after the merger began, this system was recognized as a health care network with accreditation and commendation by the Joint Commission on Accreditation of Healthcare Organizations. Although each hospital earned commendation, it is perhaps even more significant that they were able to achieve distinction as a model network system.

In this particular case the senior administrative staffs of the hospitals were reconstituted so that members from both organizations shared roles in the management and oversight of the transitional process and the ongoing management of the new enterprise. Unfortunately, the particular circumstances that made this transformation successful are not always present in every situation.

Generally, the optimal structure for successful blending includes a team (or several teams) of individuals representing multiple functions, such as clinical and administrative services, from each participating organization. Figure 33.1 illustrates an organizational model for team structure that reflects a balance of strategic, process, and organizational change. This merger and acquisition transition management team will report to the most senior leadership of the new entity; however, it will have responsibility and accountability for overseeing the process. Team members will accept specific roles and responsibility for certain areas—that is, clinical services, marketing, operations, human resources, and so on.

A review of the normative crises following a merger, described earlier, will show the advantages of this approach to the blended organization. For example, the challenges of dealing with new structures and

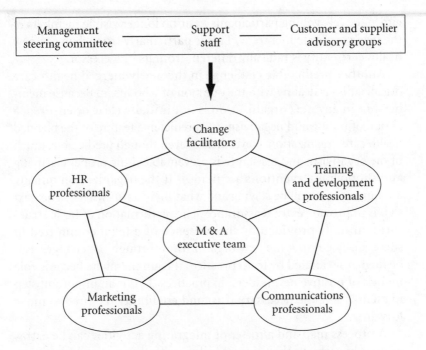

Figure 33.1.   Merger and Acquisition Transition Management
Team Structure in the Blended Organization.

systems can be quickly addressed by the team, whose responsibilities include providing immediate clarity about the basic structures and processes that need to be in place during the transition to ensure operational continuity. The problem of the power of outsiders is less when a successful team involves all significant parties and tries to avoid the we-they mentality that can impede the transition to a more integrated organization. This inclusive team membership can also alleviate the territorial battles that ensue after a merger. Old loyalties do not disappear readily, nor should they. There is a legitimate need to mourn the loss of the old ways and the previous leaders. Clear, strong transition management allows the feeling of loss, the sadness, and the power of past attachments to be given appropriate expression without endangering the new organization. The transition is further facilitated and old loyalties are more easily redirected when employees see leaders of the past organizations involved in creating the new one. Realigning commitments is easier when the leaders of the old organizations are either actively willing participants in or no longer visible members of the new corporate hierarchy. This is particularly true when the new health care entity is radically different from its predecessor.

Another predictable challenge in the newly merged health care organization is dealing with the question of who fits in. Because membership in any new organization is not initially clear or ensured, a period of testing and negativism is a predictable feature of the blended health care organization. Nevertheless, even though predictable, much of the negativism and resistance is preventable if the proper clarifying and support interventions are made—if the organization quickly announces who will be staying and what their status will be. The next step is to provide extra reassurance. The reaffirmation of basic structures, initially provided by the presence of a team committed to successfully guiding the new organization through the changes, can be further facilitated by team practices if team members become role models of positive new leadership practices. This is an important step in establishing the necessary trust and credibility required to move forward.

A process map and a roster of integrating activities can be extraordinarily useful to the team in dealing with the predictable start-up problems of a new blended organization. Because there is insufficient time to develop a culture and history to support the new organization, transitional ideologies and mediations have to be developed instead. The steps and activities required to initiate and manage this transitional process are depicted in Figure 33.2.

In the earliest stages of the change process, the individual entities involved in the new relationship create the essential infrastructure to orchestrate the transition from separate to blended organizations. This step includes identifying those who will oversee and carry out the merger. Once the basic structures for coordinating the merger and communicating its progress are in place, the team can begin to develop the new organization's leadership capacity and vision. This effort rests on the foundation of the available pool of leadership talent, the processes previously used to develop that leadership, and the vision and rationale for the merger identified during the acquisition. A successful vision is one that draws upon the strengths and talents of all participating organizations and defines the intended synergies and capacities that should result.

Once a basic level of structure and clarity has been created, involving key customers and other stakeholders is very beneficial. These

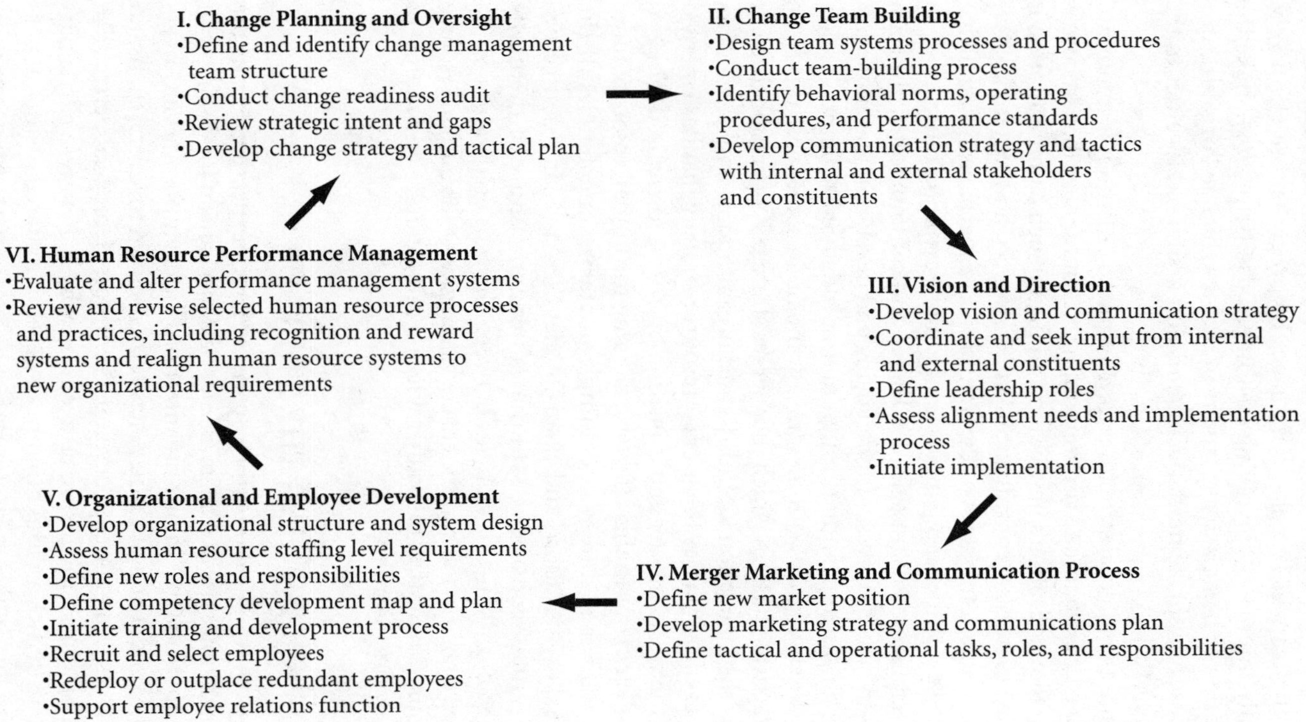

I. Change Planning and Oversight
•Define and identify change management team structure
•Conduct change readiness audit
•Review strategic intent and gaps
•Develop change strategy and tactical plan

II. Change Team Building
•Design team systems processes and procedures
•Conduct team-building process
•Identify behavioral norms, operating procedures, and performance standards
•Develop communication strategy and tactics with internal and external stakeholders and constituents

III. Vision and Direction
•Develop vision and communication strategy
•Coordinate and seek input from internal and external constituents
•Define leadership roles
•Assess alignment needs and implementation process
•Initiate implementation

IV. Merger Marketing and Communication Process
•Define new market position
•Develop marketing strategy and communications plan
•Define tactical and operational tasks, roles, and responsibilities

V. Organizational and Employee Development
•Develop organizational structure and system design
•Assess human resource staffing level requirements
•Define new roles and responsibilities
•Define competency development map and plan
•Initiate training and development process
•Recruit and select employees
•Redeploy or outplace redundant employees
•Support employee relations function

VI. Human Resource Performance Management
•Evaluate and alter performance management systems
•Review and revise selected human resource processes and practices, including recognition and reward systems and realign human resource systems to new organizational requirements

Figure 33.2. Scope of Transitional Activities (with Six Process Areas).

constituencies provide valuable reality checks and insights that support the team as it seeks to manage the process more effectively. Equally important, involving customers also helps *them* make the transition to being active partners of the new, blended organization. It helps them make new attachments and assign old loyalties to the new entity.

Once the internal structures have begun to emerge, it is important to begin developing and communicating a clear message that articulates the new organization's new vision and focus. Such communication is directed to external constituencies and customers; however, it may have greater value at this stage of the transition as a mechanism for rallying internal constituencies (employees) around a common cause.

After alignment strategies are defined and communicated, the team needs to create processes for deploying and developing the employees of the new organization through mutually defined structures and in ways closely aligned with the strategic intent. In some sense this is the core tactical phase, in which the merger strategy is operationalized. It creates the foundation for broad-based organizational implementation.

In the final phases the human resource strategy that has emerged from the entire merger and transition process is formalized. The two critical elements in this effort are aligning the human resource functions with the strategy and complementary competencies of the blended organizations and ensuring that these human resource systems remain consistent with the values and culture of the newly merged entity. Inconsistencies between the espoused values of the merged organization and the enacted strategies of the human resource function can destroy the vulnerable emerging culture and morale of the new organization.

MANAGING THE START-UP

Strong communication efforts sponsored, if not spearheaded, by the CEO and other senior leaders are a critical mechanism for dealing with start-up problems. In one organization, for example, the CEO oversaw the production of a film that was then shown to several thousand employees in an effort to develop a common ideological perspective among them on the historical events in which they were participating. This self-conscious attempt to develop a shared historical perspective and build a new culture is a necessary part of the transition process for the blended organization. A variety of means are available for developing a common new culture. Among them is the use of management education and communication forums to further the socialization and acculturation process.

Firms have used massive educational and training programs successfully to bring about a cultural change that emphasizes common objectives and shared values. At Tenet, for example, all employees attend a program on ethics developed by the company. In addition to the information and education offered, seminars like these give managers an opportunity to meet their counterparts from different parts of the aligned organizations; they get a better perspective on each other and begin necessary networking.

As an empowered force, those responsible for guiding the change should have access to a broad array of intervention strategies to alleviate the adjustment pains of employees in the blended corporate family. To communicate these strategies, leaders and those overseeing the alignment of the merged organizations may use, for example, change readiness workshops, role-definition techniques, interviews and surveys, town hall meetings, and organizational maps.

A newly blended health care organization needs a clear interpretation of its current situation so its members can gain a vision of the intermediate future, the time before the final consolidation into a functional unit. Communicating the structure and processes that will be used to manage the transition helps create this intermediate vision and alleviates uncertainty about the current situation. When an organization interprets and clarifies the transition process and outlines the immediate steps and inevitable uncertainties associated with each step, it can offer support and prevent declining morale and postmerger drift.

References

Fulmer, R.M., and Gilkey, R. W. "Blending Corporate Families: Management and Organization Development in a Postmerger Environment." *Academy of Management Executive*, 1988, *2*(4), 275–284.

Sager, C., and others. *Treating the Remarried Family.* New York: Brunner/Mazel, 1983.

PART SEVEN

Managed Care: Answers and Questions

CHAPTER THIRTY-FOUR

Regaining the Public's Trust in Managed Care

David M. Lawrence

*David M. Lawrence is chairman and CEO of Kaiser
Foundation Health Plan and Hospitals, the country's
oldest and largest nonprofit health plan, serving 9.1 million
people in nineteen states and the District of Columbia.
In a career devoted to public health and providing care
to large populations, he previously directed public health
services for Multnomah County, Oregon, oversaw medical
programs and trained physicians for the Peace Corps, and
served as a health adviser to Chile's minister of health.*

As Max De Pree (1992, p. 219) has noted, to cata-
logue the attributes of a leader is like fighting the Hydra. In examining one aspect of leadership, one soon discovers something else of
equal importance. Certainly the leadership attributes De Pree and others, such as John Gardner (1990), cite are necessary for managed care

leaders now and in the future. The job of leading the emerging health care institutions is complicated, however, by the fact that in the history of U.S. economics there is no precedent for what is occurring in health care today. We are in the midst of a profound, substantial, and complete transformation of *a sector.* There is no end in sight.

An example of what rapid change has wrought is the confusion of terms, the lack of a consistent and clear vocabulary to discuss the evolving forms of care delivery. The term *managed care* entered the lexicon during the bottom-line-focused 1980s, and although opinion polls consistently show the public neither understands nor likes the phrase, its use continues unabated. At first, managed care was shorthand for a vast spectrum of arrangements designed to solve the problems caused by unmanaged fee-for-service. The term encompassed everything from utilization review companies (on the less managed end of the spectrum) to health maintenance organizations (on the highly managed end). Today it more often refers to organizations focused on making a coherent whole of the fragmented parts of our health care.

It is impossible to know whether the term managed care will survive in the new millennium. One thing is certain, however. Systems that organize, coordinate, and integrate the components of health care, no matter what we call them, are in fact "the new American health care system" (Millenson, 1997, p. 20) and have the potential to endure and flourish in the next decade and beyond if those who are chosen or aspire to run them can meet the leadership challenges.

Many topics requiring discussion spring from the managed care leadership Hydra—changes in medical care technology, genetic engineering, the right to die, caring for our aging population, and so on. Managed care leaders must, of course, be players in the national debate on these external issues. As Peter Drucker wrote some years ago, executives must be part of the world (Drucker, 1985; first edition 1966). But the ability of managed care leaders to affect any such debate is predicated on the internal strength and stability of individual organizations and the industry as a whole and, just as important, on the trust the public has in these leaders.

The leadership challenges I focus on in this chapter reflect the observations of University of Chicago physician and bioethicist John D. Lantos (1997): "The ongoing national discussion about the future of medicine seeks solutions within the enterprise—reorganizations, new corporate entities, better health services research. But there is no 'solution' that avoids the need for ongoing moral choices" (p. 193). Those choices are crucial to the future of the new American health care system. The greatest challenge leaders must meet today and in the new millennium is building a deep and enduring trust with patients, members, purchasers, providers, and the public. Managed care as a movement has failed to establish that trust thus far. Trust is a deeply subjective matter and a requirement for optimum care and appropriate outcomes and also peace of mind. People are frightened when they are sick or injured and are often worried when well. They usually are concerned about the welfare of their families. *Insurance* must be *assurance* that care will be there when necessary, that families will get what they require to maintain health, and that they will not be bankrupted in the process. When health care is needed, it must be provided by the health care professionals and institutions patients and families depend on, in a place where the patient feels safe and comfortable. No outcomes data, no Health Plan Employer Data and Information Set (HEDIS) or National Committee for Quality Assurance (NCQA) score, no assurances about licensure can create trust.

Trust develops as a result of many factors. One of the most important is how we in health care manage ethical expectations in three closely linked relationships—between the physician (or caregiver) and the patient and family, between the health care organization and the beneficiary or member of that organization, and between the health care organization and the community. The following leadership challenges address these issues further.

PATIENT RIGHTS AND PROTECTIONS

The most basic ethical expectation we have is that the physician will act in our interest when we are patients. The physician is expected to protect us from unnecessary and inappropriate care and ensure that needed care is given. This advocacy relationship is centuries old. It is deeply rooted in ethical traditions that inform our contemporary thinking about how doctors must act and whom they serve. Ensuring that those who are ill or injured get the care they need is, after all, the primary task of medicine.

The managed care plan can aid in preserving the doctor-patient relationship by taking steps to avoid placing clinicians in a double-agency role, one in which they must balance the needs of patients and of the health plan. When a physician has to make trade-offs between what is necessary and appropriate for the patient and what will affect his or her own economic welfare, those trade-offs introduce a difficult calculus into the relationship. The health plan should not engage in clinical decision making. The physician, in partnership with the patient, should be the arbiter of the appropriate care and setting.

MEMBER RIGHTS

Members enrolled in a health care organization have a right to distributive justice. The second ethical expectation is that the institution responsible for allocating scarce resources on behalf of members will do so fairly. To achieve fairness, health care providers and institutions must manage the resources entrusted to them so that they can serve the most needy enrollees well, must improve the health of all enrollees, must make consistent and defensible decisions, and must involve members in the process of determining the trade-offs to be made in carrying out these, at times, conflicting duties.

At Kaiser Permanente, and particularly in the case of our partner, Group Health Cooperative, we believe strongly in the importance of including consumer voice in the management of our organization. Having an ongoing dialogue and involvement with members and consumer advocacy groups to shape policies and decisions related to benefits, coverage, and other concerns is invaluable for creating trust.

BALANCING PUBLIC GOOD
AND PRIVATE GAIN

The third ethical expectation derives from the prevailing historical view, deeply embedded in public policy, that health care is a public rather than private good. People expect health care professionals and institutions to act in the public interest rather than for personal gain. Information about where the resources go and how effective they are in addressing the needs of patients and communities has long been used to measure of social purpose. Health institutions, especially hospitals, have deep roots in charity and religious activities directed to serving those disadvantaged by illness or socioeconomic circumstance, to training future health care professionals, and to carrying out research to improve care.

These three expectations—patient rights, member rights, and the balancing of public good and private gain—are linked. When an organization does not act in the public interest, trust in the physicians associated with that organization is eroded. When a health care organization's distribution of limited resources is perceived as unfair, flawed, driven by the wrong incentives, or controlled through gate-keeping systems, it is difficult to believe that the organization acts in the interest of the patient or the public. When physicians benefit by reducing care, it is hard to convince the public that these physicians do not also benefit by avoiding the ill and undertreating the sick or injured. When doctors and executives make lots of money, people worry about whether that wealth has been created at their expense.

Increasingly, managed care organizations can be expected to carry the heavy weight of the three ethical expectations as these organizations take greater responsibility for providing care to larger segments of the population. If these organizations are to assume this mantle successfully, leaders must ensure that the organizations promote trust between physician and patient by providing appropriate and sensitive care to those who are sick; leaders must ensure that organizational approaches to distributing finite resources are fair, consistent, accessible to members and result in improved health for those they serve; and leaders must demonstrate that their organizations act in the public interest, helping solve rather than exacerbate the growing health-related social problems with which this society is confronted.

Many practices in the managed care field today are inconsistent with these expectations, however. For example, reimbursement methods that cause doctors to worry about how much money they will lose by treating someone appropriately or that they might lose their contract should they fail to follow a managed care company's guidelines are troublesome for patients and families. Donald Berwick, M.D., argues (1996) that managed care financial incentives probably do not affect the behavior of most physicians. Yet it is difficult to explain to a patient or family why a particular clinical approach is recommended when that discussion is contaminated by the patient's perception that economic gain influences the professional advice. This is especially true when the recommendation is for less care or more conservative care than the patient has learned to expect from traditional fee-for-service practices or when the physician expresses concern with what the managed care company is willing to cover.

Barriers to care, difficult or confusing requirements for getting care, requirements to check with third parties for care appropriateness, and gag rules can further poison physician-patient trust. Similarly, narrow and restrictive benefit coverage decisions, significant hassles over claims payments, and inconsistent or apparently capricious decisions to extend or withhold benefits raise concerns among members about the fairness of their insurance coverage and erode confidence that coverage and care will be there when needed.

Finally, significant profit taking, coupled with efforts to attract the healthy and avoid the sick, unwillingness to invest in a community health and social services infrastructure, refusal to publicly share research findings on how better to care for individuals or groups of patients, and unwillingness to fund research and education in health care and to subsidize care for the uninsured and underinsured undermine public confidence that managed care operates in the best interest of this society.

PHYSICIAN AND EMPLOYEE RIGHTS

Managed care leaders must also address the rights, privileges, and protections of those who make their careers in health care, whether physicians, nurses, aides, or office workers. These individuals have committed themselves to keeping the U.S. health care system up and running. However, the practice of medicine is rapidly changing, driven by new technology, more effective drugs, and less invasive procedures. These changes are having a profound impact on all health care professionals. Building a community among an organization's physicians and employees and facilitating ongoing dialogue with all levels of the organization should occupy a substantial amount of a managed care leader's time. Organizations that find ways to make this happen will succeed in the new millennium. Organizations can improve the delivery of quality health care and expand their competitiveness by engaging people's creativity and dedication. Again, this builds trust between the workforce and management, trust that is conveyed to members and to the public at large.

A VALUES HIERARCHY

Obviously, managed care leaders and organizations cannot weigh all moral choices case by case. The leader needs to help the organization develop a values hierarchy so that everyone in the company has a foundation on which to make day-to-day decisions. This involves clarifying the organization's mission, vision, and values and making it explicit who among the stakeholders comes first—the patient, the member, the purchaser, the stockholder, the physician, the employee, or the community.

I have not yet addressed the need for intestinal fortitude and thick skin as leaders experience unfair bashing and rampant regulation. The slings and arrows are not new and were faced by managed care's pioneers, who risked censure from the American Medical Association and their local medical societies to bring affordable quality health care to the public.

We would do well to reflect on the wisdom of those who went before us. According to the authors of *Built to Last,* an envisioned future helps an organization only so long as that future has not yet been achieved (Collins and Porras, 1997). Clifford Keene, M.D., one of the early leaders of Kaiser Permanente, understood that when he said: "We don't see ourselves as a panacea. We do see [managed care] as one valid solution to some long standing problems. We see it as an evolving method of organizing and delivering medical care which is intended to be responsive to the changing needs of the people it serves" (1986, p. 134).

As the new American health care system continues to evolve, trust, it seems to me, should be the overarching concern and priority. Trust lies at the root of whether health care organizations will be successful at treating people with compassion and at managing their care appropriately, in ways that deliver the best possible outcomes. Trust will determine whether they will be able to build the kinds of ongoing, long-term relationships among caregivers, health plans, the members who seek care, and the communities served. The moral choices leaders make will determine the level of trust the new American health care system receives and therefore its success and lasting influence.

References

Berwick, D. M. "Quality of Health Care." Part 5: "Payment by Capitation and the Quality of Care." *New England Journal of Medicine,* 1996, *335,* 1227–1231.

Collins, J. C., and Porras, J. I. *Built to Last: Successful Habits of Visionary Companies.* New York: Harper Business, 1997.

De Pree, M. *Leadership Jazz.* New York: Dell, 1992.

Drucker, P. F. *The Effective Executive.* New York: HarperCollins, 1985.

Gardner, J. W. *On Leadership.* New York: Free Press, 1990.

Keene, C. *An Oral History of the Kaiser Permanente Medical Care Program.* Berkeley, Calif.: Regents of the University of California, 1986.

Lantos, J. D. *Do We Still Need Doctors?* New York: Routledge, 1997.

Millenson, M. *The New American Health System: A Report to the American Association of Health Plans.* New York: Mercer, 1997.

CHAPTER THIRTY-FIVE

The New
Health Economics

Merrill Matthews Jr.

*Merrill Matthews Jr. is vice president of domestic policy
and director of the Center for Health Policy Studies at
the National Center for Policy Analysis. His articles have
appeared in the* Wall Street Journal, Investor's Business
Daily, National Review, *and several other periodicals.
He was a contributor to* Physician-Assisted Suicide:
Expanding the Debate *(edited by Margaret P. Battin,
Rosamond Rhodes, and Anita Silvers, 1998).*

—〜〜—

Managed care in its more restrictive forms is
dying a painful and ignominious death. It will never survive the turn
of the century. Who is killing it? Patients who demand more choices
and politicians who want to ensure those choices by regulating or
modifying managed care's cost-reducing practices.[1] In addition, the
media are hastening this demise with tales of people who claim their
health plans have harmed them or denied them care.

Of course, not *all* forms of managed care are dying, just the more restrictive practices such as closed-panel HMOs and gatekeepers. And capitation as a form of reimbursement will likely fade for all but the poorest segments of the population, who get their health insurance through Medicaid. In contrast, less restrictive forms of managed care, including networks of approved physicians, hospitals, and other providers and negotiation of discounted rates by large employers and insurers are flourishing.[2] The challenge for leaders in the managed care industry as we enter a new millennium will be to create a managed care system that meets patients' demands for increased choices and information as it continues to control costs and maintain quality. Meeting that challenge will not be easy, because it means a fundamental change in the way industry leaders think about managed care.

THE SYSTEM PROBLEMS

The growing tension between the current and future health care systems explains the existence of many of the problems we now face. The hallmarks of the current system—the way health insurance is treated under the tax law, the role of third-party payers, the limited choices, the government-imposed mandates, and the lack of good consumer information—have created a crisis of high costs, limited access, and a growing number of uninsured (for an analysis of health care cost and financing trends, see Thorpe, 1997a, 1997b). If the health care system is going to work efficiently, Congress and the state legislatures will have to address each of those problems.

Health Insurance Tax Treatment

Because of federal tax policy, many employees tend to prefer health insurance to taxable wages. Under current law, every dollar of health insurance premiums paid by an employer escapes federal income tax, the 15.3 percent Social Security (FICA) tax, and in most cases state and local income taxes. Thus the government is in effect paying up to half of some employees' premiums, a generous subsidy that encourages these employees to overinsure.

In contrast, the self-employed, the unemployed, and the people who work for an employer who does not provide health insurance get little or no tax break. Is it any wonder then that the U.S. health insurance system has evolved into an employer-based one and that nearly

90 percent of people under age sixty-five with private health insurance get their coverage through an employer (McDonnell and others, 1997, p. 218, table 26.4)? And because the employer owns the policy, the employee loses his health insurance during a job transition, which exacerbates the numbers of the uninsured. In fact among the uninsured, half lack coverage for six months or less, usually because they are changing jobs (Swartz, 1994).

Third-Party Payers

The primary reason health care spending is out of control is that most of the time, people who enter the medical marketplace are spending someone else's money. Economic studies—as well as common sense—confirm that people are less likely to be prudent, careful shoppers when someone else is paying the bill (Brook and others, 1984; Manning and others, 1987). Although polls show that most people fear they will not be able to pay their medical bills from their own resources, the reality is that few will have to. On the average (Robbins, Robbins, and Goodman, 1994, p. 2):

- Every time patients spend a dollar in a hospital, they pay only five cents out of pocket whereas ninety-five cents is paid by a third party (employer, insurance company, or the government).

- Every time patients spend a dollar on physicians' fees, they pay less than nineteen cents out of pocket.

- In the health care system as a whole, people pay only twenty-three cents out of pocket every time they consume a dollar's worth of services.

Managed care, especially in early versions of HMOs, exacerbated the problem by trying to further insulate patients from service costs. The prevalence of third-party payments has led to an adversarial relationship: patients who bear almost no out-of-pocket costs have an incentive to consume everything their health plan can provide, whereas their health plan has an economic incentive not to provide it.

Limited Choices

Large employers who provide health insurance often give their employees a choice of policy types, including a health maintenance organization (HMO) and a more traditional insurance policy, which in most cases includes a network of physicians and other providers known as a preferred provider organization (PPO). In contrast, small employers usually offer only one health insurance option. For their employees the choice is to take it or leave it. For example, a 1996 survey conducted by KPMG Peat Marwick and analyzed by the Barents Group for the American Association of Health Plans found that of 1,789 firms offering health insurance about 96 percent of the employees working for small businesses (1 to 49 employees) were offered only one health insurance plan, but 64 percent of employees working for firms with 1,000 to 4,999 employees, and 77 percent of employees of firms of 5,000 employees or more, had more than one health plan option (Barents Group, 1997).

With every other type of insurance (auto, fire, home, and so on), consumers choose among a wide range of competing plans. Not so in health insurance—especially not for employees of small firms. As a result many people feel that they are stuck in a system they would not have chosen had the decision been theirs, and such a feeling can only lead to dissatisfaction.

Health Insurance Regulation

For more than thirty years state legislatures have passed laws driving the cost of health insurance higher. Known as mandated health insurance benefit laws, they force insurers, employers, and managed care companies to cover—or at least offer—specific providers, such as chiropractors and podiatrists, and specific services, such as mental health care or in vitro fertilization, that might not be included in basic health care plans. There were only seven state-mandated benefits in 1965; there are nearly one thousand today (Laudicina and others, 1997). And although these mandated benefits make insurance more comprehensive, they also drive up the cost. As a result, young, healthy, and lower-income people often cancel their policies, increasing the number of uninsured.[3]

Besides passing mandates, states—and increasingly the federal government also—have been trying to regulate access to health insurance, which also leads to increased health insurance costs. As sick people move into the insurance pool, premiums go up, driving out lower-income families and young, healthy people who think they are being charged too much. Besides, they reason that if they can get health insurance at any time regardless of their health status, why not just wait until they get sick to buy insurance?

A perfect example of the unintended consequences of regulation is a result from a 1992 New Jersey law requiring what is known as *guaranteed issue*. Guaranteed issue makes health insurance available to anyone, regardless of her health. Such laws are based on good intentions: legislators want people—especially people with medical conditions—to have better access to health insurance at affordable prices. But according to New Jersey's own published figures, the average cost of a family health insurance policy purchased in the individual market with a $500 deductible and 20 percent copayment (generally known as a Plan D policy) is almost $27,000 a year (New Jersey Individual Health Coverage Program Board, 1997). That is the average cost of twenty plans, with the lowest annual premium being $9,960 and the highest $50,724. A similar policy in most states would cost about $5,500 a year (Health Insurance Association of America, 1997).

Uninformed Patients

Another problem that arises when a third party is paying the health care bill is that those who receive the care have little reason to be informed about the costs or benefits and physicians see little need to inform them. When insulated from information about the cost of care, patients tend to want more care, whether necessary or not, and physicians are often willing to provide it. A recent analysis of hospital stays for the under–sixty-five population found that about 54 percent of "unmanaged inpatient care is potentially medically unnecessary" (Axene, Doyle, and van der Burch, 1997, table 2). For those sixty-five years of age and over, the study found 53 percent of unmanaged inpatient care to be potentially medically unnecessary. However, insurers' and employers' attempts to limit medically unnecessary care has led to the charge that health care is being rationed, which is often true, though rationed care is bad care only when a patient is denied *needed* treatment.[4] Nevertheless, as health economist Henry Aaron of the Brookings Institution has pointed out, "Denying any form of beneficial care is an extraordinarily divisive and emotionally wrenching thing to do" (Anders and Winslow, 1997, p. A1).

THE CHANGES NEEDED

The convoluted nature of the U.S. health care system, driven by the tax system and employers' interests, has led to widespread dissatisfaction and desire for change. Because there is very little political support for a national health insurance program (along the lines of the Canadian system, for example), health care reform will come through legislation meant to restrict managed care practices, or it will seek to restructure the system so people will have more choices and more information. The latter direction is the one health care reform should take.

Individually Owned Insurance

The tax system should be changed so that employees who do not want the health insurance policy provided by their employer can opt out and receive either a tax deduction or a tax credit. Both approaches could be *revenue neutral* (that is, structured so the government neither gains nor loses tax money); the tax break would simply go directly to the individual rather than through the employer.

If Congress chose the tax credit approach, employees who elected not to take their employer's health insurance plan would receive a tax credit (say, $750 for each adult and $500 for each child, up to a maximum of $2,000) for the purchase of health insurance. Such a fixed-sum tax credit would cover most of the cost of a basic policy, and any additional costs arising from the purchase of a *Cadillac plan* (that is, one loaded with options) would be borne by the purchaser, not the taxpayer. This proposal could also be expanded so that everyone purchasing health insurance, including the self-employed and others who do not get health insurance through an employer, would get a comparable tax break.

This one change, which a number of economists and policy groups advocate, could revolutionize the health insurance system. It would unbundle health insurance from the employer because people could get a tax break whether the employer paid or they paid for insurance themselves. Of course, employees might still prefer employer-provided insurance, either because the employer might still pay for the policy or because employees might get a lower group rate. But enough people might eventually choose to purchase their own policies that employer-provided insurance would die of neglect. Then all health insurance would become personal and portable (that is, individuals would own their own policies, and those policies would go with them during job transition), just like other types of insurance.

Medical Savings Accounts

As part of the 1996 Kassebaum-Kennedy health insurance reform bill, Congress approved a limited number of medical savings accounts (MSAs) (Matthews, 1996; for a comprehensive examination of MSAs, see Goodman and Musgrave, 1992). It took the next step in 1997, when it passed legislation as part of the Balanced Budget Act that will make MSAs available for seniors on Medicare (in 1999).

Medical savings accounts give people the opportunity to move from a traditional low-deductible health insurance plan to one with a high deductible (say, $2,000 to $3,000) and to deposit the premium savings in a personal savings account. People use the account to pay for routine and preventive medical care, and the high-deductible policy pays major expenses. If money is left over in the MSA at the end of the year, the account holder can withdraw it or roll it over to grow with interest. For example, a family with employer-provided health insurance might receive a $2,000 contribution to its MSA and a $3,000 deductible policy. The employee would pay for health care expenses with the $2,000, usually provided by the employer and easily enough to cover most families during a year. If the family exhausted the $2,000 MSA deposit, the employee would pay the next $1,000 out of pocket, and insurance would pay everything over $3,000. If funds remain in the account, they belong to the employee.

Medical savings accounts reduce the impact of third-party payers as they give individuals more health care options, because the individuals, rather than insurers and health plans, control much of the money. In addition, MSAs blend well with the forms of managed care most likely to survive in the future. For example, patients could still choose from a network of providers and use their MSA money to pay the discounted rates. If they wanted to go outside the network and pay the additional cost or have a procedure not covered by the managed care plan, they could do that with their MSA (Goodman, 1998).

Thus MSAs give patients the incentive to be prudent health care shoppers for routine care. And if patients in managed care do not like their choices, they have a pool of funds to purchase what they need (for an analysis of the progress of the MSA legislation, see U.S. General Accounting Office, 1997).

Medicare

The Medicare program is heading toward bankruptcy. According to Medicare's own trustees the Medicare trust fund would have been depleted by the year 2000 (Board of Trustees of the Federal Hospital Insurance Trust Fund, 1997). Medicare reform proposals in the recently passed balanced budget agreement have postponed the crisis until 2010. But this reform only masks the program's future problems. By the year 2045, when today's high school graduates retire, almost 53 percent of the U.S. taxable payroll will be needed to fund the Social Security and Medicare benefits promised under current law (Goodman and Cordell, 1998). Congress knows changes are needed and has started to implement them. For example, for several years some seniors have had the option of taking their share of Medicare dollars and joining a private HMO. New legislation significantly expands that option, letting seniors choose from a wide range of health plans, including HMOs, PPOs, PSNs (provider sponsored networks), Medicare MSAs, and traditional fee-for-service insurance. Seniors who choose to stay in traditional Medicare or to return to it after trying one of the private plans will be able to do so.

Members of Congress have concluded that giving seniors more private sector options—and thus encouraging competition between plans—will reduce Medicare spending. They are probably right, but that is not the revolutionary aspect of the legislation. What the legislative change means is that people will increasingly perceive Medicare not as a defined benefit, a government guarantee that people will receive certain benefits regardless of what they paid into the system, but as a defined contribution, a set amount of money given to people to purchase health insurance. The new program, known as Medicare = Choice, operates as a defined contribution. This is also precisely the direction in which private sector benefit plans are moving. From 1975 to 1995, the number of private sector employees in defined-benefit plans grew less than 10 percent, from thirty-three million to thirty-six million employees. Defined-contribution plans grew by about 300 percent, from eleven million to forty-three million employees, over the same time period (Ferrara, 1997).

By moving to defined contributions, employers encourage workers to make their own decisions. As a result, employees begin to perceive *themselves,* not their employers, as responsible for their future financial security. That change in perception will make working Americans much more open to full privatization of Medicare in the future. Why spend a lifetime depositing Medicare payroll taxes in a common pool when that same money could go into a private account that would provide even more money for health insurance at retirement? Thus Medicare, like health insurance for those under age sixty-five, will gradually give people more control over their money, more choices among competing providers, and an incentive to be prudent health care shoppers.

Medicaid

For years Medicaid has been one of the fastest-growing programs in state budgets. State legislators, like employers faced with exploding health care costs, had to act, and they have taken the same route as employers: managed care. According to the Health Care Financing Administration, Medicaid managed care enrollment grew from 2.7 million people in 1991 to 13.3 million people in 1996, about 38 percent of the 35.2 million people in the Medicaid program (American Association of Health Plans, 1998a). By the year 2000, almost all Medicaid recipients will likely be in managed care.

State legislators had another reason for moving from fee-for-service insurance to managed care: fraud. Pre–managed care Medicaid had serious problems with fraudulent billing, especially in urban areas (see, for example, "Medicaid: System in Chaos," 1993). Politicians faced tremendous pressure to change the system so as to eliminate *Medicaid mills.* Capitated managed care contracts have significantly reduced the financial incentive for health care providers to overprovide care, but they also have raised ethical concerns about the possible new incentive to underprovide care.

Most states have experienced problems with the quality of Medicaid managed care, and this has led state legislators to pass consumer protection laws. The irony is that to the extent legislators undermine managed care's utilization and cost controls, they inhibit managed care's ability to save the state money. Even so, Medicaid managed care is a political win-win situation, because legislators can claim to be providing comprehensive coverage as they also cut costs. Because the poor who are Medicare's beneficiaries usually have little voice in these matters, Medicaid managed care is probably here to stay.

THE INFORMED PATIENT

One of the most significant changes in the health care field is the explosion of information available to patients. This fact alone may have the most significant impact on managed care and the health care system of the future. Increasingly, patients want to know about their choices and options, and they want to make decisions for themselves, in consultation with their physicians. If their physicians do not provide them with needed information, patients can turn to a range of other sources—the Internet, the media, and even call-in services such as Dial-a-Nurse. (Of course information access can also lead to problems; see Jadad and Gagliardi, 1998.) In addition, employers are providing information and services that facilitate employee learning about the best and most cost-effective physicians, hospitals, or pharmaceuticals.

This desire for information means that insurers and employers must bring people into the decision-making process and give them a financial stake in it. When someone else is footing the bill, most patients choose the most expensive service, drug, or medical device. But Information Age patients will find it easy to learn about all of their options. Either employers and insurers will have to increasingly limit the care covered by their plans (a strategy that has already led to the expansion of anti–managed care laws), or they will have to give patients a financial stake in health care decisions. That is why medical savings accounts, or some similar innovation that makes patients more cost conscious, in conjunction with less restrictive forms of managed care likely will constitute the health care reimbursement system of the future.

Notes

1. According to the National Conference of State Legislatures, seventeen states enacted comprehensive health care consumer rights laws in 1997, and many more are expected to do so in the future (see Kilborn, 1998; American Association of Health Plans, 1998c).
2. Between 1990 and 1996, HMO membership grew 85 percent, from 36.5 million people to 67.5 million, and PPO membership grew 154 percent, from 38.1 million people to 97.8 million (American Associa-

tion of Health Plans, 1998b). However, 67.9 percent of HMOs offered a point of service option, which accounted for 43.2 percent of enrollment growth (Hoechst Marion Roussel, 1997).

3. An analysis of the costs of twelve of the most common mandates found that collectively they could increase the cost of insurance by as much as 30 percent (Goodman and Matthews, 1997). In addition, according to an estimate from the Congressional Budget Office (1996), a 1 percent increase in health insurance premiums leads to 200,000 people canceling their coverage. Thus a 30 percent increase could lead to 6 million more uninsured.

4. One of the objects of managed care is to reduce or eliminate medically unnecessary care. However, what should be considered medically necessary care is often open to debate.

References

American Association of Health Plans. *Enrollment Trends in Medicaid Managed Care, Jan. 1998.* Policy brief. Washington, D.C.: American Association of Health Plans, Feb. 1998a.

American Association of Health Plans. *Managed Care Facts.* Washington, D.C.: American Association of Health Plans, Jan. 1998b.

American Association of Health Plans. *The Regulation of Health Plans: A Report from the American Association of Health Plans.* Washington, D.C.: American Association of Health Plans, Feb. 1998c.

Anders, G., and Winslow, R. "HMOs' Woes Reflect Conflicting Demands of American Public." *Wall Street Journal,* Dec. 22, 1997, p. A1.

Axene, D. V., Doyle R. L., and van der Burch, D. *Analysis of Medically Unnecessary Inpatient Services.* [n.p.]: Milliman & Robertson, 1997.

Barents Group. *Characteristics of Health Plan Choices Available to Employees Through Employer-Based Health Benefits, 1996.* Washington, D.C.: American Association of Health Plans, June 1997.

Board of Trustees of the Federal Hospital Insurance Trust Fund. *1997 Annual Report of the Board of Trustees of the Federal Hospital Insurance Trust Fund.* Washington, D.C.: Federal Hospital Insurance Trust Fund, Apr. 1997.

Brook, R. H., and others. *The Effect of Coinsurance on the Health of Adults.* Santa Monica, Calif.: Rand Corporation, 1984.

Congressional Budget Office. *Estimates of the Impact on Employers of the Mental Health Parity Amendment in H.R. 3103.* Washington, D.C.: Congressional Budget Office, May 1996.

Ferrara, P. J. *Pension Liberation: A Proactive Solution for the Nation's Public Pension Systems.* Washington, D.C.: The State Factor, American Legislative Exchange Council, Aug. 1997.

Goodman, J. C. *Solving the Problems of Managed Care.* Brief Analysis No. 254. Dallas: National Center for Policy Analysis, Jan. 1998.

Goodman, J. C., and Cordell, D. E. *The Nightmare in Our Future: Elderly Entitlements.* Policy Report No. 212. Dallas: National Center for Policy Analysis, Jan. 1998.

Goodman, J. C., and Matthews, M., Jr. *The Cost of Health Insurance Mandates.* Brief Analysis No. 237. Dallas: National Center for Policy Analysis, Aug. 1997.

Goodman, J. C., and Musgrave, G. L. *Patient Power: Solving America's Health Care Crisis.* Washington, D.C.: Cato Institute, 1992.

Health Insurance Association of America. *Sourcebook of Health Insurance Data, 1996.* Washington, D.C.: Health Insurance Association of America, 1997.

Hoechst Marion Roussel. *Managed Care Digest HMO/PPO Edition 1997 and SMG Marketing.* Kansas City, Mo.: Hoechst Marion Roussel, Nov. 1997.

Jadad, A. R., and Gagliardi, A. "Rating Health Information on the Internet: Navigating to Knowledge or to Babel?" *JAMA,* 1998, *279,* 611–614.

Kilborn, P. T. "In Managed Care, 'Consumer Laws' Benefit Doctors." *New York Times,* Feb. 16, 1998.

Laudicina, S. S., and others. *State Legislative Health Care and Issues: 1997 Survey of Plans.* Washington, D.C.: Blue Cross and Blue Shield Association, State Services Department, Dec. 1997.

Manning, W., and others. "Health Insurance and the Demand for Health Care: Evidence from a Randomized Experiment." *American Economic Review,* June 1987.

Matthews, M., Jr. "Medical Savings Account Legislation: The Good, the Bad and the Ugly." Brief Analysis No. 211. Dallas: National Center for Policy Analysis, Aug. 19, 1996.

McDonnell, K., and others. *EBRI Databook on Employee Benefits.* Washington, D.C.: Employee Benefit Research Institute, 1997.

"Medicaid: System in Chaos." Nine-part series. *Chicago Tribune,* Oct. 31–Nov. 9, 1993.

New Jersey Individual Health Coverage Program Board. *Rate Comparison Sheets.* Dec. 1997.

Robbins, G., Robbins, A., and Goodman, J. C. *Inefficiency in the U.S. Health Care System: What Can We Do?* Policy Report No. 182. Dallas: National Center for Policy Analysis, Apr. 1994.

Swartz, K. "Counting Uninsured Americans: Background Memorandum." Kaiser Health Reform Project. Menlo Park, Calif.: Henry J. Kaiser Family Foundation, Jan. 1994.

Thorpe, K. E. *Changes in the Growth of Health Care Spending: Implications for Consumers.* Washington D.C.: National Coalition on Health Care, Apr. 1997a.

Thorpe, K. E. *The Rising Number of Uninsured Workers: An Approaching Crisis in Health Care Financing.* Washington D.C.: National Coalition on Health Care, Sept. 1997b.

U.S. General Accounting Office. *Medical Savings Accounts: Findings from Insurer Survey.* GAO/HEHS-98–57. Washington, D.C.: U.S. General Accounting Office, Dec. 1997.

CHAPTER THIRTY-SIX

Managed Care and the Black Physician

Randall C. Morgan Jr.

*Randall C. Morgan Jr. is the immediate past president of
the National Medical Association and current president
of the Indiana Orthopedic Society. He practices medicine
in northwest Indiana, specializing in pediatric orthopedics
and surgery for arthritic conditions. Awarded an honorary
doctor of science degree by Grinnell College in 1995, he
holds faculty appointments at Northwestern, Indiana,
and Howard Universities.*

Many new challenges lie in store in the future for
traditional providers in the African American community. Managed
care has had a pervasive effect on even the most minute components
of the present-day delivery system, and providers have been motivated
to keep ahead of the curve in order to be profitable. In fact there are
few traditional modes of practice still present in many communities,
and those that have survived are endangered species. Another factor

that has complicated the adjustment of entire communities to health care changes is the pervasive influence of urbanization and population growth on medical decisions and treatment choices.

MANAGED CARE MANAGES COSTS

As we consider the role of managed care, it becomes obvious that the *fundamental* reason for its existence is to manage cost and not to manage care. The early forms of managed care involved decreased cost to the employer and to the insured because they limited access to health care services for patients. During this stage of managed care, patients were forced to see primary care physicians who acted as gatekeepers, guarding the financial interests of the payer through a savings or incentive plan that rewarded physicians who limited patient access to care.

Through physician selectivity and patient selectivity, insurers who offer a managed care product have been able to pass savings on to both the employer and the employee. However, the National Medical Association is aware that black physicians have unfortunately limited involvement as providers and members of governing boards in managed care systems nationwide. Of greatest significance now in the association's view are several important shifts in the managed care industry. The first change is an abrupt increase in the enrollment of Medicaid and Medicare patients in managed care networks nationwide. The second change is that the health care policies affecting these patients are within the jurisdiction of the individual states as opposed to the federal government. The third change is the emergence of disease management technology as one of the basic measures of a managed care company's clinical and financial success. Simply stated, this means that as sicker patients become enrolled in managed care plans, proficiency in disease management will be the primary basis for managed care plan and physician compensation. This represents a true challenge for all physicians.

In 1996, health maintenance organization (HMO) enrollees increased to fifty-six million—a sixfold increase since 1980. Coupled with this statistic is the fact that 32 percent of Medicaid beneficiaries and 10.5 percent of Medicare beneficiaries are now enrolled in managed care products, most of which are HMOs. The major group of beneficiaries enrolled in Medicaid managed care consists of low-income minority residents of central cities.

The pros of Medicaid managed care in urban communities are an improvement in *access* to primary care and a major step toward guaranteed health *services,* rather than only guaranteed health *insurance coverage.* However, studies of Medicaid managed care in urban communities, dating back to the 1970s, also illustrate several cons:

- Deceptive marketing and enrollment practices
- Pervasive underservice in communities
- Inadequate access to primary and specialty care physicians
- Insufficient provider networks
- Low-quality care
- Outright fraud

Though pros as well as cons exist in Medicaid managed care programs, the overwhelming evidence is that managed care has adversely affected black physicians in the following ways:

- Many black physicians are being excluded from managed care networks; they are then experiencing professional and monetary loss from diminished patient bases and negative shifts in referrals.
- The exclusion of black physicians is decreasing access to, availability of, and quality of service among the underserved populations that black physicians typically serve.
- The Medicare and Medicaid patients traditionally a part of black physicians' practices are often being removed from those physicians' care and enrolled by decree in new managed care plans, under different ownership.

The National Medical Association has written a study proposal that it has submitted to the Health Care Financing Administration. Through this study the association hopes to replace anecdotal data on the effects of managed care with scientifically obtained data from a large cross-section of the black physician provider base. The objective is to understand the impact of managed care on black physicians through preliminary assessment based on a nationwide survey, regional focus groups, interviews, and site visits. The study will identify key factors affecting black physicians. It will, for example, investigate these questions:

- What market characteristics have had an effect on the availability and accessibility of black participation in managed care?

- To what extent are black providers involved in managed care?

- How do Medicaid managed care waiver programs and managed care provider network strategies affect black physicians?

- What impacts, if any, have black physicians experienced as a result of managed care?

- How has managed care affected black physicians' patients and the services the physicians provide?

- How are black physicians' affiliations, structures, compensation arrangements, and clinical practice and referral patterns affected by managed care participation?

THE URBAN HEALTH PENALTY

Although many physicians find profit in leaving the urban patient and hospital, those who stay and provide care—from Detroit to Watts—require the support of hospitals and multiple funding sources, including the federal government. Ultimately, universal coverage for health care will be the only solution. The number of those uninsured must decrease.

The urban health penalty, as it has been dubbed by the American College of Physicians, is the aggregate condition, familiar to us all, in which the urban health care infrastructure is called upon to serve not only the urban population but patients from the suburbs as well, even though it is typically funded from urban resources alone. The entire nation feels the consequences of what befalls inner-city health care clients; yet good medicine and good provision of medical care is only a partial solution to the health care needs found in our cities.

By virtually any measure of health status, minority populations suffer greater morbidity, mortality, and disability. Low-income individuals, people living in impoverished neighborhoods, minority persons, and other special populations all experience substantially greater levels of premature death and disability due to preventable accidents and disease. For example, the death rate for heart disease among African

Americans averages half again what it is for whites, with black women significantly more likely to contract heart disease than the other three groups identified by combination of race and gender.

Diabetic nephropathy is six times higher in minorities than in the general population. The death rate for strokes among African Americans is essentially twice that of the general population. The infant mortality rate is still at least twice that of other ethnic groups, a statistic that has been resistant to myriad interventions over the past thirty years.

This is *indeed* the urban penalty—and sadly these statistics exist in most major urban areas of this country, in many cases in close proximity to some of the leading medical centers, educational centers, and research centers in America. This is what we need to consider as we plan for the Medicare and Medicaid populations as our national health system evolves.

The hospital in the urban community also faces a very difficult task. It first must remain financially solvent. It must provide facilities for state-of-the-art health care delivery. At a time of downsizing, it must have efficient ambulatory services. In many urban communities the hospitals are the major employers of the citizens. African American physicians, facing shrinking hospital numbers and sizes in the community, must maintain influence on the active staff, serve on committees, and steer the actions of the boards and executive committees to favorable action for their patients. The teaching hospitals, including black hospitals, must survive so they can continue providing medical education to minority communities. Hospitals are the strongest potential allies for African American physicians. (Pharmaceutical companies also are potentially strong allies.)

In spite of the trend to freestanding, outpatient facilities, hospitals must be supported and must be influenced heavily by community physicians. Giving physicians compensation for the care of the uninsured is a major way that hospitals should share resources and support financially those physicians who bear the brunt of the cost of uninsured care.

As health care leaders search for common ground upon which to build a better U.S. health care system (and make quantum changes in health care delivery), we must realize that racial residential segregation in U.S. society, which perpetuates urban poverty, also contributes to the challenge of building health care delivery systems that provide access to high-quality health services for all Americans. If segregation is permitted to continue, poverty will inevitably deepen and become more persistent within a large share of the black community. With such concentrated poverty and lack of education we will be hard pressed to continue to provide quality health care where our society needs it most, and it will prove difficult to implement the new technologies to improve patient outcomes. If segregation can be ended, then and only then can our society even begin to eliminate the manifold social and economic problems that follow from its persistence.

THE POTENTIAL OF PARTNERSHIPS

I strongly believe in the potential and the necessity of partnerships between organizations. As Medicaid and Medicare recipients are increasingly enrolled in managed care plans, these plans will be controlled at the state level. The National Medical Association (NMA) recognizes this and looks to communicate with every state and local elected official to improve the care of the patient. In addition, it is a feasible and viable option for the NMA to partner with academic health centers and institutions that traditionally serve many of the same populations as NMA physicians.

The real opportunity for partnership between the NMA and other providers servicing the minority and underserved communities is coming as this country goes forward into the next phase of the health care delivery system—*value-based care.* Simply put, competition is based much more on value than on cost. Aspects of the value-based system have been in use for several years in Minnesota with good reviews. Value-based care is characterized by

- Meaningful outcomes data
- Consistent use of best medical practices
- Team-based health care delivery
- Effective prevention and population health programs
- Patient-centered health care
- Quality-based health care competition

Value-based care is the realization of an integrated management system. The *payer,* the *physician,* and the *hospital* must work together closely to provide the best care. This is the vertically integrated system that undoubtedly will be the model for the future of community health care delivery. In anticipation of these changes, in 1996 the National Medical Association formed the Task Force on Integrated Health and Managed Care. Its mission is "to protect, advocate, and assure fairness for minority, other medically underserved patient populations, and minority business providers by empowering minority physicians, minority health-related businesses and those who seek to provide health services in the African-American community."

The NMA has also begun to establish corporate partnerships with major providers of medical goods and services. In its evolving relationship with the American Medical Association (AMA), the NMA is now a voting member with a voice in the AMA House of Delegates. The two associations have found they agree on far more than they disagree, and they maintain many parallel economic and other interests.

To promote health reform that takes minority communities' interests into account, minority organizations must collaborate. They have a distinct need for bridge building. However, because community interests overlap but do not completely coincide, the separate ethnic-focused minority organizations are also needed. It is often easier to induce physicians to join these separate organizations rather than a broader organization, and as these minority organizations grow in membership and strength, the organizations themselves can begin to pool their resources. This is the key to ensuring that minority interests are addressed in the health system.

Although many urban and the rural health care issues face this country, I charge each physician to go out and make a difference in his or her own community. There are four major challenges for physician leaders:

- *Enhance the communication skills of physicians so they can deal with multiple constituencies.* The articulate physician, one who can communicate effectively with patients, payers, and the public, will be critical to the effort to solve this nation's health care problems. And it will be necessary for physicians to help in the development of a common language for addressing management issues in health care. In this way we can work effectively with others as business partners, capable of speaking the language of finance, human resource management, and strategic planning.

- *Develop an understanding of the economics of medicine and health care.* Without the ability to think as health care managers and provide proactive leadership, physicians will have to function, not on the basis of what they are trained to do, but on the basis of what they are forced to do.

- *Become more effective at promoting public health initiatives and influencing public policy.* In the past, physicians have sometimes been their own worst enemies.

- *Assume a more active role as educators, building public awareness and supporting community efforts to promote health and wellness.* One of the most critical issues we must address in this context is giving the public more information about confronting the problem of violence and the factors leading to violence. Because violence is often rooted in social and economic conditions, most health care providers, including physicians, have avoided dealing effectively with it. Pediatricians have provided great leadership in this area; now we all need to become involved.

We physicians working together, thinking together, communicating together, breaking bread together can make a difference. We can be that nonpartisan engine that begins to drive segregation and separation from our communities, our offices, and even our hospitals.

The fact that in 1998, thirty years after the civil rights movement, little has changed in our communities does not generate optimism. Nevertheless, new partnerships will help motivate change. Partnerships among physicians and with hospitals and other providers of health care are our links to success in the future. I believe that with a willingness to work together to solve communities' health care problems, the health care professionals in this country possess the necessary skills and resources to succeed. It will require sophisticated vertical integration, and it will also mean creating cooperative *racial* integration as a characteristic of this complex partnership.

CHAPTER THIRTY-SEVEN

Leading Behavioral Health Services

Keith Dixon

Keith Dixon is president of United Behavioral Health, a national managed behavioral health care company headquartered in San Francisco and covering mental health care for more than 13 million Americans through employers, health plans, and governmental agencies. Active in health care policy issues, Dixon served in 1997 as chairman of the American Managed Behavioral Health Care Association, which represents eighteen behavioral health care organizations covering 150 million Americans.

S everal decades of research conducted under the auspices of the National Institute of Mental Health and other groups suggests that perhaps as much as one-quarter of the U.S. population experiences a major mental health problem in any given year (Regier and others, 1993; Kessler and others, 1994). The economic cost of mental illness is staggering. Treatment costs alone are $90 billion per year. However, lost productivity in the U.S. workforce (for example, absenteeism, turnover, and poor performance) and other "indirect" costs in our society (for example, accidents, jail incarceration, divorce, suicide, and preventable medical costs) are, for all intents and purposes, economically incalculable but generally estimated to be in the monetary range of $270 billion annually (Rice, Kelman, and Miller, 1991).

At present many of the costs of mental illness in our health care system are incurred because people do not get correct and appropriate treatment—or do not get treatment at all. In addition, because these costs are shifted or hidden, their importance is not considered; they are in effect invisible. For example, perhaps as many as 60 percent of all primary care office visits scheduled by consumers that are meant to deal with physical complaints and ailments have an underlying mental illness at the source that is rarely addressed appropriately, if addressed at all (Simon and Vonkorff, 1995; Rost, Smith, Matthews, and Guise, 1994).

We are not accustomed to thinking about mental illness as a *contagion*. Although mental illness, as far as we know, is not transmitted like the flu or AIDS, it is indeed transmitted. One need spend only a few moments with a family that has had a member with schizophrenia, depression, or a substance abuse problem to sense the profound "collateral damage" these conditions exert on social systems and their devastating impacts on the psychological well-being of others at home and at work. In this sense, mental illness is indeed contagious and broadly destructive and would meet the standard for an epidemic. Moreover, although modern treatments are effective and readily available, mentally ill individuals are often reluctant to access services because of the stigma such services are perceived to carry, and these individuals' families frequently feel too emotionally depleted to help them. The same sense of helplessness can often characterize coworkers and managers in the workplace when they are faced with managing employees with mental illness.

When it comes to providing insurance coverage for mental illness treatment, it is common for employers to cover only what one might call (to borrow an insurance colloquialism) "fender-benders." Most people are just plain out of luck if they are "totaled." In its most catastrophic forms, mental illness requires treatment and rehabilitation resources beyond the coverage typically found in policies sponsored by many employers and health maintenance organizations. Special limits on mental health benefits (that is, higher copays and deductibles and lower annual and lifetime dollar maximums than those applied to physical care) leave many beneficiaries high and dry in a catastrophe (for example, needing coverage of treatment for a child with schizophrenia).

Employers and government payers often fear that benefits covering mental health care will be susceptible to what Harvard health economist Richard Frank calls "moral hazard." This is the tendency for beneficiaries to use the benefit simply because it is there rather than because it is needed (Frank, Huskamp, McGuire, and Newhouse, 1996; Frank and McGuire, 1994). Many employers fear that mental health professionals will tend to *medicalize* people's problems in living. Therefore employers have tried to control any potential abuse of mental health benefits by imposing large copayments and low dollar maximums to discourage unnecessary utilization and prolonged hours "on the couch."

Coverage of catastrophic mental illness has traditionally been the responsibility of public mental health systems, many of which have been badly strained by cutbacks in public funding and the onus of caring for the ever growing number of citizens who have exhausted their assets or private benefits for care. The shifting of the costs for chronic and severely ill patients onto a poorly financed public system is a national tragedy and considered by many to be a form of institutionalized discrimination against the mentally ill. This practice, whether intentional policy or an unintentional consequence of employer-based insurance purchasing, is nonetheless disturbing in its immediate effects on the mentally ill and its long-term effects on our society at large.

The good news is that we are now entering a new age in mental health services. A revolution in psychopharmacology has demonstrated enormous promise for improving the functioning and quality of life for the mentally ill and for preventing lifelong institutionalization. This revolution also points the way to the large part genetics and brain biochemistry play in severe mental illness (though they appear not to be the sole cause), linking these disorders more closely with our concepts of "real" disease and medical care. Also, the link between physical illness and mental illness is now more widely understood. Societal stigma has also lessened, due in part to the efforts of patient and family advocacy groups and the willingness of such famous persons as Mike Wallace, Rod Steiger, Betty Ford, and William Styron to share openly their personal struggles with mental conditions.

The leadership challenge in mental health care in this new era is to seize on these developments and bring mental health care fully into the mainstream of U.S. health care delivery. The goal is to broaden population access to preventive and therapeutic forms of intervention that have a demonstrable effect on outcome. In the following sections, I discuss two examples of leadership important to this new era: leadership in enacting new laws that mandate *parity* between physical and mental health care coverage in private health plans, and leadership in incorporating managed care principles and practices into health plans.

LEADERSHIP AND PARITY

Parity in the mental health field refers to the elimination of differences between how a health plan covers physical and mental illness. To achieve parity, leaders must overcome harmful attitudes about the mentally ill and must reduce the social stigma associated with mental illness. They must also confront stereotypes about mental health treatments and professionals and overcome resistance from employers and health plans who abhor any governmental mandate in benefit plan design and fear a cost explosion from expanded use of mental health treatments by beneficiaries.

The fight for parity illustrates two key attributes of leadership: a willingness to take personal risk, and a willingness to collaborate with others with whom one is usually in conflict, in order to achieve a broader goal. Taking personal risk is best illustrated by the example of Senator Peter Domenici. A conservative Republican from New Mexico, Domenici was asked in 1996 by mental health consumers and advocates to support a parity amendment to the health care portability act sponsored by Senators Kennedy and Kassebaum, whose main intent was to allow beneficiaries to carry over coverage from one health plan to another. Resistance to the parity amendment came primarily from business groups such as the Chamber of Commerce, the National Association of Manufacturers, and the insurance industry— all very powerful Washington lobbies.

Although lobbyists were successful in getting the parity amendment dropped, Senator Domenici and others were successful in ensuring its separate passage in the Mental Health Parity Act of 1996. Domenici was instrumental in changing the mind-set and attitudes of his congressional colleagues by going public with his personal story of dealing with a mentally ill child in his own family. He soon had the company of another unlikely backer of mental health parity, Senator Alan Simpson of Wyoming, who told a similar story, but one that ended in a suicide. It took the advocacy of two conservative Republicans friendly to business and supportive of limited government to revolutionize congressional perspectives on mental illness and on the benefits of a measure fiercely opposed by the business community. To mental health advocates, these events were analogous to President Nixon's opening to China.

The Mental Health Parity Act, however, is a weak law. It merely requires that employers sponsor plans that eliminate differences in physical and mental health care coverage with respect to copayments, annual maximums, and lifetime maximums. Employers may impose hospital stay and outpatient visit limitations. Indeed, employers do not have to provide mental health coverage at all, and if they do provide coverage and the costs escalate more than 1 percent, they are allowed to return to a discriminatory benefit. However, the importance of the act lies less in its actual content than in its symbolic value. It is helping to shatter the stigma attached to mental illness extant in political circles that shape U.S. health care policy.

A second characteristic of leadership illuminated by the parity fight is the willingness to reach out over differences to find common ground with antagonists and a broader vision. During the year of legislative battles over parity, the leadership of the American Psychiatric Association and the American Psychological Association had declared war on privately managed behavioral health care companies. However, despite the deep antipathy between managed care companies and mental health professional associations, both sides agreed to put aside their differences to form the Fairness Coalition, which lobbied for the Mental Health Parity Act. They were joined by major consumer groups, most notably the National Mental Health Association and the National Alliance for the Mentally Ill (NAMI). Despite consumer wariness of managed care, NAMI and other groups readily recognized the valuable contribution of the managed behavioral health care industry in supplying the Fairness Coalition with data on the projected costs of parity, derived from the vast databases owned by these companies. These data, analyzed by the Congressional Budget Office and others, were critical in weakening the argument that parity would result in a cost explosion for employers. Senators Domenici's and Simpson's compelling personal stories, data from the managed care industry, and political support from consumer and provider groups combined to overcome resistance to the Mental Health Parity Act.

Looking to the future, the passage of the Mental Health Parity Act has made it more likely that the public will come to see less difference between mental and physical illness, an outcome that will help reduce stigma. Eliminating stigma should encourage more individuals to seek preventive and ameliorative interventions. If organized correctly under managed care (our next challenge), such interventions show great promise to reduce health care and societal costs and improve the quality of life in our communities and the productivity of our workforce.

LEADERSHIP AND RESPONSIBLE MANAGED CARE

According to a 1997 report from the American Managed Behavioral Health Care Association, more than 144 million Americans have benefits for mental health treatment that are under the management of private managed behavioral health care companies. Perhaps ominously, 80 percent of these Americans are covered by no more than seven national managed behavioral health care companies. Further mergers and acquisitions characterize this multibillion-dollar industry—an industry that barely existed a mere decade ago.

Within the next two years, fewer than four national companies may control up to 90 percent of the market for mental health services in the United States. Whether or not this industry will go through some future cycle of divestiture and decentralization is a speculation fueled by comparisons to older industries such as banking, telecommunications, and airlines. At the present time, consolidation among managed mental health care companies is the norm.

Managed care is controversial generally and in mental health care in particular. Managed care challenges the basic right of a provider to be isolated from the economic effects of his or her professional practices, if these practices are paid for by a private or public third party. As such, managed care arrangements that break down this isolation inevitably come into conflict with traditional values regarding professionalism, autonomy, privacy, locus of accountability for good and bad clinical practices, and providers' expectations of financial remuneration for years of rigorous professional training.

In mental health care, we are rapidly moving away from a pre-industrial cottage industry of disconnected professionals working in isolation in private practices, into conglomerates of networks and group practices organized by private managed care companies of growing size, capitalization, and management sophistication. Despite recent calls for increased government regulation of managed care companies, the public, and certainly employers, have nonetheless embraced market-based competition between these large enterprises as a means to ensure the quality of mental health care and simultaneously keep costs under control.

The central leadership challenge in managing mental health care is providing effective *stewardship* of a scarce resource to meet the critical mental health needs of a defined population. Stewardship implies a populationwide perspective on health problems and a public health orientation to the assessment of need. Stewardship implies a commitment that resources will not be wasted on those who will not benefit from them and that inappropriate resource use by a few will be prevented and will not result in irrational scarcities for others.

The concept of scarcity in the mental health field is a complex one, even though it is typically expressed simply as the maximum amount of money an employer or government payer is willing to spend on mental health treatment in any given year for a defined population. However, any notion of scarcity in mental health care is often anathema to consumers and providers who believe one or more of the following: businesses and government have *never* allocated sufficient resources to mental health care and have in fact discriminated against the mentally ill, who deserve more, not less; an affluent society should resist *any* notion of limits, particularly when it comes to the health needs of individuals; and the most rational allocation of a health resource—abundant or scarce—is the one that occurs within the hermetically sealed confines of an individual doctor's conversation with an individual patient, carried out in total privacy on a case-by-case basis.

The controversies engulfing managed mental health care derive from fundamental disagreements over these basic concepts. Someone exercising stewardship has to allocate a scarce resource in a rational way, with an eye on both the individual's requirements for care and the population's total needs and available resources. Effective stewardship obviously entails a major attribute of leadership—the willingness to be held publicly accountable for accomplishing a necessary, difficult, and controversial task. Not infrequently, the task requires saying no to a demand for a particular service desired by a patient and a provider when the need, clinical value, or cost-benefit of the service is questionable. In mental health care, there are an inordinate number of questionable needs and great doubt about the value of many services.

Private professional practice in mental health care is highly variable from clinician to clinician and overly dependent on subjective "clinician judgment." Many practitioners do not know how to develop and follow a treatment plan with explicit goals and objectives, let alone monitor and measure patient progress toward goal accomplishment. It is obviously difficult for anyone to be held accountable for the use of a resource when there are no standards or benchmarks for performance.

Contrary to popular myth, the pioneer leaders of managed mental health care were not Wall Street entrepreneurs or insurance executives on a quest for profit, but individuals (primarily psychiatrists) extensively involved in patient care and concerned about the economic and clinical value of mental health services. Some were among the first to develop explicit criteria and practice guidelines pertaining to mental health procedures and practices covering defined populations. The development of criteria and uniform guidelines by managed care companies came at a time in the late 1980s when many employers, distressed by the rising costs of mental health care and the lack of standards for practices in the field, were considering elimination of mental health benefits entirely. Therefore, the emergence of specialized managed mental health care enterprises came at an opportune time and was a market response to employers interested in preserving benefits while achieving accountability for the costs, quality, and outcomes of mental health interventions.

The current size of managed mental health care companies, their rapid consolidation, and the prospect of monopolies in the industry have recently instilled fear in consumers and practitioners. Indeed, the industry is currently experiencing a very public indictment by anecdote in the popular press. Consumers are fearful of large, faceless private enterprises that have access to information about individuals' highly intimate problems. Practitioners share this fear and often resent their loss of autonomy in making clinical decisions on behalf of their patients. These are legitimate fears and concerns that responsible companies must address. Though large, these companies will be increasingly challenged to embrace the concept of *mass customization*. As industry leaders steward resources for very large populations, their challenge will be to provide highly customized solutions to individual mental health problems and situations, yet organized on a mass scale. Their ability to provide humane and highly personalized service to people will be, as it always has been, the determinant of their success.

Looking to the future, we are likely to see leadership in managed mental health care emerge in the following three areas:

- The transformation of academic medical centers and training programs to produce a new generation of practitioners able to work effectively in an environment of rigorous clinical and financial accountability

- The emergence of a commitment by leading companies to principles and practices of corporate social responsibility, philanthropy, and community service as their capital assets continue to grow over the coming years

- The development and implementation of populationwide preventive interventions that will reduce demand for expensive, tertiary mental health services and empower consumers with information and resources so they can take better care of themselves

These present exciting leadership challenges for all of us.

References

Frank, R. G., Huskamp, H. A., McGuire, T. G., and Newhouse, J. P. "Some Economics of Mental Health 'Carve-Outs.'" *Archives of General Psychiatry*, 1996, *53*, 933–937.

Frank, R. G., and McGuire, T. G. "Health Care Reform and Financing of Mental Health Services." In R. Manderscheid and M. Sonnenschein (eds.), *Mental Health, United States, 1994.* Washington, D.C.: U.S. Government Printing Office, 1994.

Kessler, R. C., and others. "Lifetime and 12-Month Prevalence of DSM-III-R Psychiatric Disorders in the United States: Results from the National Comorbidity Survey." *Archives of General Psychiatry*, 1994, *51*, 8–19.

Regier, D. A., and others. "The De Facto U.S. Mental and Addictive Disorders Service System: Epidemiological Catchment Area

Prospective One-Year Prevalence Rates of Disorders and Services." *Archives of General Psychiatry*, 1993, *50*, 85–94.

Rice, D. P., Kelman, S., and Miller, L. S. "Estimates of Economic Costs of Alcohol and Drug Abuse and Mental Illness, 1985 and 1988." *Public Health Report*, 1991, *106*, 250–292.

Rost, K., Smith, R., Matthews, D. B., and Guise, B. "The Deliberate Misdiagnosis of Major Depression in Primary Care." *Archives of Family Medicine*, 1994, *3*, 333–337.

Simon, G. E., and Vonkorff, M. "Recognition, Management, and Outcomes of Depression in Primary Care." *Archives of Family Medicine*, 1995, *6*, 99–105.

Name Index

A

Aaron, H., 359
Adler, N. E., 56, 67
Aesop, 24
Albert, S., 310, 314
Aly, I. T., 51*n*
Amler, R. W., 56, 57, 67
Amundson, B., 213, 214
Anders, G., 359, 365
Appleby, C., 16, 19
Ardell, D. B., 3, 19
Armey, R., 9
Axene, D. V., 359, 365
Ayanian, J. Z., 56, 67

B

Baker, E. L., 144, 148
Baker, W. G., 293, 298
Banthin, J. S., 53, 72
Baraff, L. J., 65, 72
Barbakow, J. C., 93
Bayer, R., 58, 67
Beaulieu, L., 211, 214, 215
Beckham, D., 7
Beckhard, R., 110
Bedell, S. E., 65, 67
Bell, R., 327, 329
Bellack, J. P., 291*n*
Bennis, W., 156, 157
Benson, H., 19
Berenson, R. A., 65, 72
Berry, L. L., 326, 329–330
Berwick, D. M., 64, 70, 351, 353
Beyers, M., 278
Biddle, R. M., 308
Bor, D. H., 56, 67

Bovbjerg, R. R., 63, 70
Boyd, M. S., 327, 329
Bradford, D. R., 155, 157
Brandenburger, A. M., 5, 19
Brock, D. W., 54, 58, 68
Brook, R. H., 62, 68, 357, 365
Brown, L. D., 56, 68
Bueler, J., 57, 68
Burg, M. A., 174, 177
Burns, J. M., 209, 214
Burstin, H. R., 56, 68
Butts, C. Q., 57, 68

C

Casey, M., 208, 215
Cassel, C. K., 187, 197
Chow, M. P., 290
Christianson, J. B., 205
Clancy, C. M., 54, 69
Cleary, P., 65, 68
Codman, E. A., 220–221, 227, 229–230
Coffman, J. M., 270, 277, 290
Cohen, A. R., 155, 157
Cohen, J. J., 112, 116
Coile, R. C., Jr., 3, 5, 19
Collins, J. C., 293, 298, 322, 353
Cook, R., 206, 208, 214
Cordell, D. E., 362, 366
Cornelius, L. J., 57, 68
Corrigan, K. V., 17–18, 20
Cretin, S., 65, 72

D

Daniels, N., 54, 55, 58, 68
Davidson, J., 233, 240
Davidson, S., 26, 37

Davidson, W. H., 232, 240
Davis, K., 53, 68
Davis, S., 102, 110
Davis, S. M., 232, 240
Degas, E., 102–103
DePalma, A. F., 221, 230
DePree, M., 347, 353
Deutsch, H., 107, 110
Dixon, K., 376
Dodson, E. S., 219, 227, 230
Domenici, P., 379–380
Donabedian, A., 65, 68
Donaho, B. A., 293, 298
Donelan, K., 53, 68
Dougherty, C. J., 55, 69
Dower, C., 291n
Doyle, R. L., 359, 365
Droste, T. M., 5, 7, 19
Drucker, P. F., 307, 348, 353
Dubler, N. N., 62, 69
Dull, H. B., 56, 57, 67

E

Einhorn, T., 63, 69
Eisenberg, D. M., 30–31, 37, 173, 177
Ellwood, P. M., 65, 69
Elstad, J., 63, 69
Emanuel, E. J., 62, 69
Emanuel, L., 266
Enthoven, A., 11, 19
Epstein, A. M., 56, 67
Epstein, P. R., 56, 67
Erikson, E. H., 104, 192, 197
Eyler, J. M., 56, 69

F

Feder, J., 54, 56, 69
Feinstein, J. S., 55, 69
Feldt, G., 161
Ferguson, T., 238, 240
Ferrar, P. J., 362, 366
Findlay, S., 15, 21
Flower, J., 22
Foege, W. H., 85
Folkman, J., 25, 37
Ford, B., 378

Fralic, M. F., 292, 298
Frame, C. D., 323
Frank, R. G., 378, 384
Franklin, E., 316
Franklin, S., 322
Franks, P., 54, 69
Freudenheim, M., 8, 20
Fronstin, P., 133, 141
Fulmer, R. M., 335, 343

G

Gable, L., 51n
Gagliardi, A., 364, 366
Gandhi, M., 105
Gardner, J. W., 347, 354
Gilkey, R. W., 101, 331, 335, 343
Ginsburg, P. B., 7–8, 20
Glenzer, K., 74
Gold, M. R., 54, 69
Golden-Biddle, K., 308, 310, 314
Goldman, E. F., 17–18, 20
Goldsmith, M., 110, 301
Goodman, J. C., 357, 361, 362, 365, 366, 367
Gostin, L. O., 51, 57, 69
Greene, J., 13, 15, 20
Greenleaf, R., 312, 314
Grudin, R., 272, 277
Grumbach, K., 62, 63, 72
Guise, B., 377, 385
Gutmann, A., 58, 69

H

Hadley, J., 54, 56, 69
Hafner-Eaton, C., 69
Halverson, P. K., 142
Hamel, G., 322
Hamer, R. L., 7, 8, 9, 10n, 11, 12, 20
Hastings, K. E., 65, 72
Hays, P. G., 124
Henry, J. D., Sr., 101, 318
Herzlinger, R., 304
Hesselbein, F., 102, 110
Hewitt, M., 206, 215
Hiebeler, R., 284, 288
Hippocrates, 268

Hobbs, D., 208, 214, 215
Holm, C. E., 13, 20
Hornung, K., 16, 20
Huskamp, H. A., 378, 384

I

Israel, G., 211, 214, 215

J

Jadad, A. R., 364, 366
Japsen, B., 12, 20
Jenner, E., 86
Johns, M., 117
Jones, W. K., 171
Jost, T. S., 65, 70
Joyce, G., 26, 38

K

Kaluzny, A. D., 149, 150, 153, 154, 155, 157
Kanter, R. B., 152, 154, 157, 293–294, 298
Kassebaum, N., 361, 379
Keeler, E. B., 47, 50
Keene, C., 353, 354
Kelly, T. B., 284, 288
Kelman, S., 377, 385
Kennedy, E. M., 361, 379
Kessler, R. C., 376, 384
Ketteman, C., 284, 288
Kilborn, P. T., 6, 11, 20, 57, 70, 364, 366
Kinney, E. D., 60–61, 70
Kirch, D. G., 111
Kohles, M. K., 293, 298
Krampf, R. F., 327–328, 330
Krein, K., 200, 204
Krein, S., 208, 215
Krivich, M. J., 327, 329

L

Laffel, G., 64, 70
Lagnado, L., 15, 19, 20, 21
Lantos, J. D., 348–349, 354
Larsen, R., 307
Latham, S. R., 250
Laudicina, S. S., 358, 366

LaVeist, T. A., 56, 70
Lawley, T. J., 117
Lawrence, D. M., 347
Leavenworth, G., 234, 240
Levit, K. R., 52, 70, 118, 123, 235, 240
Lewis, J., 155, 157
Lieberman, G. R., 331
Lohr, S., 16, 20
Long, S. H., 54, 70
Longo, D. R., 62, 65, 70
Lopez, A. D., 75, 84
Lowes, R. L., 14, 20
Lutz, W., 33, 38

M

Manning, W., 357, 366
Mariner, W. K., 65, 70
Marquis, M. S., 54, 70
Marsteller, J. A., 63, 70
Matthews, C., 133, 141
Matthews, D. B., 377, 385
Matthews, M., Jr., 355, 361, 365, 366
McCall, C. W., 219
McCarthy, D., 63, 70
McDonald, C. J., 236, 240
McDonnell, K., 357, 366
McGraw, D. C., 66, 70
McGuire, J., 8, 20
McGuire, T. G., 378, 384
McKinney, M., 155, 157
McLaughlin, C. P., 153, 157
McNerney, W. J., 153, 157
McSteen, M. A., 178
Meade, M. S., 206, 215
Mechanic, D., 63, 71
Merton, V., 56, 71
Mertz, B., 291*n*
Meyer, H., 5, 6, 12, 20
Meyerson, M. H., 231
Middleberg, M. I., 74
Millenson, M., 348, 354
Miller, L. S., 377, 385
Miller, T., 238, 241
Minnix, W. L., Jr., 186
Monroe, S., 12, 14, 21

Montague, J., 16, 19, 21
Moore, R. M., 316
Morath, J., 285, 288
Morgan, R. C., Jr., 368
Morjikian, R. L., 290
Moscovice, I., 208, 212, 215
Moses, E. B., 292, 298
Murdaugh, C. L., 280, 281, 289
Murphy, E. C., 294, 298
Murray, C.J.L., 75, 84
Musgrave, G. L., 361, 366

N

Nalebuff, B. J., 5, 19
Nanus, B., 156, 157
Nelms, S., 86
Neuhauser, D., 221, 230
Newhouse, J. P., 378, 384
Nichols, L. M., 63, 70
Nixon, R. M., 166, 380
Noe, T., 124*n*
Normanno, N., 25, 38

O

O'Haren, M., 133*n*
Ohmae, K., 153, 155, 157
Olson, R., 23, 25, 26, 38
O'Neil, E., 269, 270, 277, 291, 298
O'Neil, J., 272, 277
O'Neill, T. P., 133
O'Rourke, R. A., 280, 281, 289

P

Parasuraman, A., 326, 329–330
Parsons, M. L., 280, 281, 289
Pear, R., 52, 71
Peterson, P. G., 187, 197
Peterson, S., 19, 21
Petrila, J., 61, 71
Phipps, J., 86
Pickreign, J. D., 20
Pinto, C., 18, 21
Pitman, H., 16, 21
Pooley, E., 208, 215
Porras, J. I., 293, 298, 322, 353

Prahalad, C. K., 322
Priester, R., 55, 71

Q

Quesenberry, C. P., 62, 63, 72

R

Randall, V. R., 57, 71
Rao, H., 310, 314
Rawls, J., 58, 60, 72
Reardon, T. R., 261
Reed, W. L., 57, 72
Regier, D. A., 376, 384–385
Reinhardt, W. E., 52, 72
Ricci, R. J., 242
Rice, D. P., 377, 385
Ricketts, T., 150, 157
Robbins, A., 357, 367
Robbins, G., 357, 367
Rodrigue, G., 9, 21
Rogers, W. H., 65, 72
Rosenberg, C. E., 56, 72
Rosenberg, M., 85
Rosenblatt, R., 213, 214
Rost, K., 377, 385
Rubin, H. R., 63, 72

S

Sage, W. M., 65, 72
Sager, C., 335, 343
Sanger, M., 161, 162, 170
Sashkin, M., 322
Saxton, J. F., 118*n*
Schaeffer, L. D., 132
Schein, E. H., 152, 157
Schieber, G. J., 52, 72
Schlesinger, M., 63, 71
Schmittdiel, J., 62, 63, 72
Schriger, D. L., 65, 72
Schroeder, S. A., 53, 72
Scott, L., 210, 212, 215
Scott, R., 19
Seago, J. A., 291*n*
Selby, J. V., 62, 63, 72
Senft, J., 25, 38
Senge, P., 156, 157, 193, 198, 311, 315

Shaha, S., 238
Shalowitz, J., 39
Sharpe, A., 15, 21
Short, P. F., 53, 72
Shortell, S. M., 144, 148
Simon, G. E., 377, 385
Simpson, A., 380
Slepin, R. E., 14, 16, 21
Smith, R., 11–12, 377, 385
Steiger, R., 378
Steinberg, E. P., 54, 56, 69
Stewart, F., 167, 170
Stoddard, J. J., 72
Styron, W., 378
Sutcliffe, I., 247, 249
Swartz, K., 53, 72, 357, 367

T

Tarnove, L., 199
Taylor, J., 271, 277
Temkin-Greener, H., 63, 72
Thorpe, K. E., 52, 72, 356, 367
Turner, V., 309, 315

V

van der Burch, D., 359, 365
van der Griff, D., 133*n*
Vandewater, D., 19
Verrilli, D. K., 63, 70
Vladeck, B., 200
Volpe, L. C., 132
Vonkorff, M., 377, 385

W

Wacker, W., 271, 277
Wagner, E. H., 66, 73
Walker, T., 15, 21
Wall, P., 12, 21
Wallace, M., 378
Walzer, M., 54, 73
Ward, T., 5, 21
Warnecke, R. B., 154, 155, 157
Watson, S. D., 57, 73
Wechsler, J., 10, 21
Weick, K. F., 154, 157
Wellever, A. L., 205
Wennberg, J.M.D., 235, 241
Wenneker, M. B., 55, 56, 73
Weyrauch, K., 62, 63, 73
Whetten, D., 310, 314
White, J. B., 15, 21
Wills, G., 209, 215
Winchell, M., 63, 72
Winslow, R., 359, 365
Wise, P. H., 56, 73
Wojcik, S., 133*n*
Woodyard, C., 15, 21
Wyden, R., 199–200, 204

Z

Zaleznik, A., 108, 110
Zeithaml, V. A., 326, 329–330
Zeng, D., 25, 38
Zifko-Baliga, G. M., 327–328, 330
Zuckerman, H., 149, 150, 152, 153, 157
Zuza, D. J., 13, 20

━✐━ Subject Index

A

Academic health centers: aspects of, 111–123; change agents for, 121; department chairs in, 122–123; development of, 111–112, 118–119; economic reality for, 113; identity of, 310–311; and leadership development, 317–322; leadership of, 114–116, 117–123; medical schools in, 112, 122–123; mission of, 118; number of, 112; organizational issues for, 113–114, 119–121; and risk management, 121; roles in, 120

Academic Leadership Workshop, 296

Access: and choice, 62–63; concerns over, 30; equity of, 55–57; ethical value of, 52–57; and freedom of choice, 48; policy challenges of, 46–47; for underinsured, 53; universal, 54–55

Accountability: and information, 220; and nurses, 286–287; and physicians, 264–266

Accreditation, of physicians, 265

Acknowledge-create-empower paradigm, 320

Acquisitions, alliances distinct from, 275

Administration, technology for, 28

Aetna US Healthcare, 17, 19, 332

Agency for Health Care Policy and Research, 43, 47, 50, 265

Agency for Toxic Substance and Disease Registry, 144, 148

Aging population: aspects of, 34, 178–204; axioms for care of, 188, 189, 190; background on, 178–179,

186–187; caring for, 178–185; changes in, 178–181, 201–202; chronic care perspective for, 194–197; ego integrity or despair for, 192; and family dynamics, 189–190; geriatric care for, 186–198; geriatric team for, 190–191; geriatricians needed for, 182–183, 184, 190–191; and insurers, 129; leadership for, 183–184, 197; learning organization for, 192–194; long-term care for, 199–204; medicines for, 187–188, 189; organizational culture for, 191–192; philosophy f or, 191–192; professional services for, 188; resource and research needs of, 181–182, 197; stories of, 187–190; strategies for, 190–198

Aid to Families with Dependent Children, 45

Alaska, Medicare HMOs lacking in, 7

Alliance for Aging Research, 182, 185

Alliances: acquisitions distinct from, 275; aspects of, 149–157; challenges for, 152–153; in delivery systems, 96; functions of, 150–151; future for, 155–156; limitations of, 156; management guidelines for, 153–155; opportunities for, 151–152; for rural health systems, 212; strategic, 83. *See also* Partnerships

Allina Health System, 247–248

Allina HealthVillage, 247–248

Alternative medicine: in health care, 18–19; mainstreaming of, 30–31; and women's health, 173–174

Altruism, narcissism in balance with, 107

American Academy of Medical Colleges, 169, 170

American Airlines, Sabre system of, 232

American Association of Colleges of Nursing, 287, 288; Executive Development Series of, 296

American Association of Health Plans, 134, 141, 363, 364–365

American Association of Nurse Anesthetists, 294

American Board of Nursing Specialties, 286

American College of Healthcare Executives, 151

American College of Physicians, 371

American College of Surgeons, 220–221

American Electronics Association, 16

American Geriatrics Society, 129

American Healthcare Systems, 150

American Hospital Association, 94, 151

American Internet Users Survey, 238

American Managed Behavioral Health Care Association, 381

American Medical Accreditation Program, 265

American Medical Association, 250n; and aging population, 184; and black physicians, 374; and clinical leadership, 262, 264, 265, 266, 267; and cost control efforts, 44; and managed care, 353; and physician dissatisfaction, 31

American Nurses Association, 294

American Organization of Nurse Executives, 283, 288, 294, 296

American Psychiatric Association, 9–10, 380

American Psychological Association, 380

America's Health Network, 19

Antibiotics, decline in effectiveness of, 27

Anticipatory learning, 321–322

Anxiety, and mergers, 334

Any willing provider legislation, 49, 63

APACHE, 23

Ask-a-nurse service, 234, 285, 364

Assisted suicide, ethical issues of, 257

Atlanta Senior Care, 196

Attention, in leadership, 106

Australia, aging population in, 34

Automated teller machine (ATM), impact of, 243

Automation, in information technology, 223–224

B

Balanced Budget Act of 1997, 44–45, 361

Bangladesh, management assessment in, 83

Banking, and information technology, 243, 247

Barents Group, 358, 365

Barnes Jewish, merger of, 244

Behavioral health services. *See* Mental and behavioral health services

Best-practice models, and information technology, 243–244

Bipartisan Commission on Comprehensive Health Care, 53, 67

BJC Health System, Project Spectrum of, 244

Black physicians: and advent of managed care, 368–375; adverse impacts on, 370; and cost management, 369–371; issues for, 371; and partnerships, 373–374, 375; and urban health penalty, 371–373

Blended organizations: aspects of, 331–343; changing environment for, 332–333; dimensions of, 335–337; integrating activities for, 340–342; interventions for, 338–342; issues for, 336; psychological challenge for, 333–335; start-up management for, 342–343

Blue Cross and Blue Shield Association, 6, 129

Board of Trustees of the Federal Hospital Insurance Trust Fund, 362, 365

Booz-Allen & Hamilton, 247

Boren Amendment of 1981, 45
Boston Women's Health Book
    Collective, 171–172
Boundaries, and empowerment,
    102–104
Boundary spanners, for alliances, 155
Brown & Toland Medical Group, 14
Burden of disease, causes of, 76
Buyers Health Care Action Group
    (BHCAG), 5, 11

C

California: and for-profit conversions,
    15; Knox-Keen license in, 14; HMOs
    in, 6, 8; managed competition in,
    11; market consolidation in, 12, 99;
    and Medicare fraud, 15; provider
    sponsored organizations in, 5; small
    business cooperatives in, 303
California at San Francisco, University
    of: Center for the Health Professions
    at, 296–297; and mergers, 333
California Pacific Medical Center, 14
California Public Employee Retirement
    System (CalPERS), 11, 15
Canada, aging population in, 34
CARE, 78, 83
Care managers role, 128–129
Case management, in geriatric care, 196
Catholic Health Association, 151
Celebration, for innovations, 147
Censorship, and women's health,
    165–166
Center for Health Leadership, 286, 288,
    319–320
Center for Health Management
    Research, 115
Center for Nursing Leadership, 296
Center for the Health Professions,
    296–297
Centers for Disease Control, 144, 148,
    233, 240
CEO rounds, 105, 106
Certification, for nurses, 286–287
Chamber of Commerce, 379
Change: agents of, 121; in aging
    population, 179–181, 201–202;

aspects of managing, 308–315;
    background on, 309; for blended
    organizations, 332–333; in con-
    sumer satisfaction, 324–325; in
    delivery system, 22–23; in econom-
    ics, 360–363; in health care, 4–6;
    managed, by physicians, 276–277;
    management of, for leadership, 297;
    in nursing, 291–292, 293; as oppor-
    tunity, 293; and organizational
    identity, 310–311; and partnerships,
    311–312; and structural participa-
    tion, 313–314; sustaining, 314; and
    trust, 312–313
Choice: ethical value of, 61–64; freedom
    of, and HMOs, 48–50; and health
    economics, 357–358; of product,
    133–136
Christian Health Services, merger of,
    244
Chronic illnesses: and aging popula-
    tion, 194–197; and insurers, 128
Clinical decisions, technology for,
    234–237
Clinical leaders: aspects of, 259–298;
    nurses as, 278–298; physicians as,
    261–277
Clinical pathways, information tech-
    nology for, 235–236
Clinical practice, technology for, 29
Clinton administration, 9, 10, 32, 36, 43
Coaching: and leadership, 108; for
    leadership development, 319–321
Coalition for Healthier Cities and
    Communities, 151
Coalition of Not-for-Profit Health
    Care, 150
Coalitions, for public health, 90
College of Healthcare Information
    Management Executives, 233, 240
Colorado Trust, 213
Columbia/HCA, 15, 19, 332
Columbia, South Carolina, partnership
    in, 212
Commission on Graduates of Foreign
    Nursing Schools, 288
Commitment, in alliances, 153

Communication: and practice alignment, 273–274; skills in, 374

Communities: dialogue with, 311–312; empowerment of, 78; and nursing leaders, 295; partnerships in, for geriatric care, 194–197; rural, 213–214; and trust, 350–352; and violence, 375

Community access management, and information technology, 229

Community care centers, nurses in, 281

Community Care Networks, 151

Community Health Corp., 332

Community health systems: aspects of, 142–148; background of, 143–144; characteristics of, 145–148; described, 144–145

Competencies: in leadership, 271–277, 297; for physicians, 269–277. *See also* Skills

Competition: managed, 11; and network leadership, 306–307

Complementary medicine, 18–19

Computer Motion, 24, 37

Computing, for strategic health care, 242–249. *See also* Information technology

Confidentiality: and information technology, 247, 252–253; and physicians, 266

Congressional Budget Office, 235, 240, 365, 380

Connecticut, network in, 5

Connectivity, in information technology, 224–225

Consumer satisfaction: aspects of, 323–330; concepts of, 325–326; dimensions of, 326; forces for change in, 324–325; and quality, 326–329

Consumerism trend, 17–18

Consumers: alliances of, 302–303; care of, and physicians, 262–264; decision making by, 98; education of, 130; expectations of, 133; and information technology, 229, 234–235, 237–240; informed, 364; and insurer networks, 136–137; and insurers, 132–141; integrated solutions for, 303–304; and nursing, 285–286; and organizational blending, 342; and procedural justice, 60–61; and product choice, 133–136; and quality, 137–140; rights and protections of, 9, 265, 349–350; roles of, 313–314; technology for, 29; uninformed, 359; in value chain, 306

Continuous quality improvement, patient care model of, 327–328

Contracting, direct, 11–12

Co-opetition, 5–6

Cost control: ethical issues of, 253–255; for insurers, 140

Costs: concerns over, 30; ethical value of, 65–66; and freedom of choice, 49–50; and managed care, 369–371; and physicians, 264; policy challenges of, 42–45

Council of Economic Advisers, 65, 68

Council on Ethical and Judicial Affairs, 56, 68

Creativity: for leadership, 297; in vision, 273

Creighton University Medical Center, 96

Culture, organizational: for aging population, 191–192; in alliances, 152–153; and mergers, 343

Customer health care center, and information technology, 238–239

Customers. *See* Consumers

Cyberhealth trend, 16–17

D

Dallas, complementary medicine in, 18–19

Data-mining technology, 246

Decision making: computer-assisted, 236; by consumers, 98; in public health, 87–89

Deficit, disappearance of, 36

Defined-contribution plans, 362–363

Delivery of health care: alliances in, 96; aspects of, 22–38; changes in, 22–23;

for disease management, 95; future for, 37; industry forces on, 30–33; integrated, 94, 142–148, 285; and medical advances, 23–27; for prevention and wellness, 95–96; social forces on, 33–36; technology for, 27–29; unbundled, 284

Deloitte & Touche, 243

Demographic trends: and delivery of health care, 33–34; and fragmentation, 35; and long-term care, 201–202; policy challenges of, 40–41; and rural health systems, 208–209

Development. *See* Leadership development

Diagnostic advances, 23

Dial-a-Nurse, 364

Direct contracting, for health care, 11–12

Doc extenders, 30

Duke Endowment, 151

E

E-business, in future, 246–247

E-mail, for managed care triage, 229

Economics: and academic health centers, 113; aspects of, 355–367; changes needed in, 360–363; and information technology, 364; and physicians, 375; and systems problems, 356–359

Education: of consumers, 130; for nurses, 282, 283, 286–287

Electronic data interchange (EDI), and cyberhealth, 16

Electronic medical records, and privacy issues, 9–10

Electronic records, and results-driven medicine, 27

Emory Healthcare, 193, 195–196; Learning Council of, 317–322

Emory University Hospitals, 106, 318

Emory University School of Medicine, 193; Center for Healthcare Leadership at, 319–320

Employee Benefit Research Institute, 53, 69

Employee Retirement Income Security Act (ERISA), 11, 40, 45

Employees: empowerment of, 329; rights of, and trust, 352

Employers, coalitions of, 5, 11

Empowerment: and boundaries, 102–104; commitment to, 109–110; of communities, 78; of employees, 329; and leadership development, 320; oversight balanced with, 103; vision and strategy for, 108

End-of-life stage: decisions at, 203; ethical issues at, 256–257; and physician ethics, 266

Engagement, in leadership, 105

Equity: of access, 55–57; ethical values of, 58–59

Ernst & Young, 244

Ethics: of access, 52–57; aspects of, 51–73; and choice, 61–64; consensus lacking on, 125; and costs, 65–66; and equity, 58–59; in geriatric care, 194; and justice, 59–61; in long-term care, 203; and managed care trust, 347–354; and nursing, 288; paradoxes of, 52, 67; and physicians, 266–267; of quality, 64–65; and technology issues, 250–257. *See also* Values

Evidence-based medicine, 26–27

Expert systems, growth of, 30

Extranet, and health care, 248

F

Failure, learning from, 147

Fairness, procedural, 61

Fairness Coalition, 380

Falls Church, Virginia, information technology in, 16

Family planning, and women's health, 162–164

Federal Bureau of Investigation (FBI), 15

Feedback, 360-degree, 318–319

FICA, 44, 356

Financing of health care: and cost issues, 66; and information technology,

228–229; and justice issues, 59–60; and public health, 88

FIND/SVP, 200, 204

Florida: complementary medicine in, 19; delivery network in, 95–99; freedom of choice in, 48

Food and Drug Administration, 64

For-profit organizations, and backlash, 15

Foster Higgins, 136, 141

Foundation for Accountability (FAACT), 46, 49

Future focus, in vision, 272

Fuzzy logic, for diagnostics, 23

G

Gag rules, 9, 165–166

Genetics: and diagnostics, 23; ethical issues of, 251–252; and pharmaceuticals, 25–26

Georgia, Medicaid demonstration project in, 187

Geriatric care: stories of, 187–190; strategies for, 190–198

Geriatricians, need for, 182–183, 184, 190–191

Globalization: and delivery of health care, 34; trends in, 74–84

Goals: for physicians, 271; for rural health systems, 209–210

Group Health Cooperative, 350

H

Haiti, management assessment in, 83

Hartford Health Care Corporation, 5

Harvard University: business School at, 304; and managed care, 138, 141; School of Public Health at, 75, 234

Health: basic importance of, 54–55, 58; revolution in, 231–241

Health awareness trend, 36

Health care: aspects of system of, 1–90, 270; changes in, 4–6; clinical leaders for, 259–298; complementary medicine in, 18–19; consumerism trend in, 17–18; delivery of, 22–38; direct contracting for, 11–12; ethical values in, 51–73; and global transitions, 74–84; issues in, 3–21, 130–131; and managed care issues, 345–385; market consolidation in, 12–13; needs-based system for, 59; options expanded in, 262; organizations for, 91–157; policy challenges in, 39–50; pricing model and cost structure of, 234–235; as public good, 350–352; and public health issues, 85–90; revolution in, 125–126; skills needed for, 299–343; for special populations, 159–215; spending for, 7–9, 235; technology leaders for, 217–257

Health Care Financing Administration: and delivery, 32, 37; and information technology, 246; and long-term care, 200, 203; and managed care, 99, 363, 370; and quality, 265

Health Care Purchasing Organization, 11

Health institutions, capacity of, 78

Health Insurance Association of America, 9, 359, 366

Health maintenance organizations (HMOs): and complementary medicine, 18; and cost control, 33; extent of, 5, 11; and freedom of choice, 48–50; and insurance pricing cycle, 8; and Medicare, 7–8; membership in, 6, 8, 9–10, 134–136, 364–365, 369; reinventing, 6–7; spending forecast for, 7–9

Health Plan Employer Data and Information Set, 49, 349

Health plans. See Insurance

Health professionals: and nurses, 286, 294; technology for, 28–29

Health security framework, 76–78

HealthSouth, 15

Helplessness, and mergers, 334

Henry J. Kaiser Family Foundation, 9, 15, 138, 141

Hewitt Associates, 136, 141

Hill-Burton Act of 1946, 200

Hoechst Marion Roussel, 365, 366

Holy Cross Health System, 16
Hospital Research and Educational
Trust, 151
Hospital Standardization Program,
220–221
Hospitals: and community benefit,
143–144; mergers of, 12–13, 32,
93–100, 150, 332; resource utiliza-
tion by, 97–98; urban, 372
Houston: cooperation in, 5; direct
contracting in, 11
Humana, 6

I

Iatrogenesis, ethical issues of, 255–256
IBM Global Network, 248
IBM/Wilkerson study, 246
Illinois: employer groups in, 11; free-
dom of choice in, 48, 49; HMOs
in, 7
Imaging: advances in, 24; optical, and
storage, 226
Incentives: in alliances, 154–155; finan-
cial, 351; performance-based,
127–129
Inclusiveness, in community health
system, 145–146
Independent practice associations
(IPAs), 14, 332
Indian Health Service, 66
Indianapolis, information technology
in, 17
Industry: and delivery system, 30–33;
information across, 223–228
Industry/University Cooperative
Research Center, 151
Information: collecting, 221, 222–223;
conclusion on, 229–230; industry-
wide, 223–228; in leadership,
106–107; for restructuring,
221–223; vision of, 220–221. *See
also* Information technology
Information appliances, 233
Information system: in geriatric care,
196–197; of insurers, 127
Information technology: barriers to,
227–228; and consumers, 229,

234–235, 237–240; and customer
health care center, 238–239; and
economics, 364; essential elements
in, 224–227; evolving role of, 219–
230; funding for, 228–229; in future,
237, 246–248; growth of, 16–17;
integration of, 245–246; need and
capability for, 243–244; network
challenges in, 244–245; and network
leadership, 303, 306–307; opportunities and lessons of, 249; and
privacy and confidentiality, 247,
252–253; for strategic health care,
242–249. *See also* Information;
Technology
Informed consent, and choice, 63–64
Innova Health System, 16
Innovation: for community health
system, 146–147; cycle of, 231–232
Institute for Alternative Futures (IAF),
25, 26
Institute for Ethics, 266–267
Institute of Medicine: and aging population, 182, 185; and ethics, 54, 55, 56,
57, 65, 69–70; and nursing, 285, 288
Insurance: and aging population, 129;
aspects of, 124–141; and chronic illnesses, 128; and clinical outcomes,
127–129; and consumers, 132–141;
and delivery system, 32; future for,
140; hybrid products in, 134–136;
individually owned, 360–361;
information systems for, 127; issues
for, 124–131; lack of, 52–54, 57;
and member rights, 350; and mental
illness, 377–378, 379–381; networks
in, 136–137; policy challenges for,
40; pricing cycle in, 8; and product
choice, 133–136; and quality, 137–
140; and regulatory system, 129,
358–359; roles of, 126; and rural
residents, 207; and tax policies,
356–357
Integrated delivery systems, providers
as, 6
Integrity, for community health
systems, 147–148

Intensity of care, and cost issues, 42–43

International health care nongovernmental organizations (IHNGOs): aspects of challenges for, 74–84; and health transition, 75–76; and organizational missions, 79–82; programming for, 76–78; reinventing, 82–83; structural changes for, 81–82

Internet: and cyberhealth, 16; and delivery systems, 28, 29, 30, 37; and health information, 229, 232, 238, 247–248, 263, 285, 364; and virtual rounds, 248; and women's health, 176

InterStudy, 7, 8, 9

Iowa, employer groups in, 11

Istituto Nazionale per lo Studio e la Cura dei Tumori, 248

Italy, health care computing network in, 248

J

Jet Propulsion Laboratory, 24, 38

Johnson & Johnson, and leadership development, 307

Johnson & Johnson-Wharton Fellows Program in Management for Nurse Executives, 296

Joint Commission on Accreditation of Healthcare Organizations, 221, 265, 338

Justice: and ethical values, 59–61; procedural, 60–61

K

Kaiser Permanente, 6, 350, 353

Kansas City, HMOs in, 6

Kansas Health Foundation, 213

Kassebaum-Kennedy health insurance reform bill of 1996, 361, 379

Kellogg Foundation, W. K., 151, 213

Kershaw County Memorial Hospital, 212

Knowledge: clinically useful, 30; workers in, and networks, 304–305, 307

KPMG Peat Marwick, 135, 141, 358

L

Leadership: of academic health centers, 114–123; for aging population, 183–184, 197; aspects of, 101–110; attention in, 106; clinical, 259–298; competencies in, 271–277, 297; cosmopolitan, 294; dispersed, 102–104, 145–146; distributive, 102; engagement in, 105; and goals, 209; and individual development, 107–109; information in, 106–107; of integrated community health system, 144–146; issues for, 99–100; and managed care issues, 345–385; and mental health services, 376–385; for network, 301–307; in nursing, 290–298; and parity for mental health services, 379–381; and responsbile managed care, 381–384; for rural health systems, 210–214; and self-knowledge, 109, 297; skills needed for, 299–343; specialized and generalized, 211, 214; strategies for, 102–104; for technology, 217–257; transformational, 293; for women's health, 169, 176–177

Leadership development: aspects of, 316–322; learning modes in, 321–322; need for, 317–318; for nursing, 295–298; process for, 318–321

Learning, modes of, 321–322

Learning organizations: for aging population, 192–194; alliances as, 156

Legitimized trust, 312

Lewin/VHI for Families USA Foundation, 53, 70

Liminality phase, 309

Long-term care: for aging population, 199–204; background on, 199–200; and continuum of services, 202; data source for, 203–204; and demographic trends, 201–202; ethics in, 203; and regulatory barriers, 201

Louisiana, and Medicare fraud, 15

Loyalties, and mergers, 334, 339

M

Maintenance learning, 321

Managed behavioral health companies, and leadership, 381–384

Managed care: aspects of, 345–385; and black physicians, 368–375; concept of, 348; and costs, 369–371; and economics, 355–367; evolution of, 126; and financial incentives, 351; information technology in, 225, 227–228, 229; and mental health services, 376–385; and physicians, 263; and procedural fairness, 61; regulation of, 9–11; responsible, 381–384; and rural residents, 207–208; trust in, 347–354; and urban health penalty, 371–373; vision of, 163; and women's health, 175

Managed competition, and direct contracting, 11

Management Capacity Assessment Tool, 83

Marketing: and consolidation, 12–13; relationship, 196; in rural areas, 212; strategies for, 17–18

Massachusetts General Hospital, 220

McJob, rise of, 35–36

Medicaid: demonstration project of, 187; and direct contracting, 11; and ethical values, 53, 56, 59, 66; and HMOs, 9; and information technology, 234; and managed care, 363, 369–370, 373; and medical mega-group, 14; and rural residents, 207–208; waivers of, 43, 44–45; and women's health, 166, 172

Medicaid Access Study Group, 56, 71

Medical advances, and delivery system, 23–27

Medical loss ratios, rising, 6, 8

Medical mega-groups, physician organizations as, 13–14

Medical savings accounts, 361

Medical schools, in academic health centers, 112, 122–123

Medicare: changes needed in, 362–363; and cost control, 33; and direct contracting, 11; and ethical values, 59, 66, 253; and fraud, 15, 184; and long-term care, 203; managed, 7–8, 9, 99, 369–370, 373; and medical savings accounts, 361; and policy challenges, 40, 43–44, 48; and provider sponsored organizations, 5; and rural residents, 207–208

Medicare–Choice, 362

Medicare Hospital Trust Fund, 43–44

MediConsult.com, 247

Medpartners, 333

Mental and behavioral health services: aspects of, 376–385; background on, 376–379; developments in, 378–379; future for, 384; parity for, 379–381; and responsible managed care, 381–384; scarcity and stewardship in, 382–383

Mental Health Parity Act of 1996, 379–381

Mental illness: costs of, 377; and insurance, 377–378, 379–381

Mentoring, and leadership, 107

Mergers, and organizational blending, 332–343

Milwaukee, medical mega-group in, 14

Minerva, 24

Minnesota: employer group in, 5, 11; value-based care in, 373

Minority population: and access inequity, 57; health status of, 371–372

Missouri, Medicare HMOs lacking in, 7

Modern Healthcare, 18

Motorola, 6

Mullikin, 33

N

Nanotechnology, for surgery, 25

Narcissism, altruism in balance with, 107

NASA, 24

NASDAQ, 16

National Academy of Sciences, 182

National Advisory Council on Nurse Education and Practice, 287, 288–289

National Alliance for the Mentally Ill, 380

National Association of Manufacturers, 379

National Blue Initiative for Quality Senior Care, 129

National Center for Children in Poverty, 56, 71

National Center for Health Statistics, 56, 71

National Committee for Quality Assurance, 17, 49, 265, 349

National Conference of State Legislatures, 364

National Federation of Specialty Nursing Organizations, 294

National Heart, Lung, and Blood Institute, 56, 71

National Institute of Mental Health, 376

National Institute of Nursing Research, 288, 289

National Institute on Disability and Rehabilitation Research, 56, 71

National Investment Conference for Senior Living and Long Term Care Industries, 200

National Medical Association, 369, 370, 373, 374

National Mental Health Association, 380

National Patient Safety Foundation, 265

National Science Foundation, 151

Nebraska, and for-profit conversions, 15

Network for Healthcare Management, 296

Network leadership: aspects of, 301–307; capabilities for, 305–307; challenges of, 302–305; in future, 307

Networks, of insurers, 136–137

New Jersey Individual Health Coverage Program Board, 359, 366

New Orleans, managed care in, 99

New York: HMOs in, 6; and Medicare fraud, 15; quality in, 46

New York City, consumerism in, 17

New York University, 333

Northwest Area Foundation, 213

Nursing: architecture of, 282–283; and ask-a-nurse services, 234, 285, 364; aspects of, 278–298; assumptions about, 278–279; change in, 291–292, 293; cosmopolitan outlook for, 293–295; education in, 282, 283, 286–287; forces shaping, 283–286; future of, 278–289; and health professionals, 286, 294; initiatives for, 286–288; leadership development for, 295–298; leadership in, 290–298; perspectives for, 292–295; practice in, 279–281, 287–288; professional organizations for, 294; workforce in, 283, 287, 292

Nursing Home Reform Act of 1987, 203

Nursing homes. *See* Long-term care

Nursing Organization Liaison Forum, 294

O

Office of Technology Assessment, 42–43, 64, 71, 207, 215

Open access products, 49, 50

Optical imaging and storage, in information technology, 226

Oregon, Medicaid waiver in, 43

Organizations: academic health centers as, 111–123; alliances as, 149–157; aspects of, 91–157; blended, 331–343; challenges for, 99–100; and consolidation, 93–100; cultures of, 152–153, 191–192, 343; identity of, and change, 310–311; insurers as, 124–141; integrated community health systems as, 142–148; international, 74–84; leadership in, 101–110; in nursing, 294; in public health, 89–90; trends for, 94–95

Outcomes management, 26–27

Oxford Health Plans, 6, 8

P

Pacific Business Group on Health, 5
PacifiCare, 5
Partnerships: for alignments, 274–275; and black physicians, 373–374, 375; and change, 311–312; in communities, 194–197; of consumer and provider, 314; forming, 305–306; as networks, 301–307. *See also* Alliances
Patient Bill of Rights, 9, 265
Patients. *See* Consumers
Pennsylvania, quality in, 46
Pennsylvania, University of, Medical Center at, 23
Pennsylvania Health Care Cost Containment Council, 41
Performance standards, in alliances, 155
Person identification, in information technology, 225–226
Pharmaceutical firms: advances for, 25–26; and black physicians, 372; formularies for, 43; mergers of, 332; in networks, 302
PhyCor, 15, 333
Physician groups: and cost control, 33; health plans from, 262, 264; and information technology, 16; as management companies, 333; as medical mega-groups, 13–14
Physicians: and accountability, 264–266; advocacy role of, 349; black, 368–375; challenges to, 261–268, 374–375; change management by, 276–277; competencies for, 269–277; and costs, 264; dissatisfaction of, 31–33; and ethics, 266–267; mission of, 263; and patient care, 262–264; performance-based incentives for, 127–129; and power base, 270–271; rights of, and trust, 352; roles of, 313–314; and vision for future, 267–268
Planned Parenthood Federation of America, 162–163, 167
Point of service (POS) plan: and freedom of choice, 50; in hybrid products, 134–136; and information technology, 226–227, 228; self-insured, 7
Policy challenges: of access, 46–47; aspects of, 39–50; conclusion on, 50; of costs, 42–45; of demographics, 40–41; for insurance, 40; for international organizations, 78; paradoxes of, 47–50; and physicians, 375; and quality, 46; of value, 41–42
Politics, and women's health, 164–165
Population. *See* Demographic trends; Special populations
Power base, and physicians, 270–271
Practice: guidelines of, in mental health services, 383; models of, and information technology, 243–244; in nursing, 279–281, 287–288; results-driven, 26–27; technology for clinical, 29; vision aligned with, 273–274
Preferred provider organizations (PPOs): appeal of, 6; and freedom of choice, 49–50; in hybrid products, 134–136; membership in, 364
Premier, Inc., 150–151
Premier Health Alliance, 150
Presidential Commission on Quality in Health Care, 265
President's Commission for the Study of Ethical Problems in Medicine and Biomedical and Behavioral Research, 54, 71
Prevention and wellness: delivery system for, 95–96; in women's health, 174–175
Primary care centers, nurses in, 280
Privacy: and electronic medical records, 9–10; and information technology, 247, 252–253
Private Health Care Systems, 6
Provider sponsored organizations (PSOs): and direct contracting, 11–12; networks of, 5
Psychological quit, 335
Public health: aspects of, 85–90; concepts of, 87; decision making in,

87–89; leadership for, 86–87; organizations in, 89–90; workforce for, 89

Public Health Service Act of 1970, Title X of, 166

Q

Quality: and consumer choice, 137–140; and consumer satisfaction, 326–329; and cost, 66; and ethics, 64–65; and freedom of choice, 48–49; measures of, 138; perceived, 328; and policy challenges, 46

R

Rand Corporation, 47, 235, 241
Reagan, Weaver v., 64
Reagan administration, 43
Regenstrief Institute for Health Care, 236
Regulation: and insurance, 129, 358–359; and long-term care, 201; of managed care, 9–11; of technology applications, 42–43
Relationship marketing, for geriatric care, 196
Reproductive health care: components of, 167; ethical issues of, 256; primacy of, 162–170
Research: and aging population, 181–182, 197; ethical issues of, 251; and nursing, 283
Resident Assessment Minimum Data Set (MDS), 203
Resource-based relative value schedule (RBRVS), and costs, 44
Resources: and aging population, 181–182, 197; and ethical issues, 254–255
Rhode Island, and for-profit conversions, 15
Richland Memorial Hospital, 212
Risk analysis, in global health, 77, 82
Risk management, and academic health centers, 121
Robert Wood Johnson Foundation, 151, 194–195, 198; Executive Nurse Fellows Program of, 296–297

Robodoc, 24
Robots, and surgery, 24–25
Rolling Meadows, Illinois, 7
Rural health systems: aspects of, 205–215; background on, 206–207; and demographic trends, 208–209; and diverse populations, 207–209; future for, 213–214; goals for, 209–210; leadership for, 210–214

S

Sachs seal of excellence, 17
St. Joseph Medical Center, 96
St. Louis, information technology in, 244
Saint Louis University Hospital, 96
San Francisco: coalition in, 5; medical mega-group in, 14
Satisfaction: of consumers, 323–330; and physicians, 31–33
Self-knowledge, and leadership, 109, 297
SERVQUAL scale, 326
Setting Priorities for Retirement Years (SPRY) Foundation, 183
Sex education, and women's health, 164, 166
Sherlock Company, 8
Shock learning, 321
Sigma Theta Tau, Leadership Institute of, 296
Sinai Medical Center, 333
Skills: aspects of gaining, 299–343; for change management, 308–315; for consumer satisfaction, 323–330; and leadership development, 316–322; in network leadership, 301–307; in organizational blending, 331–343. See also Competencies
Small wins, in alliances, 154
Smithville, Missouri, hospital ownership in, 210, 212
Social Security, 36, 356, 362
Social structure: change in, 35; and delivery system, 33–36
South Bend, Indiana, information technology in, 16

South Carolina, Medicare HMOs lacking in, 7

Southern California, University of (USC), School of Medicine at, 96

Special populations: aging, 34, 178–204; aspects of, 159–215; rural, 205–215; women as, 161–177

Specialized care centers, nurses in, 280–281

SRI International, 24, 38

Stanford University, 333

States: mandated benefits in, 358; Medicaid management for, 45

Stewardship, in managing mental health care, 382–383

Strategic alliances, for international organizations, 83

Strategies, for international organizations, 79–81

Structural participation, and change, 313–314

Structured data, and information technology, 227

SunHealth, 150

Surgery advances, 24–25

Survivor's guilt, 335

Systems thinking, for learning organization, 193–194

T

Task Force for Aging Research, 181, 185

Task Force on Integrated Health and Managed Care, 374

Tax policies, and insurance, 356–357

Teams: in academic health centers, 115, 123; geriatric, 190–191; in health care system, 127; for inclusiveness, 146; nurses on, 280, 281; for organizational blending, 338–340

Technology: aspects of, 217–257; assessment consortium for, 43–44; for clinical decisions, 234–237; for competitive advantage, 306–307; for delivery system, 27–29; diagnostic, 23; and ethics, 250–257; for health revolution, 231–241; and improvements, 232–233; and information, 219–230; innovation cycle for, 231–232; and nursing, 284–285, 288; regulating application of, 42–43; for strategic health care computing, 242–249. *See also* Information technology

Temporary Assistance for Needy Families, 45

Tenet Healthcare Corporation, 15, 95–99, 332, 343

Tennessee, Medicare HMOs lacking in, 7

Texas: employer groups in, 11; malpractice legislation in, 139

Texas, University of: M. D. Anderson Cancer Center of, 243–244; Southwest Medical School of, 19

Therapeutic oasis, in geriatric care, 194

Third-party administrator (TPA), 6–7

Third-party payers, and economics, 357

TriBrook/AM&G, 12

Trust: in alliances, 153; aspects of, in managed care, 347–354; background on, 347–349; and change, 312–313; and communities, 350–352; and community health systems, 148; and patient rights and protections, 349–350; and physician and employee rights, 352; and values hierarchy, 352–353

U

Unconventional therapies. *See* Alternative medicine

United Healthcare, 7

U.S. Bureau of the Census, 180, 185, 207

U.S. Department of Defense, 24

U.S. Department of Health and Human Services: and aging population, 184; and ethical issues, 52, 56, 57, 72–73; and women's health, 172

U.S. Department of Justice, 15

U.S. General Accounting Office, 54, 56, 73, 361, 367

U.S. Public Health Service, 172

Urban health penalty, and black physicians, 371–373

USC University Hospital, 96, 98

Utilization review and prior authorization, and quality, 138–139

V

Value-based care, 373–374

Values: conflicting, and mergers, 335; and nursing, 293; policy challenge of, 41–42; shifting concepts of, 125; and trust, 352–353; in vision, 272–273. *See also* Ethics

Veterans Administration, 66

VHA, Inc., 248, 332

VHAseCURE.net, 248

Violence, and communities, 375

Vision: competency in developing, 271–273; for empowerment, 108; for inclusiveness, 146; of information, 220–221; of managed care, 163; and physicians, 267–268; practice aligned with, 273–274; values in, 272–273

Voluntary Hospitals of America, 151

W

Weaver v. Reagan, 64

Wellpoint, 8

Wesley Woods Center on Aging, 186–190, 193, 195–196; SOURCE program of, 187

Whitman Corporation, 7

William N. Wishard Memorial Hospital, 17

Wisconsin, employer groups in, 11

Wisconsin Independent Physicians Group, 14

Withdrawal, and mergers, 334–335

Women's health: agenda for, 171–177; and alternative medicine, 173–174; aspects of, 161–177; and censorship, 165–166; challenges for, 161–170; choices in, 166–167; context of, 163, 172–173; and family planning, 162–164; future for, 169–170, 177; issues in, 172–174; leadership for, 169, 176–177; and politics, 164–165; prevention and wellness in, 174–175; providers for, 167–168; underserved segments of, 168, 172

Women's Research and Education Institute, 162, 170

Workforce: models of, 103–104; in nursing, 283, 287, 292; for public health, 89

World Health Organization, 75, 84

World Wide Web, 28, 238, 244, 246–247, 248

X

Xenographic transplantation, ethical issues of, 256